Chapman & Hall/CRC Biostatistics Series

Published Titles

Adaptive Design Methods in Clinical Trials, Second Edition
Shein-Chung Chow and Mark Chang

Adaptive Designs for Sequential Treatment Allocation
Alessandro Baldi Antognini and Alessandra Giovagnoli

Adaptive Design Theory and Implementation Using SAS and R, Second Edition
Mark Chang

Advanced Bayesian Methods for Medical Test Accuracy
Lyle D. Broemeling

Analyzing Longitudinal Clinical Trial Data: A Practical Guide
Craig Mallinckrodt and Ilya Lipkovich

Applied Biclustering Methods for Big and High-Dimensional Data Using R
Adetayo Kasim, Ziv Shkedy, Sebastian Kaiser, Sepp Hochreiter, and Willem Talloen

Applied Meta-Analysis with R
Ding-Geng (Din) Chen and Karl E. Peace

Applied Surrogate Endpoint Evaluation Methods with SAS and R
Ariel Alonso, Theophile Bigirumurame, Tomasz Burzykowski, Marc Buyse, Geert Molenberghs, Leacky Muchene, Nolen Joy Perualila, Ziv Shkedy, and Wim Van der Elst

Basic Statistics and Pharmaceutical Statistical Applications, Second Edition
James E. De Muth

Bayesian Adaptive Methods for Clinical Trials
Scott M. Berry, Bradley P. Carlin, J. Jack Lee, and Peter Muller

Bayesian Analysis Made Simple: An Excel GUI for WinBUGS
Phil Woodward

Bayesian Designs for Phase I–II Clinical Trials
Ying Yuan, Hoang Q. Nguyen, and Peter F. Thall

Bayesian Methods for Measures of Agreement
Lyle D. Broemeling

Bayesian Methods for Repeated Measures
Lyle D. Broemeling

Bayesian Methods in Epidemiology
Lyle D. Broemeling

Bayesian Methods in Health Economics
Gianluca Baio

Bayesian Missing Data Problems: EM, Data Augmentation and Noniterative Computation
Ming T. Tan, Guo-Liang Tian, and Kai Wang Ng

Published Titles

Published Titles

DNA Microarrays and Related Genomics Techniques: Design, Analysis, and Interpretation of Experiments
David B. Allison, Grier P. Page, T. Mark Beasley, and Jode W. Edwards

Dose Finding by the Continual Reassessment Method
Ying Kuen Cheung

Dynamical Biostatistical Models
Daniel Commenges and Hélène Jacqmin-Gadda

Elementary Bayesian Biostatistics
Lemuel A. Moyé

Emerging Non-Clinical Biostatistics in Biopharmaceutical Development and Manufacturing
Harry Yang

Empirical Likelihood Method in Survival Analysis
Mai Zhou

Essentials of a Successful Biostatistical Collaboration
Arul Earnest

Exposure–Response Modeling: Methods and Practical Implementation
Jixian Wang

Frailty Models in Survival Analysis
Andreas Wienke

Fundamental Concepts for New Clinical Trialists
Scott Evans and Naitee Ting

Generalized Linear Models: A Bayesian Perspective
Dipak K. Dey, Sujit K. Ghosh, and Bani K. Mallick

Handbook of Regression and Modeling: Applications for the Clinical and Pharmaceutical Industries
Daryl S. Paulson

Inference Principles for Biostatisticians
Ian C. Marschner

Interval-Censored Time-to-Event Data: Methods and Applications
Ding-Geng (Din) Chen, Jianguo Sun, and Karl E. Peace

Introductory Adaptive Trial Designs: A Practical Guide with R
Mark Chang

Joint Models for Longitudinal and Time-to-Event Data: With Applications in R
Dimitris Rizopoulos

Measures of Interobserver Agreement and Reliability, Second Edition
Mohamed M. Shoukri

Medical Biostatistics, Third Edition
A. Indrayan

Meta-Analysis in Medicine and Health Policy
Dalene Stangl and Donald A. Berry

Mixed Effects Models for the Population Approach: Models, Tasks, Methods and Tools
Marc Lavielle

Modeling to Inform Infectious Disease Control
Niels G. Becker

Modern Adaptive Randomized Clinical Trials: Statistical and Practical Aspects
Oleksandr Sverdlov

Monte Carlo Simulation for the Pharmaceutical Industry: Concepts, Algorithms, and Case Studies
Mark Chang

Multiregional Clinical Trials for Simultaneous Global New Drug Development
Joshua Chen and Hui Quan

Multiple Testing Problems in Pharmaceutical Statistics
Alex Dmitrienko, Ajit C. Tamhane, and Frank Bretz

Noninferiority Testing in Clinical Trials: Issues and Challenges
Tie-Hua Ng

Optimal Design for Nonlinear Response Models
Valerii V. Fedorov and Sergei L. Leonov

Published Titles

Patient-Reported Outcomes: Measurement, Implementation and Interpretation
Joseph C. Cappelleri, Kelly H. Zou, Andrew G. Bushmakin, Jose Ma. J. Alvir, Demissie Alemayehu, and Tara Symonds

Quantitative Evaluation of Safety in Drug Development: Design, Analysis and Reporting
Qi Jiang and H. Amy Xia

Quantitative Methods for Traditional Chinese Medicine Development
Shein-Chung Chow

Randomized Clinical Trials of Nonpharmacological Treatments
Isabelle Boutron, Philippe Ravaud, and David Moher

Randomized Phase II Cancer Clinical Trials
Sin-Ho Jung

Sample Size Calculations for Clustered and Longitudinal Outcomes in Clinical Research
Chul Ahn, Moonseong Heo, and Song Zhang

Sample Size Calculations in Clinical Research, Second Edition
Shein-Chung Chow, Jun Shao, and Hansheng Wang

Statistical Analysis of Human Growth and Development
Yin Bun Cheung

Statistical Design and Analysis of Clinical Trials: Principles and Methods
Weichung Joe Shih and Joseph Aisner

Statistical Design and Analysis of Stability Studies
Shein-Chung Chow

Statistical Evaluation of Diagnostic Performance: Topics in ROC Analysis
Kelly H. Zou, Aiyi Liu, Andriy Bandos, Lucila Ohno-Machado, and Howard Rockette

Statistical Methods for Clinical Trials
Mark X. Norleans

Statistical Methods for Drug Safety
Robert D. Gibbons and Anup K. Amatya

Statistical Methods for Healthcare Performance Monitoring
Alex Bottle and Paul Aylin

Statistical Methods for Immunogenicity Assessment
Harry Yang, Jianchun Zhang, Binbing Yu, and Wei Zhao

Statistical Methods in Drug Combination Studies
Wei Zhao and Harry Yang

Statistical Testing Strategies in the Health Sciences
Albert Vexler, Alan D. Hutson, and Xiwei Chen

Statistics in Drug Research: Methodologies and Recent Developments
Shein-Chung Chow and Jun Shao

Statistics in the Pharmaceutical Industry, Third Edition
Ralph Buncher and Jia-Yeong Tsay

Survival Analysis in Medicine and Genetics
Jialiang Li and Shuangge Ma

Theory of Drug Development
Eric B. Holmgren

Translational Medicine: Strategies and Statistical Methods
Dennis Cosmatos and Shein-Chung Chow

Chapman & Hall/CRC Biostatistics Series

Applied Surrogate Endpoint Evaluation Methods with SAS and R

Ariel Alonso
Theophile Bigirumurame
Tomasz Burzykowski
Marc Buyse
Geert Molenberghs
Leacky Muchene
Nolen Joy Perualila
Ziv Shkedy
Wim Van der Elst

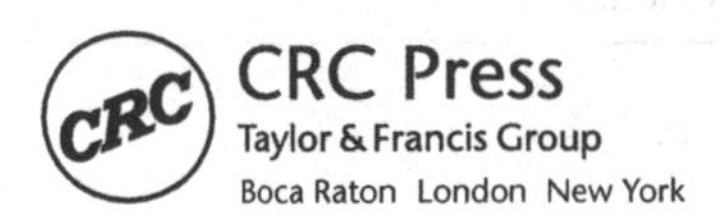

CRC Press is an imprint of the
Taylor & Francis Group, an informa business
A CHAPMAN & HALL BOOK

CRC Press
Taylor & Francis Group
6000 Broken Sound Parkway NW, Suite 300
Boca Raton, FL 33487-2742

First issued in paperback 2020

ISBN-13: 978-1-4822-4936-1 (hbk)
ISBN-13: 978-0-367-73655-2 (pbk)

Library of Congress Cataloging-in-Publication Data

Names: Alonso, Ariel (Statistician)
Title: Applied surrogate endpoint evaluation methods with SAS and R / Ariel Alonso [and eight others].
Description: Boca Raton : CRC Press, 2017. | Includes bibliographical references and index.
Identifiers: LCCN 2016033893 | ISBN 9781482249361 (hardback)
Subjects: LCSH: Clinical trials--Statistical methods. | Medicine--Research--Methodology. | SAS (Computer file) | R (Computer program language)
Classification: LCC R853.C55 A677 2017 | DDC 610.72--dc23
LC record available at https://lccn.loc.gov/2016033893

Visit the Taylor & Francis Web site at
http://www.taylorandfrancis.com

and the CRC Press Web site at
http://www.crcpress.com

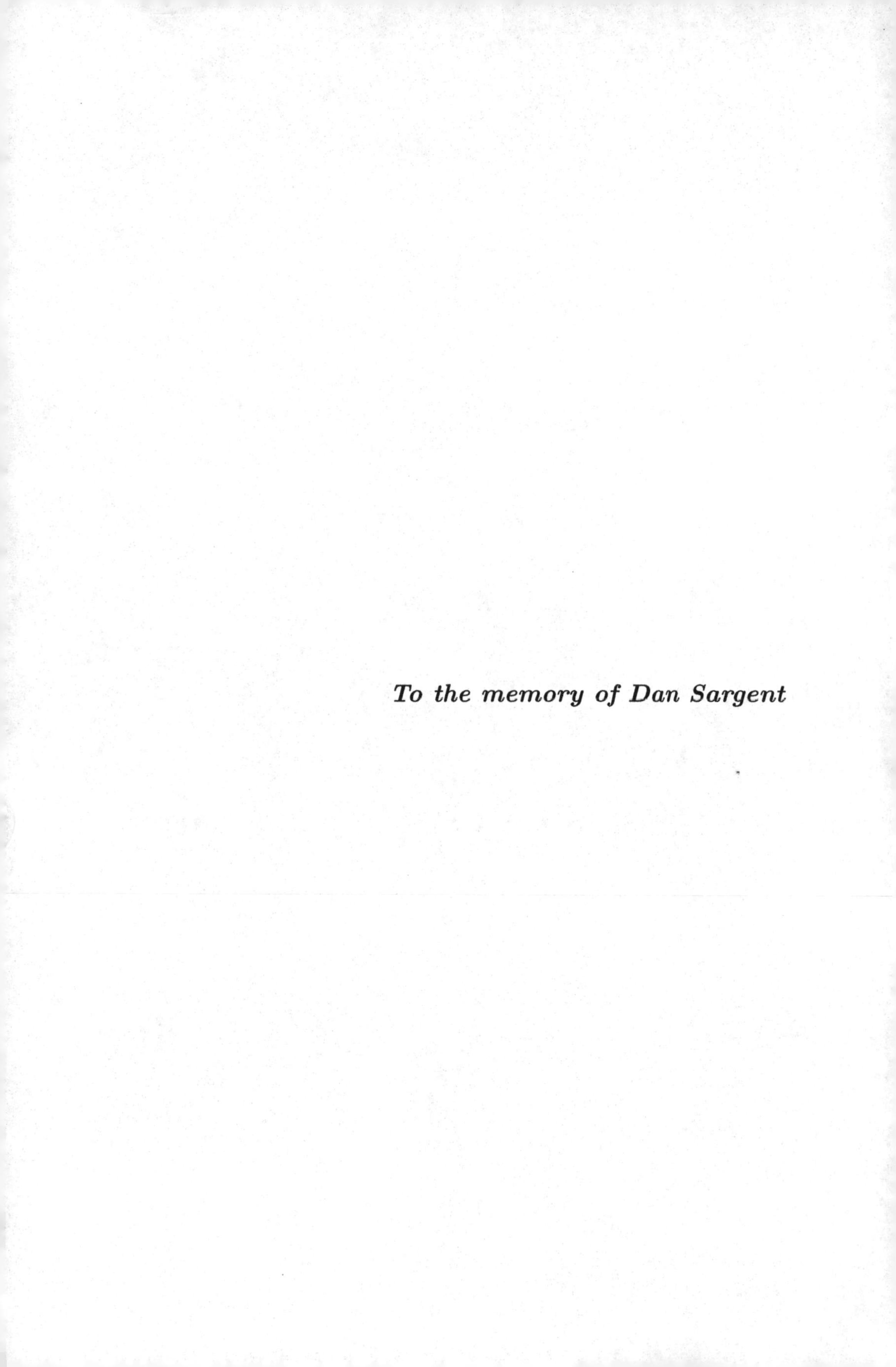

To the memory of Dan Sargent

Contents

III Software Tools 157

List of Contributors

Ariel Alonso Abad	KU Leuven, Belgium
Theophile Bigirumurame	Hasselt University, Belgium
Luc Bijnens	Janssen Pharmaceutica, Belgium
Astrid Bottelbergs	Janssen Pharmaceutica, Belgium
Tomasz Burzykowski	Hasselt University, Belgium & IDDI, Louvain-la-Neuve, Belgium
Marc Buyse	IDDI, Belgium & CluePoints, USA & Hasselt University, Belgium
Hannah Ensor	BioSS, United Kingdom
W.H. Göhlmann	Janssen Pharmaceutica, Belgium
Tom Jacobs	Janssen Pharmaceutica, Belgium
Adetayo Kasim	Durham University, United Kingdom
Nikolay Manyakov	Janssen Pharmaceutica, Belgium
Geert Molenberghs	Hasselt University, Belgium & KU Leuven, Belgium
Leacky Muchene	Hasselt University, Belgium
Darrell Pemberton	Janssen Pharmaceutica, Belgium
Nolen Joy Perualila	Hasselt University, Belgium
Jelle Praet	University of Antwerp, Belgium
Mark Schmidt	Janssen Pharmaceutica, Belgium
Rudradev Sengupta	Hasselt University, Belgium
Ziv Shkedy	Hasselt University, Belgium
Willem Talloen	Janssen Pharmaceutica, Belgium
Tom Van De Casteele	Janssen Pharmaceutica, Belgium
Wim Van der Elst	Janssen Pharmaceutica, Belgium & Hasselt University, Belgium
Annemie Van der Linden	University of Antwerp, Belgium
Bie Verbist	Janssen Pharmaceutica, Belgium
Marleen Verhoye	University of Antwerp, Belgium
Christopher J. Weir	University of Edinburgh, United Kingdom

Preface

Surrogate endpoint evaluation has been a very active area of research ever since the seminal papers by Ross Prentice, Laurence Freedman, and their co-authors, in the late 1980s and early 1990s. The original singe-trial work was followed by meta-analytic developments. Later, information-theoretic methodology was introduced. Research followed both the path of association as well as causal inference. Recently, efforts have been undertaken to study similarities and differences between these strands. However, methodological development is worth very little in the absence of two crucial resources.

The first resource is data. It is now broadly accepted that surrogate endpoint evaluation in practice is best done from a multi-trial perspective, implying that large volumes of data are needed. Arguably, data should be made available by a variety of companies and other sponsors to provide the necessary critical data volume. The second resource is software. No matter how appealing a model or other methodological approach is user-friendly software in broadly accessible platforms is needed to allow for and to promote its use.

Starting from a general methodological overview, covering a variety of situations in terms of (true and surrogate endpoint) outcome types and therapeutic areas, contemporary surrogate endpoint evaluation tools are described. These are accompanied by software implementations. This book focuses on both SAS and R; for the latter Shiny Apps are also developed. Software is described in a tutorial fashion, illustrated by means of real examples, and made available via the authors' web pages.

The authors gratefully acknowledge contributions from a number of additional chapter-specific authors. We would also like to thank John Kimmel, Statistics Editor at Chapman & Hall/CRC Press, for his encouragement and expert advice throughout all stages of this project.

Financial support from the IAP research network #P7/06 of the Belgian Government (Belgian Science Policy) is gratefully acknowledged. Part of the research reported in this book was supported by funding received from the European Seventh Framework programme FP7 2007–2013 under grant agreement Nr. 602552 and by funding from the IWT-SBO ExaScience grant.

Ariel Alonso, Theophile Bigirumurame, Tomasz Burzykowski, Marc Buyse, Geert Molenberghs, Leacky Muchene, Nolen Joy Perualila, Ziv Shkedy, Wim Van der Elst

Preface

Part I

Introductory Material

1

Introduction

Marc Buyse
IDDI, Belgium, CluePoints, USA, and Hasselt University, Belgium

CONTENTS

1.1 Overview of Surrogate Endpoint Evaluation

In clinical research, interest typically focuses on the most clinically relevant endpoints such as survival (in cancer), myocardial infarction (in cardiovascular disease), loss of vision (in ophthalmic diseases), performance on some rating scale (in psychiatry), and so on. The objective of therapy is to improve clinical endpoints that are considered most relevant to patients. However, these endpoints may be difficult to use in prospective trials for a number of reasons:

1. clinical endpoints may require a very long follow-up time (e.g., survival in early stage cancers), such that the assessment of new therapies using these endpoints would be unduly delayed and potentially confounded by other therapies;

2. clinical endpoints may require a large sample size if the event of interest has low incidence (e.g., cytotoxic drugs may have rare but serious side effects, such as leukemias induced by topoisomerase inhibitors);
3. clinical endpoints may be difficult to measure (e.g., quality-of-life assessments involve multi-dimensional instruments that are hard to validate);
4. clinical endpoints may be costly to measure (e.g., cachexia, a condition associated with malnutrition and involving loss of muscle and fat tissue, is assessed using expensive equipment that measures the levels of nitrogen, potassium and water in the patient's body).

A potential strategy in these cases is to look for surrogate endpoints or biomarkers that can be measured earlier, more frequently, more conveniently, or more cheaply than the true clinical endpoint of interest.

The Biomarker Definitions Working Group (Biomarkers Definition Working Group, 2001) proposed formal definitions that have since been widely adopted. A clinical endpoint is considered the most credible indicator of drug response and defined as a characteristic or variable that reflects how a patient feels, functions, or survives. In clinical trials aimed at establishing the worth of new therapies, clinically relevant endpoints should be used, unless a biomarker or other endpoint is available that has risen to the status of surrogate endpoint. A biomarker is defined as a characteristic that can be objectively measured as an indicator of healthy or pathological biological processes, or pharmacological responses to therapeutic intervention. A surrogate endpoint is a biomarker that is intended for substituting a clinical endpoint. A surrogate endpoint is expected to predict clinical benefit, harm, or lack of these.

1.1.1 Individual-Level versus Trial-Level Surrogacy

Notwithstanding these formal definitions, there is a critical ambiguity about the meaning of the term "surrogate" in practice. A surrogate endpoint may be used to predict the course of the disease in an individual patient, in order to adjust the treatment accordingly. In this book, we will refer to this situation as *individual-level surrogacy*. A surrogate endpoint may also be used to predict the effect of some therapy on the clinical endpoint of interest, based on the effect of this therapy on the surrogate endpoint. We will refer to this situation as *trial-level surrogacy*. The mathematical models described in this book have been developed to address both levels of surrogacy, thus building a useful parallel between the intended use of potential surrogates, and their statistical evaluation. In these models, the two levels of surrogacy are independent from each other, at least when the surrogate and the clinical endpoint are both captured by normally distributed variables. This intriguing feature of the two levels of surrogacy has created much confusion, and continues to plague their use. We will return to this issue in Section 1.2.5.

The International Conference on Harmonisation (ICH) Guidelines on Statistical Principles for Clinical Trials reflect the distinction between these two levels of surrogacy: "In practice, the strength of the evidence for surrogacy depends upon (i) the biological plausibility of the relationship, (ii) the demonstration in epidemiological studies of the prognostic value of the surrogate for the clinical outcome, and (iii) evidence from clinical trials that treatment effects on the surrogate correspond to effects on the clinical outcome" (ICH, 1998). Condition (i) involves biological rather than statistical considerations, condition (ii) is individual-level surrogacy, and condition (iii) is trial-level surrogacy. Surrogate endpoints can be put to different uses depending on the phase of drug development. Early or "intermediate" endpoints are commonly used in phase I or phase II trials when they have been shown to be individual-level surrogates. However, very few intermediate endpoints have been shown to be acceptable trial-level surrogates that can substitute for a clinical endpoint in pivotal phase III trials.

1.1.2 Early Successes with Surrogates

Surrogate endpoints have long been used in medical research, under the implicit assumption that treatments with efficacy on the surrogates would automatically have an impact on the more important long-term clinical endpoints. In cardiovascular disease, blood pressure and cholesterol levels have been used as surrogates *de facto* for a long time, mostly because of the overwhelming epidemiologic evidence of a correlation between these markers and cardiovascular events. Such epidemiological evidence, however, only informs individual-level surrogacy. Trial-level surrogacy requires an analysis of intervention trials aimed at lowering blood pressure, for instance, to establish the level of reduction in blood pressure required to see a benefit on clinical endpoints such as stroke, cardiovascular mortality, or overall mortality. The paradox is that such an analysis is only possible when the long-term clinical endpoints have been observed, at which point the critics would argue it is too late to establish the value of the surrogate! As it turns out, using a meta-analytic approach on 18 randomized trials, blood pressure was recently shown to be an acceptable surrogate endpoint for stroke, with a benefit on stroke predicted for a reduction in systolic blood pressure of at least 7.1 mmHg, and a reduction in diastolic blood pressure of at least 2.4 mmHg (Lassere et al., 2012). The same analysis provided no evidence that this magnitude of effect on blood pressure would lead to reductions in cardiovascular or all-cause mortality. These analyses are undoubtedly informative, yet the critics would say they are only valid in the context of the types of anti-hypertensive drugs tested in all available trials. It remains to be seen (and evaluated) whether blood pressure is still a surrogate for a future anti-hypertensive treatment having a substantially different mode of action as compared with the currently available treatments. We will return to this issue in another clinical context in Section 1.2.3.

1.1.3 Early Failures with Surrogates

Despite the potential advantages of surrogates, their use has been surrounded by controversy (Fleming and DeMets, 1996). An unfortunate precedent set the stage for heightened skepticism about surrogates in general: the US Food and Drug Administration (FDA) approved three antiarrhythmic drugs (encainide, flecainide, and moricizine) based on their major effects on the suppression of arrhythmias. It was believed that, because arrhythmias are associated with an almost fourfold increase in the rate of cardiac-complication-related death, drugs that reduced arrhythmic episodes would also reduce the death rate in all patients. However, the Cardiac Arrhythmia Suppression Trial (CAST), a multicenter, randomized, placebo-controlled study, showed that the suppression of asymptomatic or mildly symptomatic ventricular arrhythmias with antiarrhythmic drug therapy after myocardial infarction did not reduce the death rate due to arrhythmia (CAST, 1989). Contrary to expectation, in the patient population studied in the CAST trial, the death rate was more than twice higher for patients receiving antiarrhythmic drugs than for patients receiving placebo. The main reason for this unexpected result was the incorrect assumption that surrogacy followed from the association between a potential surrogate endpoint and the corresponding clinical endpoint, which seemed a very reasonable assumption. But, as emphasized above, the association between arrhythmias and cardiovascular mortality establishes individual-level surrogacy, but does not imply an association between treatment-induced *changes* in arrhythmias and corresponding *changes* in cardiovascular events, the condition required to establish trial-level surrogacy. In addition, the CAST trial recruited patients with asymptomatic or mildly symptomatic arrhythmias, while encainide and flecainide had been approved for patients with life-threatening arrhythmias. At any rate, this dramatic episode led to negative opinions about the use of surrogates in the assessment of the efficacy and safety of new treatments (Fleming, 1994; Ferentz, 2002; Schatzkin and Gail, 2002).

1.1.4 Why Surrogate Endpoints Are Important Today

The development of new drugs is facing unprecedented challenges today, with more molecules than ever available for clinical testing, a better targeting of the populations likely to respond, but a very slow, costly and inefficient clinical development process. An important factor influencing the duration and complexity of this process is the choice of endpoint(s) used to assess drug efficacy. The pressure to increase the speed with which new drugs are approved creates a need to use surrogate endpoints measured early and reliably, rather than long-term clinical endpoints that may be confounded by successive lines of active therapies (Saad and Buyse, 2015).

This trend is especially clear in oncology, where the increased knowledge about the genetic mechanisms operating in cancer cells leads to a large number of novel therapies with specific molecular targets. These therapies are likely to exhibit larger effects than conventional cytotoxic agents, and if so, one would like to detect these effects (or lack thereof) as soon as possible. The ability to predict clinical benefits on long-term endpoints such as survival from benefits observed on earlier endpoints could be enormously useful, hence the acute interest in surrogate endpoints. Shortening the duration of clinical trials not only decreases the cost of the evaluation process; it may also limit potential problems with non-compliance, missing data, and attrition, all of which are more likely in longer studies (Verbeke and Molenberghs, 2000).

Alongside the increased pressure for a speedier clinical development, the rapid advances in molecular biology, in particular the -omics revolution and the advent of new drugs with well-defined mechanisms of action at the molecular level, dramatically increase the number of biomarkers available to define surrogate endpoints (Lesko and Atkinson, 2001). We will discuss illustrative examples of biomarker-based surrogates in Section 1.2.4. Surrogate endpoints also hold potential for the earlier detection of safety signals that could point to toxic problems with new drugs. The duration and sample size of clinical trials aimed at evaluating the therapeutic efficacy of new drugs are often insufficient to detect rare or late adverse effects (Jones, 2001); using surrogate endpoints or biomarkers in this context might allow one to obtain information about such effects even during the clinical testing phase.

1.1.5 The Need for Statistical Evaluation of Surrogates

The unfortunate precedent of anti-arrhythmic drugs made it plain that a statistical evaluation of potential surrogates was required before they were used in clinical research. The seminal paper of Ross Prentice sparked interest in using statistical methods to validate potential surrogates (Prentice, 1989). Prentice suggested definitions and criteria for the validation of surrogates (see details in Section 3.2). At the surge of the AIDS epidemic, the impressive early therapeutic results obtained with zidovudine, and the pressure for accelerated approval of new antiviral therapies, led to the use of CD4+ T-lymphocyte counts as a surrogate endpoint for time to clinical events and overall survival (Lagakos and Hoth, 1992). Yet concerns were expressed about the limitations of CD4+ counts as a reliable predictor for clinical endpoints. Modeling of the effect of treatment and CD4+ counts on survival suggested that CD4+ counts did not fulfill the Prentice criteria (Lin et al., 1993; DeGruttola and Tu, 1994). CD4+ counts were also found to be an incomplete surrogate for clinical progression in individuals with asymptomatic HIV infection taking zidovudine (Choi et al., 1993). These analyses led to a great deal of skepticism about the evaluation and use of surrogate endpoints in general (DeGruttola et al., 1997). However, all these assessments were done using data from single trials, an approach that has serious intrinsic limitations (Molenberghs et al., 2002;

Alonso et al., 2004b, 2006). Shortly after the results of several trials carried out by the AIDS Clinical Trials Group were analyzed simultaneously and a meta-analytic approach was proposed to inform the evaluation of CD4+ as a surrogate endpoint (Daniels and Hughes, 1997).

The present book makes a clear distinction between surrogacy analyses in a single trial and those that require a meta-analysis of multiple trials. When a single trial is available, only individual-level surrogacy can be investigated, unless the trial is very large and can be broken down in smaller units such as countries, regions, or investigational sites. When a meta-analysis of several trials is available, a full evaluation of individual-level as well as trial-level surrogacy can be investigated (Gail et al., 2000). The basic concepts for such analyses have been covered in detail in a previous book (Burzykowski, Molenberghs, and Buyse, 2005). Our purpose here is three-fold:

1. to build on the approach published previously to present more recent methodological developments,
2. to describe software available in SAS and R to implement the methods presented, and
3. to illustrate use of these methods on actual datasets that are available for readers to perform their own analyses.

This book will hopefully contribute to making the methods for surrogate evaluation readily available to anyone familiar with the SAS or R environment.

1.1.6 Surrogate Evaluation and Data Transparency

Initial attempts to validate a surrogate endpoint using data from a single trial have been largely unsuccessful, and today, much of the attention has shifted to the meta-analytic setting in which data are available from several trials. Getting individual patient data from multiple trials was, up until today, a tall order. The principal investigators of the trials had to be convinced to share their data, the protection of patient anonymity was often an insurmountable barrier to data access, and hence there were only rare opportunities to perform the analyses described in this book (Buyse, 2009). The last few years have seen a welcome and timely shift toward making patient-level data from clinical trials available for further analysis. The pharmaceutical industry led this initiative (Nisen and Rockhold, 2013), and implemented a system that is attracting a fast-growing number of research proposals (Strom et al., 2014). The European Medicines Agency (EMA) will soon require that patient-level data be made available for all drugs approved in Europe (Bonini et al., 2014). The International Committee of Medical Journal Editors now mandates that a data sharing plan be available for the trials published in their journals (Taichman et al., 2016). These developments truly revolutionize clinical research, by making it possible to conduct meta-analyses that were previously arduous, hugely time-consuming, and often downright impossible.

As far as surrogacy analyses are concerned, a key limitation of the analyses performed so far is that they were performed as a "one-off" exercise in the context of a specific treatment comparison. But, as mentioned above, a leap of faith is required to apply current knowledge to future treatments that have substantially different modes of action, and in clinical environments that evolve rapidly. The near real-time availability of individual patient data from randomized clinical trials will facilitate updates of previously performed meta-analyses, and an on-going evaluation of surrogate endpoints.

1.2 Typical Uses of Surrogate Endpoints

1.2.1 Earlier Clinical Endpoints

The evaluation methods described in this book can be used in the straightforward situation where a clinical endpoint is repeatedly measured over time, and the treatment effect is assessed at a pre-specified time such as one year after treatment initiation. A natural question in such situations is whether an earlier measurement of the same endpoint would essentially be equivalent to the measurement at the later time point, thus reducing time to analysis (as well as time to market for new drugs). The age-related macular degeneration (ARMD) example is typical: patients with this disease lose vision over time, and the purpose of treatment is to prevent vision loss or, hopefully, restore normal vision. The regulatory agencies commonly require the change in vision one year after starting therapy as the primary endpoint in clinical trials. The dataset described came from a trial of interferon-α, a drug that has no efficacy in ARMD (Pharmacological Therapy for Macular Degeneration Study Group, 1997). In contrast, anti-angiogenic drugs such as ranibizumab have more recently been shown to have remarkable efficacy in in ARMD, and the clinical effect of these agents is already manifest a couple of months following treatment initiation (Rosenfeld et al., 2006). It makes sense, in this setting, to investigate whether vision change at earlier time points (perhaps as early as 3 months) would be an equally good endpoint as vision change at 12 months. An earlier endpoint would considerably reduce the clinical development time of new treatments for this condition, even if the regulatory agencies would still require evidence of maintenance of benefit and absence of safety issues at 1 year and 2 years after initiation of therapy.

1.2.2 Multiple Rating Scales

A second situation in which surrogate evaluation methods are attractive is when the true endpoint is not clearly defined, such as is frequently the case in psychiatric disorders. The case of schizophrenia described in Section 2.2.2

is typical of such situations, with several scales being used to assess the patient's condition, in this case the Clinical Global Impression (CGI), the Brief Psychiatric Rating Scale (BPRS), and the Positive and Negative Syndrome Scale (PANSS). In fact any of these scales could be considered the true endpoint of interest, with the other two being surrogates for it (Molenberghs et al., 2010). Mathematically, the models are symmetric in the surrogate and the true endpoint, so either endpoint can be considered a surrogate for the other. The evaluation methods described in this book can provide valuable insight in the predictive value of one scale for another, both at the individual and trial level, and as such they can inform the choice of a preferred endpoint for future clinical trials when multiple rating scales are being used.

1.2.3 More Sensitive Clinical Endpoints

A situation that has attracted a lot of attention over the last decade is the identification of surrogates when the ultimate endpoint of interest is survival, as is frequently the case in advanced forms of cancer. Overall survival (OS) requires prolonged follow-up, except in fast progressing tumor types, and treatment effects on OS are diluted by competing causes of death, especially in elderly patient populations. In addition, the effect of a new agent on OS may be confounded by the further lines of treatment a patient is likely to receive after failing on this agent. For these reasons, progression-free survival (PFS) is often used as the primary endpoint in clinical trials, with OS being a secondary (but crucially important) endpoint. PFS is often defined as the time from randomization to an increase by more than 25% in the largest dimension of the tumor(s). The treatment effects on PFS tend to be larger than those on OS (Ciani et al., 2013). However, PFS is a controversial endpoint because some new agents (e.g., anti-angiogenic agents in advanced breast cancer) have been shown to have a marked effect on PFS but no sizable benefit on OS. The meta-analytic approach to surrogate endpoint evaluation has been extensively used to investigate PFS as a surrogate endpoint for OS, with diverging results. PFS was found to be a poor surrogate for OS in advanced breast cancer (Burzykowski et al., 2008). In contrast, PFS was a good surrogate in advanced ovarian cancer, using the dataset of Section 2.2.3 (Burzykowski et al., 2001). PFS also appeared to be a good surrogate for OS in advanced colorectal cancer treated with fluoropyrimidines, using the dataset of Section 2.2.4 (Buyse et al., 2007). However, PFS was not as good a surrogate in colorectal cancer treated with more recent therapies, perhaps because of the much larger number of lines of active therapies patients currently receive in this disease (Shi et al., 2015; Ciani et al., 2015). The value of PFS as a surrogate for OS seemed questionable in advanced non-small cell lung cancer (Laporte et al., 2013), and also in advanced cancer, using the dataset of Section 2.2.6 (Paoletti et al., 2013). All in all, PFS cannot be assumed *a priori* to be a good surrogate for OS in advanced solid tumors; each situation has to be assessed on its own merits (Ciani et al., 2014).

It is worth noting that in patients with less advanced tumors that can be resected surgically, disease-free survival (DFS) is a very good surrogate in every tumor type for which formal surrogacy analyses have been carried out, e.g., colon cancer (Sargent et al., 2005), operable or locally advanced head and neck cancer (Michiels et al., 2009), lung cancer (Mauguen et al., 2013), and gastric cancer, using the dataset of Section 2.2.6 (Oba et al., 2013). Taken together, these findings suggest that in early forms of cancer that are amenable to local treatment, DFS can be used as a reliable surrogate for OS. In contrast, in more advanced forms of cancer that are no longer amenable to local treatment, PFS cannot be used as a reliable surrogate for OS. These contrasting findings for DFS and PFS may seem counterintuitive (Buyse et al., 2016). If anything, one would expect PFS to be a better surrogate for OS than DFS, because the time between tumor progression and death is much shorter in advanced disease than after surgical resection of the tumor. However, from a biological standpoint, the reappearance of a tumor after a long disease-free period may be a far more consequential event than an increase in size of a measurable tumor mass.

1.2.4 Biomarker-Based Surrogates

Given the mixed performance of PFS as a surrogate for OS in advanced cancer, interest is currently shifting to biomarker-based surrogate endpoints, which have the potential of providing a much better read-out of the treatment efficacy than measurements of tumor size (Matsui et al., 2015). In prostate cancer, for instance, prostate-specific antigen (PSA) can easily be quantified in the blood. This biomarker has been studied for decades, with a decrease in levels of PSA generally indicating treatment benefit, and a rise in PSA predicting tumor recurrence, and calling for intensified treatment regimens. Various metrics using longitudinal measurements of PSA have been used: PSA doubling time, PSA rate of change or "velocity," PSA decline by more than 30%, PSA nadir under 0.5ng/mL, etc. Some of these metrics have been claimed to satisfy criteria for surrogacy both in early (Valicenti et al., 2006; Denham et al., 2008; Ray et al., 2009; D'Amico et al., 2012) as well as metastatic prostate cancer (Petrylak et al., 2006; Armstrong et al., 2007; Halabi et al., 2013). However, the only analyses that used the full vector of PSA longitudinal measurements and quantified individual-level as well as trial-level associations failed to demonstrate acceptable surrogacy at both levels (Buyse et al., 2003; Collette et al., 2005). The need for a rigorous evaluation of PSA and other biomarkers, including the more recently proposed circulating tumor cells, is especially acute given the long time needed to reach clinical endpoints in prostate cancer (Scher et al., 2015). Such evaluation require large meta-analyses of all randomized trials (Collette, Burzykowski, and Buyse, 2007). The Intermediate Clinical Endpoints in Cancer of the Prostate working group has recently set out to perform an exhaustive meta-analysis of all trials in prostate cancer to formally address the surrogacy of currently known biomarkers (ICECaP, 2015).

1.2.5 Regulatory Use for Accelerated Approval

Some recent targeted agents and immunotherapies for cancer have exceptional efficacy that may warrant their accelerated approval, conditional on further follow-up showing sustained tumor control and clinical benefit. When cytotoxic chemotherapy formed the bulk of anticancer drugs, tumor response (shrinkage by more than by more than 30% of the largest dimension of the tumor) was anticipated to be a reasonable surrogate for long-term benefit. As it turns out, however, while tumor response is associated with longer survival at the individual level, improvements in tumor response rates have generally not been shown to be associated with improvements in survival (Buyse et al., 2000; Burzykowski et al., 2008).

The same lack of trial-level surrogacy was recently shown in a meta-analysis carried out by the US FDA in collaboration with the principal investigators of 12 trials including close to 12,000 patients (Cortazar et al., 2014). This meta-analysis confirmed that patients with a pathological complete response also have a longer survival; however, there was no association between the effects of treatment on pathological complete response and on survival. The reason may be in the heterogeneity of the trials included in the meta-analysis, or in the modest effects of treatment on pathological complete response rates. In spite of these negative results, the US FDA has maintained its guidance on pathological complete response as an approvable endpoint in early breast cancer. The fact remains, however, that caution must be exercised in predicting the long-term benefits of new drugs approved based on pathological complete response, and for now, long-term follow-up of randomized trials is still the best way to generate a definitive answer to this question (DeMichele et al., 2015; Buyse et al., 2016; DeMichele et al., 2016). The same lack of trial-level surrogacy was recently shown in a meta-analysis carried out by the the US FDA in collaboration with the principal investigators of 12 trials including close to 12,000 patients (Cortazar et al., 2014). This meta-analysis confirmed that patients with a pathological complete response also have a longer survival; however, there was no association between the effects of treatment on pathological complete response and on survival. The reason may be in the heterogeneity of the trials included in the meta-analysis, or in the modest effects of treatment on pathological complete response rates. In spite of these negative results, US FDA has maintained its guidance on pathological complete response as an approvable endpoint in early breast cancer. The fact remains, however, that caution must be exercised in predicting the long-term benefits of new drugs approved based on pathological complete response, and for now, long-term follow-up of randomized trials is still the best way to generate a definitive answer to this question (DeMichele et al., 2015; Buyse et al., 2016; DeMichele et al., 2016).

1.2.6 Health Technology Assessment

In a review of 35 model-based cost-effectiveness analyses conducted in the UK, Taylor and Elston (2009) found that only four of them had used a surrogate endpoint. Building on previously published recommendations in the Health Technology Assessment literature (Lassere, 2008), these authors recommend evaluation of surrogacy based on meta-analyses of individual patient data, which is the approach described in this book. Consistent with ICH recommendations (ICH, 1998), they define three levels of evidence:

- level 3 (lowest), is evidence of surrogacy based only on biological plausibility
- level 2 is evidence at level 3 plus surrogacy at the individual level
- level 1 (highest) is evidence at levels 2 and 3 plus surrogacy at the trial level

Some authors (Lassere et al., 2007) and health authorities (e.g., the German Institute for Quality and Efficiency in Health Care (IQWiG, 2011)) have attempted to set thresholds that need to be met by measures of association at the individual level and at the trial level before a surrogate is considered acceptable. While such thresholds may provide useful guidance, they depend on the objective pursued as well as on clinical and other judgments involved in evaluating surrogates. Alternative approaches to simple measures of association could also play a larger role in assessing the strength of evidence in favor of candidate surrogates (Burzykowski and Buyse, 2006; Alonso and Molenberghs, 2007).

1.3 Structure of This Book

This book presents methods and software developed by our group for the evaluation of surrogate endpoints at the individual level and at the trial level. It does *not* present alternative methods that can be used for the evaluation of surrogate endpoints; in particular, very promising methods based on causal inference (Pearl, 2001; ?; Taylor et al., 2005; Li et al., 2010, 2011; Alonso et al., 2015, 2016). The interested reader is referred to Joffe and Greene (2008) for a useful taxonomy of statistical methods for surrogate validation.

The structure of this book is as follows.

Part I provides details on the illustrative examples and datasets used throughout the book (Chapter 2), and presents evaluation methods when data are available from a single trial (Chapter 3).

Part II presents the meta-analytic evaluation framework for different types of endpoints: two continuous endpoints (Chapter 4), two survival endpoints (Chapter 5), a categorical and a survival endpoint (Chapter 6), a continuous and a survival endpoint (Chapter 7), a longitudinal and a survival endpoint (Chapter 8), the evaluation of a surrogate from an information-theoretic point-of-view, both at the trial level (Chapter 9) and at the individual level (Chapter 10), to then conclude with two categorical endpoints (Chapter 11).

Part III provides software details for SAS (Chapter 12), R (Chapter 13), and cloud computing (Chapter 14), whereas Part IV explores further topics: surrogate endpoint evaluation methods in rare diseases (Chapter 15), high dimensional biomarkers (Chapter 16), and imaging biomarkers (Chapter 17).

2

Notation and Example Datasets

Wim Van der Elst
Hasselt University and Janssen Pharmaceutica, Belgium

Ariel Alonso Abad
KU Leuven, Belgium

Marc Buyse
IDDI, Belgium, CluePoints, USA, and Hasselt University, Belgium

Tomasz Burzykowski
Hasselt University, Belgium and IDDI, Belgium

CONTENTS

2.1 Notation

Let us adopt the following notation: T_j and S_j are random variables that refer to the true and the surrogate endpoints of a patient j, respectively. Z_j is a binary indicator for treatment. The present book focuses on multiple-trial surrogate evaluation methods. These methods assume that information regarding the endpoints is available from multiple clinical trials (or from multiple other relevant units in which the patients are clustered, such as the investigators who treated the patients or the countries where patients live in). When the multiple-trial surrogate validation methods are considered, the (T, S, Z) notation is supplemented with an index $i = 1, \ldots, N$ that refers to the ith clinical trial, in the ith of which there are $j = 1, \ldots, n_i$ study participants. Thus in the multiple-trial setting, T_{ij} and S_{ij} are random variables that denote the true and the surrogate endpoints for patient j in trial i, respectively. Z_{ij} is the binary treatment indicator for patient j in trial i. When S and/or T are repeatedly measured over time, an additional index $t = 1, \ldots, k$ is used to indicate the time t at which a measurement took place. For example, when S is repeatedly measured over time, S_{ijt} refers to the surrogate endpoint for patient j in trial i at time t.

2.2 Example Datasets

2.2.1 The Age-Related Macular Degeneration (ARMD) Trial

The objective of this trial was to examine the efficacy of interferon-α to treat age-related macular degeneration (ARMD). ARMD is a medical condition in which patients progressively lose vision (Pharmacological Therapy for Macular Degeneration Study Group, 1997). In the ARMD trial, visual acuity was examined using standardized vision charts that display lines with five letters of decreasing sizes (see Figure 2.1). The patients had to read these letters from top (largest letters) to bottom (smallest letters). Visual acuity was quantified as the total number of letters that were correctly read by a patient.

A total of 181 patients from $N = 36$ centers participated in the ARMD trial. There were two treatment conditions: interferon-α and placebo (coded as $1 =$ interferon-α and $-1 =$ placebo). The true endpoint (T) is the change in visual acuity 52 weeks after the start of the treatment. The candidate surrogate endpoint (S) is the change in visual acuity 24 weeks after starting the treatment. A total of 84 and 97 patients were enrolled in the placebo and interferon-α treatment conditions, respectively.

Figure 2.2 shows histograms of the changes in visual acuity after 24 and 52 weeks. As can be seen, both endpoints are roughly normally distributed. Figure 2.3 presents a scatter plot of T against S. There was a moderately strong correlation between S and T in both the placebo and the experimental treatment groups, i.e., $\widehat{r}(S, T) = 0.7693$ and 0.7118, respectively. The overall correlation combining the information of both treatment groups was $\widehat{r}(S, T) = 0.7464$.

The aim of the ARMD trial was to show that interferon-α is superior to the placebo treatment (using visual acuity as the primary endpoint). Recall that

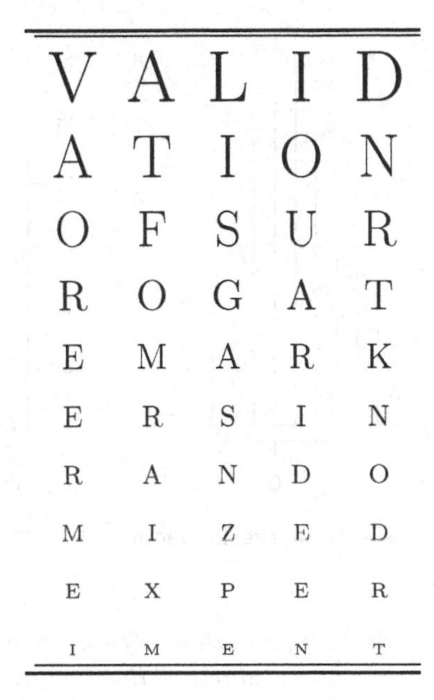

FIGURE 2.1
Age-Related Macular Degeneration Trial. Vision chart.

for a (two-sided) superiority trial, the null and the alternative hypotheses are $H_0 : \Delta = 0$ and $H_A : \Delta \neq 0$ (with Δ= the true difference in the means of the outcomes for both treatment groups). When the result of the hypothesis test is significant, it is concluded that the effect of the experimental treatment on the outcome differs from the effect of the control treatment on the outcome. When the observed result is in favor of the experimental treatment, it is concluded that the experimental treatment is performing significantly better as compared to the control treatment. Note that in case of a non-significant result, it cannot be concluded that the experimental treatment is equally good as the control treatment. The reason for this is that for each small true difference Δ, one can always establish a sample size for which H_0 will be rejected with a high probability (Lesaffre, 2008).

In the ARMD dataset, the means of the changes in visual acuity after 24 weeks (S) were −6.0309 in the placebo group and −7.8095 in the interferon-α group ($\widehat{\Delta}_S = -1.7786$, $t = -0.9352$, $p = 0.3509$; two-sided t-test). The means of the changes in visual acuity after 52 weeks (T) were −11.7423 in the placebo group and −14.6548 in the interferon-α group ($\widehat{\Delta}_T = -2.9125$, $t = -1.2372$, $p = 0.2176$; two-sided t-test). There was thus no evidence that the true differences in the means of S and T in both treatment groups differed from zero.

In the remainder of this book, this dataset will be referred to as the ARMD

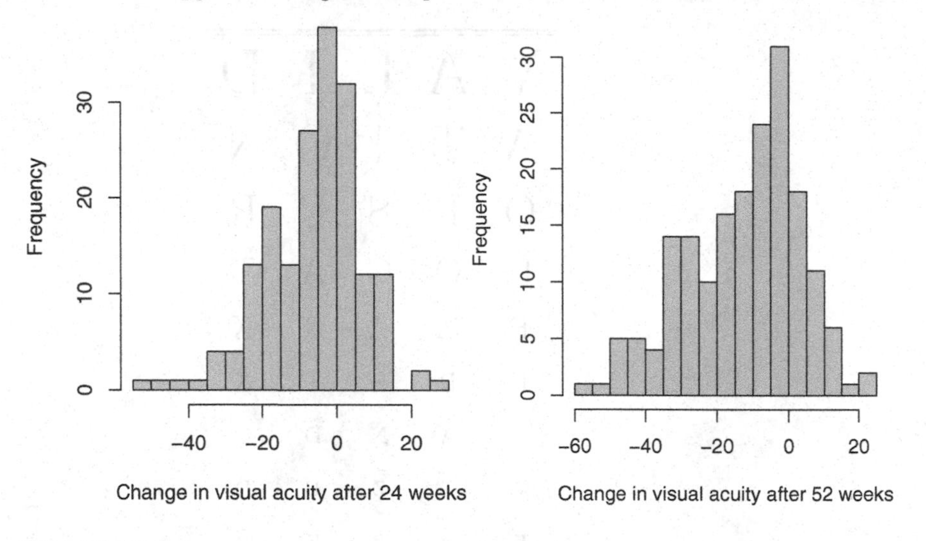

FIGURE 2.2
Age-Related Macular Degeneration Trial. Histograms of the change in visual acuity 24 *weeks after starting the treatment (the candidate surrogate; left panel) and* 52 *weeks after starting the treatment (the true endpoint; right panel).*

dataset. The ARMD dataset is included in the R library Surrogate (where it can be accessed using the command `data(ARMD)`). Alternatively, it can be downloaded from `http://ibiostat.be/online-resources` (file ARMD.txt) for use in SAS or any other software package. Table 2.1 provides a summary of the variables that are included in the ARMD dataset. The dataset is organized in the "wide" format (i.e., there is one line of data per patient). By means of illustration, Table 2.2 shows the first 5 observations in the ARMD dataset.

The data were provided by the Pharmacological Therapy for Macular Degeneration Study Group (Pharmacological Therapy for Macular Degeneration Study Group, 1997).

2.2.2 Five Clinical Trials in Schizophrenia

This dataset combines the data that were collected in five double-blind randomized clinical trials. In these trials, the objective was to examine the efficacy of risperidone to treat schizophrenia. Schizophrenia is a mental disease that is hallmarked by hallucinations and delusions (American Psychiatric Association, 2000).

In each trial, the Clinical Global Impression (CGI; Guy, 1976), the Brief Psychiatric Rating Scale (BPRS; Overall and Gorham, 1962), and the Positive and Negative Syndrome Scale (PANSS; Singh and Kay, 1975) were administered. These instruments are clinical rating scales that are routinely used to

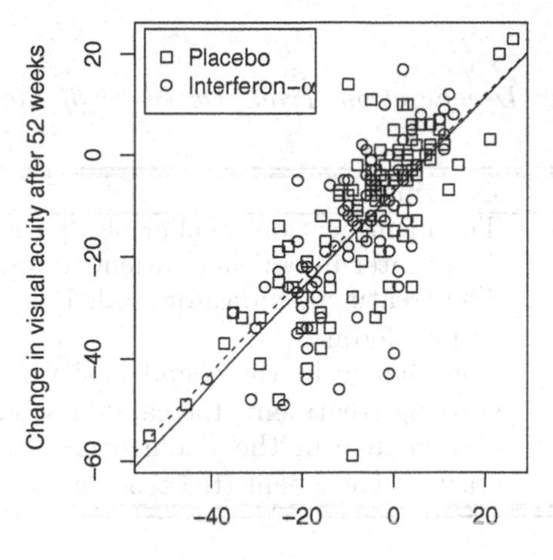

FIGURE 2.3
Age-Related Macular Degeneration Trial. Scatter plot of the change in visual acuity after 52 *weeks (T) against the change in visual acuity after* 24 *weeks (S). The full and dashed lines result from regressing T on S in the groups that were administered interferon-α and placebo, respectively.*

assess symptom severity in patients with schizophrenia (Mortimer, 2007). The patients in the different trials were administered risperidone or an active control (e.g., haloperidol, levomepromazine, or perphenazine) for four to eight weeks. The main endpoints of interest were the change in the CGI score (= CGI score at the end of the treatment − CGI score at the start of the treatment), the change in the PANSS score, and the change in the BPRS score.

A total of 2,128 patients participated in the five trials (1,591 patients received risperidone and 537 patients were given an active control). The patients were treated by a total of $N = 198$ psychiatrists. Each of the psychiatrists treated between $n_i = 1$ and 52 patients.

Figure 2.4 shows the histograms of the changes in the CGI, BPRS, and PANSS scores, respectively. As can be seen, the CGI score is a categorical outcome (score range [1, 7]) whilst the BPRS and PANSS scores can be considered (semi)continuous outcomes that are approximately normally distributed. Figure 2.5 shows scatter plots of the different combinations of the endpoints. Especially the change in the PANSS and the change in the BPRS scores were highly correlated, i.e., $\widehat{r}(BPRS,\ PANSS) = 0.9597$ and 0.9644 in the active control and the experimental treatment groups, respectively (when the information of both treatment groups is combined, $\widehat{r}(BPRS,\ PANSS) = 0.9634$). The correlations between the changes in the CGI and the changes in BPRS/PANSS scores were moderate in both treatment groups, i.e., $\widehat{r}(CGI,\ BPRS) = 0.7394$ and 0.7393 in the active con-

TABLE 2.1
Age-Related Macular Degeneration Trial. Overview of the variables in the dataset.

Variable name	Description
Id	The identification number of a patient
Center	The center in which a patient was treated
Treat	The treatment indicator, coded as -1=placebo and 1=interferon-α
Diff24	The change in the visual acuity at 24 weeks after starting treatment (the candidate surrogate)
Diff52	The change in the visual acuity at 52 weeks after starting treatment (the true endpoint)

TABLE 2.2
Age-Related Macular Degeneration (ARMD) Trial. First five observations in the dataset.

Id	Center	Treat	Diff24	Diff52
1	13395	1	0	−10
2	13395	−1	−3	1
3	13396	1	−6	−17
4	13396	−1	8	1
5	13396	−1	−2	−2

trol and the experimental treatment groups and $\widehat{r}(CGI, PANSS) = 0.7532$ and 0.7503 in the active control and the experimental treatment groups, respectively. When the information of both treatment groups is combined, $\widehat{r}(CGI, BPRS) = 0.7394$ and $\widehat{r}(CGI, PANSS) = 0.7522$.

The means of the changes in the active control and the risperidone treatment groups were 3.4465 and 3.2050 for the CGI endpoint ($\widehat{\Delta}_{CGI} = -0.2415$, $t = -3.254$, $p = 0.0012$; two-sided t-test), -6.6461 and -8.9383 for the BPRS endpoint ($\widehat{\Delta}_{BPRS} = -2.2923$, $t = -3.407$, $p = 0.0007$), and -11.4719 and -16.0151 for the PANSS endpoint ($\widehat{\Delta}_{PANSS} = -4.5432$, $t = -3.876$, $p = 0.0001$), respectively. Note that a larger positive change in the CGI score indicates deteriorated mental health (more schizophrenic symptoms), whereas a larger negative change in the PANSS or BPRS score indicates improved mental health (less schizophrenic symptoms). There was thus strong evidence that the true differences of the means for the three endpoints in both treatment groups differed significantly from zero (in favor of risperidone).

In the reminder of this book, this dataset will be referred to as the Schizophrenia dataset. In the subsequent chapters, different combinations of

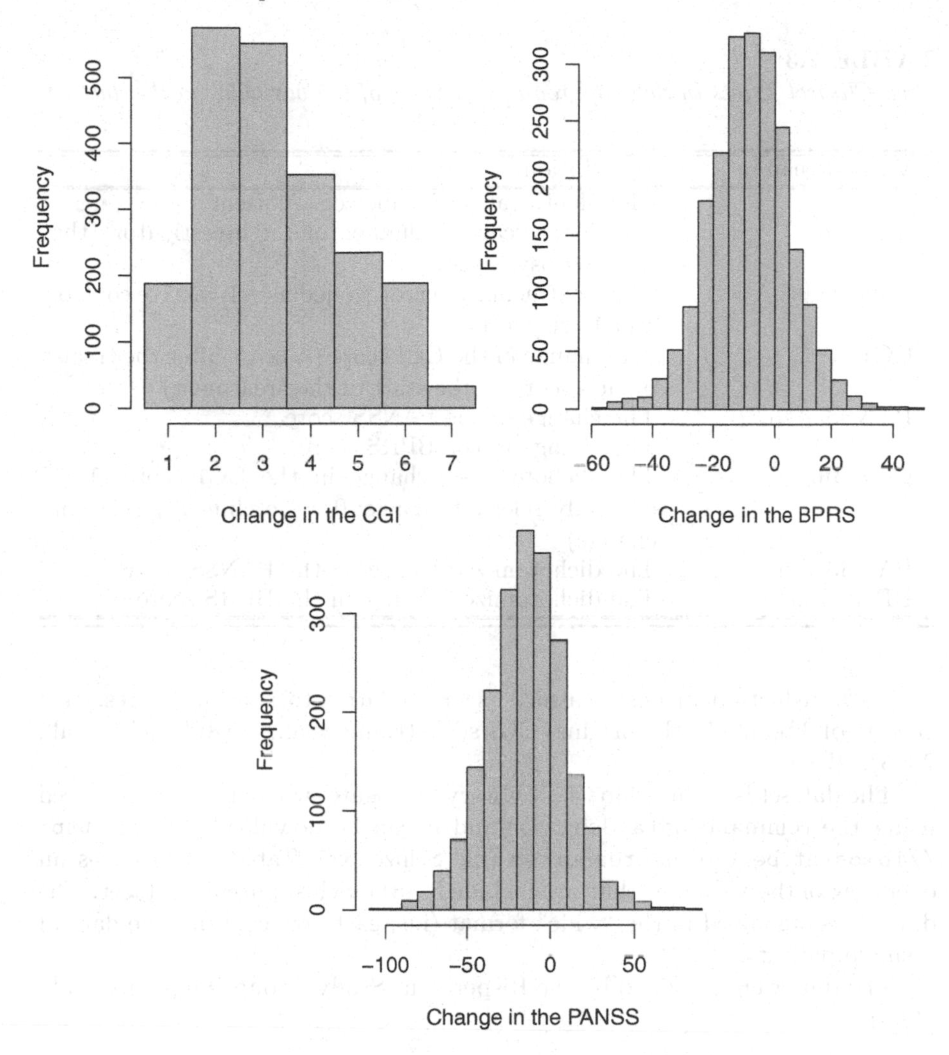

FIGURE 2.4
Five Clinical Trials in Schizophrenia. Histograms of the change in the CGI scores (upper left figure), the change in the BPRS scores (upper right figure), and the change in PANSS scores (bottom figure).
Note: CGI = Clinical Global Impression, BPRS = Brief Psychiatric Rating Scale, and PANSS = Positive and Negative Syndrome Scale.

the endpoints (CGI, BPRS, and PANSS) in various forms (binary, continuous) will be considered as the candidate surrogate and the true endpoint. The binary endpoints BPRS/PANSS/CGI reflect the presence or absence of clinically relevant change in schizophrenic symptomatology. Clinically relevant change is defined as a reduction of 20% or more in the BPRS/PANSS scores,

TABLE 2.3
Five Clinical Trials in Schizophrenia. Overview of the variables in the dataset.

Variable name	Description
Id	The identification number of a patient
InvestId	The identification number of an investigator (the treating psychiatrist)
Treat	The treatment indicator, coded as −1=active control and 1=risperidone
CGI	The change in the CGI score (= score after the treatment - score at the start of the treatment)
PANSS	The change in the PANSS score
BPRS	The change in the BPRS score
CGI_Bin	The dichotomized change in the CGI score (1 = clinically relevant change; 0 = no clinically relevant change)
PANSS_Bin	The dichotomized change in the PANSS score
BPRS_Bin	The dichotomized change in the BPRS score

i.e., 20% reduction in posttreatment scores relative to baseline scores, or a change of 3 points in the original CGI scale (Kane et al., 1988; Leucht et al., 2005).

The dataset is included in the R library Surrogate (where it can be accessed using the command `data(Schizo)`) and it can be downloaded from `http://ibiostat.be/online-resources` (file Schizo.txt). Table 2.3 provides an overview of the variables that are included in the Schizophrenia dataset. The dataset is organized in the "wide" format (i.e., each row contains the data of a single patient).

The data were provided by the Risperidone Study Group (Peuskens et al., 1995).

2.2.3 Advanced Ovarian Cancer: A Meta-Analysis of Four Clinical Trials

This dataset combines the data that were collected in four double-blind randomized clinical trials in advanced ovarian cancer (Ovarian Cancer Meta-Analysis Project, 1991). In these trials, the objective was to examine the efficacy of cyclophosphamide plus cisplatin (CP) versus cyclophosphamide plus adriamycin plus cisplatin (CAP) to treat advanced ovarian cancer. The treatments are coded as $CP = 0$ and $CAP = 1$. The candidate surrogate endpoint S is progression-free survival time, defined as the time (in years) from randomization to clinical progression of the disease or death. The true endpoint

T is survival time, defined as the time (in years) from randomization to death of any cause.

Figure 2.6 shows the progression-free survival and overall survival curves that are obtained when the data of the four available studies are combined. Overall, there was a statistically significant effect in favour of CAP for survival (i.e., estimated relative risk $= 0.8480$, $p = 0.011$) and for progression-free survival (i.e., estimated relative risk $= 0.8136$, $p = 0.0012$).

The dataset combines four trials. In two trials, information was available on the centers in which the patients were treated. In the other two trials, this information was not available but according to the investigators the patients in the latter two trials could be considered a homogeneous group. When the multiple-trial surrogate evaluation methods are used, center will be used as the unit of analysis for the first two trials and trial will be used as the unit of analysis for the last two trials. A total of 50 units were available for analysis, with a number of patients per unit ranging between 2 and 274. In total, $N = 1192$ patients participated in the trial, of whom $n = 606$ received CP and 586 received CAP.

In the remainder of this book, this dataset will be referred to as the Ovarian dataset. The dataset is included in the R library Surrogate (where it can be accessed using the command `data(Ovarian)`) and it can be downloaded from `http://ibiostat.be/online-resources` (file Ovarian.txt). Table 2.4 provides an overview of the variables that are included in the Ovarian dataset.

The data were provided by the Ovarian Cancer Meta-Analysis Project (Ovarian Cancer Meta-Analysis Project, 1991).

2.2.4 Advanced Colorectal Cancer: A Meta-Analysis of 25 Trials

This dataset comprises 3,791 patients enrolled in 25 randomized trials. The data were collected and checked by the Meta-Analysis Group in Cancer between 1990 and 1996 to confirm the benefits of experimental fluoropyrimidine treatments in advanced (metastatic) colorectal cancer (Buyse et al., 2000). The variables collected for every patient randomized in each of these 25 trials consisted of baseline clinical characteristics (patient identification, eligibility, date of randomization, age, sex, performance status, primary tumor site, site of metastases), treatment allocated by randomization, tumor response, duration of response (if applicable), date of death or last visit, survival status, and cause of death (if applicable). Four meta-analyses were carried out and published using these data (Buyse et al., 2000). In all four meta-analyses, the comparison was between a control treatment ($Z = 0$) and an experimental treatment ($Z = 1$). The control treatments were similar across the four meta-analyses and consisted of fluorouracil or floxuridine given as a bolus intravenous injection. The experimental treatments differed across the four meta-analyses: it was either fluorouracil modulated by leucovorin, fluorouracil modulated by methotrexate, fluorouracil given by continuous infusion,

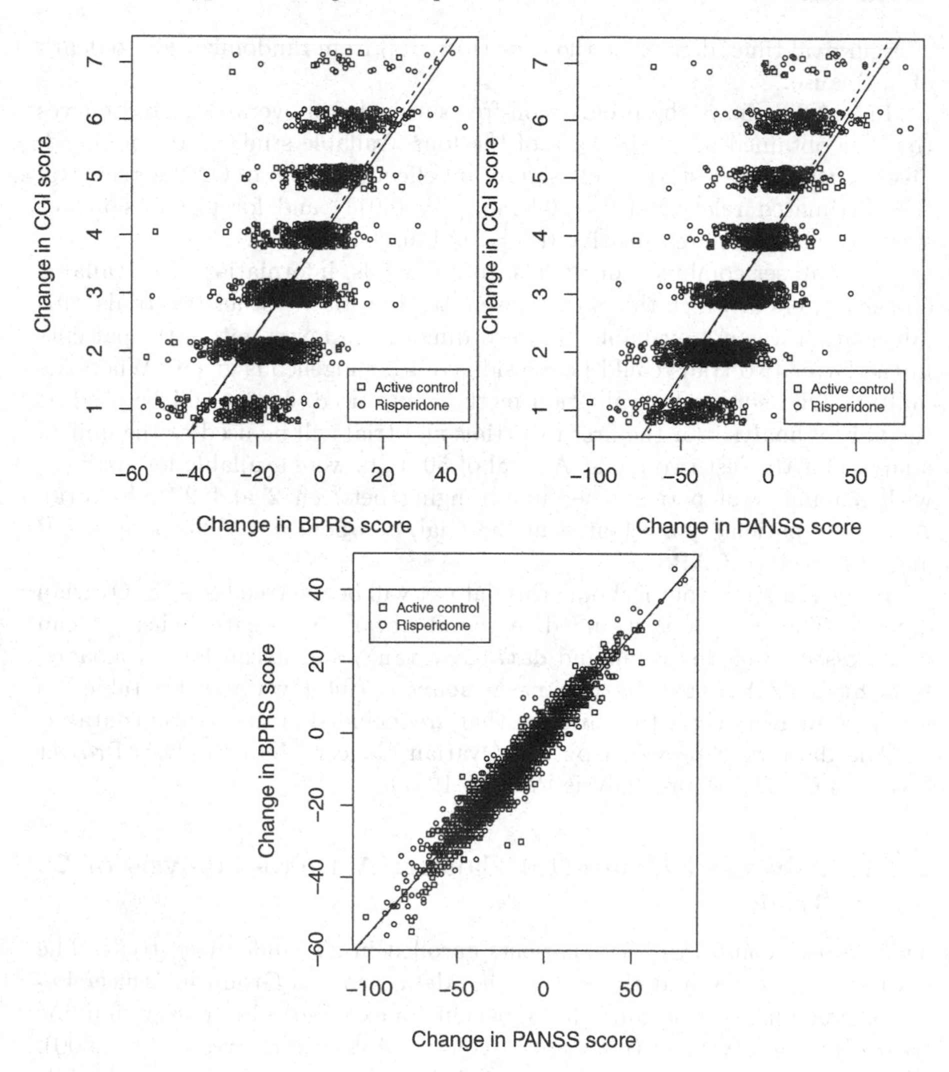

FIGURE 2.5
Five Clinical Trials in Schizophrenia. Scatter plots of the change in the CGI scores against the change in the BPRS scores (upper left figure), the change in the CGI scores against the change in the PANSS scores (upper right figure), and the change in the BPRS scores against the change in the PANSS scores (bottom figure). The full and dashed lines result from regressing the endpoint on the Y-axis on the endpoint on the X-axis in the groups that were administered risperidone and the active control, respectively. Jitter (a small amount of random noise) was added to the change in the CGI scores to prevent overplotting of the data points.
Note: CGI = Clinical Global Impression, BPRS = Brief Psychiatric Rating Scale, and PANSS = Positive and Negative Syndrome Scale.

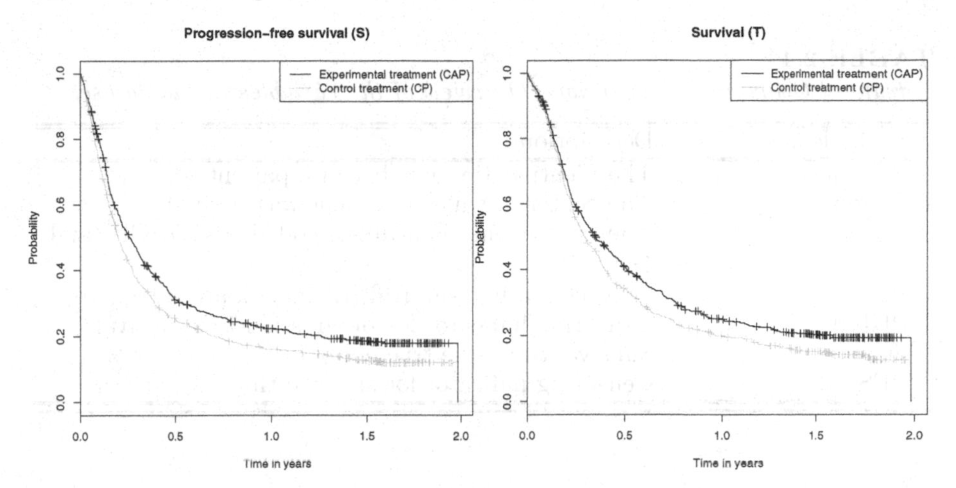

FIGURE 2.6
Advanced Ovarian Cancer Trials. Progression-free survival (S) and overall survival (T) curves (left and right panel, respectively) combining the data of the four available studies.

or hepatic-arterial infusion of floxuridine for patients with metastases confined to the liver.

In the meta-analysis of 25 trials, the response rate was 22% with the experimental treatments *vs.* 12% with the control treatments, a highly statistically significant benefit (odds ratio = 0.48, 95% CI [0.40; 0.57], $p < 0.0001$). The experimental treatments also had a significant effect on overall survival, though the magnitude of the benefit was modest, with an absolute difference of a few percentage points at all times between the Kaplan–Meier survival estimates (hazard ratio = 0.90, 95% CI [0.84; 0.97], $p = 0.003$).

For the surrogacy analyses (Buyse et al., 2000; Burzykowski, Molenberghs, and Buyse, 2004), the true endpoint (T) is survival time, calculated from the day of randomization to the day of death irrespective of the cause of death. The candidate surrogate endpoint (S) is tumor response. Tumor response is commonly defined as a categorical variable with four ordered categories: complete response (CR), partial response (PR), stable disease (SD) and progressive disease (PD). CR is defined as the disappearance of all detectable tumor. PR is defined as a decrease of 50% or more in the tumor surface area measured by CT scan (sum of the products of the largest perpendicular diameters of all measurable disease), without appearance of new lesions and a duration of at least 4 weeks. SD is defined as a decrease of less than 50% or an increase of less than 25% in the tumor surface area, without new lesions. PD is defined as an increase of more than 25% in the tumor surface area or the appearance of any new lesion. The surrogacy analyses are carried out with

TABLE 2.4
Advanced Ovarian Cancer Trials. Overview of the variables in the dataset.

Variable name	Description
Patient	The identification number of a patient
Center	The center in which a patient was treated
Treat	The treatment indicator, coded as 0=CP and 1=CAP
Pfs	Progression-free survival (the candidate surrogate)
PfsInd	Censoring indicator for progression-free survival
Surv	Survival time (the true endpoint)
PFSInd	Censoring indicator for survival time

response considered a binary outcome: $S = 1$ for patients with CR or PR and $S = 0$ for patients with SD or PD.

In the remainder of this book, this dataset will be referred to as the Colorectal25 dataset. The dataset is included in the R library Surrogate (where it can be accessed using the command data(Colorectal25)) and it can be downloaded from `http://ibiostat.be/online-resources` (file Colorectal25.txt). Table 2.5 provides an overview of the variables that are included in the Colorectal25 dataset. The data were provided by the Meta-Analysis Group In Cancer (see Buyse et al., 2000).

2.2.5 Advanced Colorectal Cancer: A Meta-Analysis of 13 Trials

This dataset comprises 3089 patients enrolled in 10 historical trials and 1263 patients enrolled in 3 validation trials that all had a fluorouracil + leucovorin group in common (Buyse et al., 2007). Historical trials compared fluorouracil + leucovorin with fluorouracil alone (7 trials, 1744 patients), or fluorouracil + leucovorin with raltitrexed (3 trials, 1345 patients). Validation trials (1263 patients in total) compared fluorouracil + leucovorin with the same + irinotecan (2 trials, 843 patients) or with the same + oxaliplatin (1 trial, 420 patients). The variables collected for every patient randomized in each of these trials consisted of patient identifier, center identifier, randomization date, treatment assigned by randomization, tumor measurability (i.e., measurable or non-measurable tumors), age, gender, performance status, primary tumor site (colon or rectum), site of metastases, overall response status with the first assigned treatment, date of response, date of progression with the first allocated treatment, date of death or last visit, survival status, and cause of death if applicable. The control group ($Z = 0$) was considered to be fluorouracil + leucovorin in all trials, and the other treatment group was considered experimental ($Z = 1$). Note that in reality fluorouracil alone was the control group

TABLE 2.5
25 Trials in Advanced Colorectal Cancer. Overview of the variables in the dataset.

Variable name	Description
Trial	The trial in which a patient was treated
Newptid	The identification number of a patient
Newtrt	The treatment indicator, coded as 0=Control and 1=Experimental
Binresp	Binary response (a candidate surrogate), coded as 0=no response and 1=response
Ordresp1	Categorical ordered response (a candidate surrogate), coded as 1=complete response (CR), 2=partial response (PR), 3=stable disease (SD) and 4=progressive disease (PD)
Ps	Performance status, a baseline categorical ordered covariate taking the values 0, 1 or 2
Surv	Survival time in days (the true endpoint)
Status	Censoring indicator for survival time (0=alive, 1=dead)

in the 7 trials that had compared fluorouracil alone with fluorouracil + leucovorin. The convention adopted here facilitates interpretation in so far as the same control group is used throughout. In the meta-analysis, the experimental group was statistically different from the control group in terms of progression-free survival and survival in both the 10 historical trials and the 3 validation trials.

For the surrogacy analyses (Buyse et al., 2007; Burzykowski et al., 2001), the true endpoint (T) is survival time, calculated from the day of randomization to the day of death irrespective of the cause of death. The candidate surrogate endpoint (S) is progression-free survival, calculated from the time of randomization to progressive disease or death from any cause. Progressive disease is defined as an increase of more than 25% in the tumor surface area measured by CT-scan or the appearance of any new lesion. In historical trials, 1760 patients (57%) progressed or died within 6 months, and 1622 (52%) died within 1 year. Hence the information would be about the same for an analysis of progression-free survival at 6 months as for an analysis of survival at 1 year.

In the remainder of this book, this dataset will be referred to as the Colorectal13 dataset. The dataset is included in the R library Surrogate (where it can be accessed using the command data (Colorectal13)) and it can be downloaded from `http://ibiostat.be/online-resources` (file Colorectal13.txt). Table 2.6 provides an overview of the variables that are included in the Colorectal13 dataset. The data were provided by the Meta-Analysis Group in Cancer, the Biostatistics and Epidemiology Unit of Institut Gustave-Roussy, AstraZeneca, Sanofi-aventis, and Pfizer (see Buyse et al., 2007).

TABLE 2.6
13 Trials in Advanced Colorectal Cancer. Overview of the variables in the dataset.

Variable name	Description
Trial	The trial in which a patient was treated
Treat	The treatment indicator, coded as 0=Control and 1=Experimental
Pfs	Progression-free survival in months (the candidate surrogate)
Pfsind	Censoring indicator for progression-free survival
Surv	Survival time in months (the true endpoint)
Survind	Censoring indicator for survival time (0=alive, 1=dead)

2.2.6 Advanced Gastric Cancer: A Meta-Analysis of 20 Trials

Two meta-analyses of randomized clinical trials were conducted by the GASTRIC (Global Advanced/Adjuvant Stomach Tumor Research International Collaboration) Group. The first meta-analysis included individual data on 3,838 patients with curatively resected gastric cancer randomized in 17 trials. This meta-analysis confirmed the benefit of adjuvant chemotherapy as compared with no adjuvant treatment in terms of both disease-free survival (DFS) and overall survival (OS) (GASTRIC Group, 2010). It was also used to show that DFS is a valid surrogate for OS in the adjuvant setting (Oba et al., 2013). The second meta-analysis included individual data on 4,245 patients with advanced or recurrent gastric cancer randomized in 22 trials. This meta-analysis confirmed the benefit of adding experimental agents to standard chemotherapy regimens in terms of both progression-free survival (PFS) and overall survival (OS) (GASTRIC Group, 2013). It was used to show that PFS cannot be used reliably as a surrogate in advanced disease (Paoletti et al., 2013). These two meta-analyses illustrate how a quantitative evaluation can inform the use of potential surrogate endpoints, since two situations that appear relatively similar at face value lead to opposite conclusions as to whether a putative surrogate can be used in practice (Buyse et al., 2016).

In this book we will focus on the situation of advanced gastric cancer. Data are available on 4,069 patients randomized in 20 trials with documented overall survival and progression-free survival (Paoletti et al., 2013). The variables available for analysis include patient identifier (pat_id), trial identifier (id_study), treatment assigned by randomization (arm), time to progression or death with the first allocated treatment (pfs), progression or death status (pfs_status), time to death or last visit (os), and survival status (last_status). Details on the coding of treatments (1=Control vs. 2=Experimental) are pro-

TABLE 2.7
Advanced Gastric Cancer Trial. Observed treatment effects [95% confidence intervals] on PFS and OS, and predicted treatment effect on OS [95% prediction intervals] in twelve validation trials in advanced gastric cancer (Paoletti et al., 2013). Asterisks mark intervals that exclude no effect.

Trial	Observed HR_{PFS}	Observed HR_{OS}	Predicted HR_{OS}
Jeung	0.63 [0.38, 1.05]	0.56 [0.35, 0.88]*	0.73 [0.46, 1.04]
AIO	0.67 [0.43, 1.04]	0.82 [0.47, 1.45]	0.76 [0.53, 1.07]
ToGA	0.71 [0.59, 0.85]*	0.74 [0.60, 0.91]*	0.80 [0.58, 1.09]
AVAGAST	0.80 [0.68, 0.93]*	0.87 [0.73, 1.03]	0.88 [0.76, 1.14]
Kang	0.80 [0.63, 1.03]	0.85 [0.64, 1.13]	0.88 [0.76, 1.14]
Park	0.86 [0.54, 1.37]	0.96 [0.60, 1.52]	0.93 [0.71, 1.18]
REAL(a)	0.92 [0.80, 1.04]	0.92 [0.80, 1.10]	0.98 [0.77, 1.22]
REAL(b)	0.92 [0.81, 1.05]	0.86 [0.80, 0.99]*	0.98 [0.77, 1.22]
Ross	0.95 [0.80, 1.08]	0.91 [0.76, 1.04]	1.00 [0.79, 1.29]
FLAGS	0.99 [0.86, 1.14]	0.92 [0.80, 1.05]	1.03 [0.81, 1.31]
Rao	1.13 [0.63, 2.01]	1.02 [0.61, 1.70]	1.14 [0.89, 1.46]
Moehler	1.14 [0.59, 2.21]	0.77 [0.51, 1.17]	1.15 [0.90, 1.48]

vided in the original meta-analysis (GASTRIC Group, 2013) and surrogate evaluation paper (Paoletti et al., 2013).

One interesting feature of this meta-analysis was that the results of the surrogate evaluation could be externally validated using twelve trials not included in the meta-analysis, using treatment effects extracted from reports published in the literature after the meta-analysis was completed (Table 2.7). The observed treatment effects on survival (HR_{OS}), along with their 95% confidence intervals, could be compared with the treatment effects on survival predicted from the treatment effects on the surrogate (HR_{PFS}) in each of these 12 trials. For reasons that are fully detailed in Section 5.3, the prediction intervals were quite wide and included one (no treatment effect on OS) in all 12 trials, which means that the observed effects on PFS would not have allowed predicting an effect on OS in any of these twelve trials. Yet, three of the twelve trials showed a statistically significant effect of treatment on survival (Paoletti et al., 2013), which provided further evidence that treatment effects on PFS were unreliable predictors for treatment effects (or lack thereof) on OS.

In the remainder of this book, this dataset will be referred to as the Gastric dataset. The dataset is included in the R library Surrogate (where it can be accessed using the command data(Gastric)) and it can be downloaded from `http://ibiostat.be/online-resources` (file gastric.txt). Table 2.8 provides an overview of the variables that are included in the Gastric dataset. The data were provided by the GASTRIC (Global Advanced/Adjuvant Stom-

TABLE 2.8
Advanced Gastric Cancer Trial. Overview of the variables in the dataset.

Variable name	Description
id_study	The trial in which the patient was treated
id_pat	The identification number of a patient
arm	The treatment indicator (1=Control, 2=Experimental)
pfs	Progression-free survival in days (the candidate surrogate)
pfs_status	Censoring indicator for progression-free survival (0=alive and progression-free, 1=with progression or dead)
os	Overall survival time in days (the true endpoint)
last_status	Censoring indicator for survival time (0=alive, 1=dead)

ach Tumor Research International Collaboration) Group (see Paoletti et al., 2013).

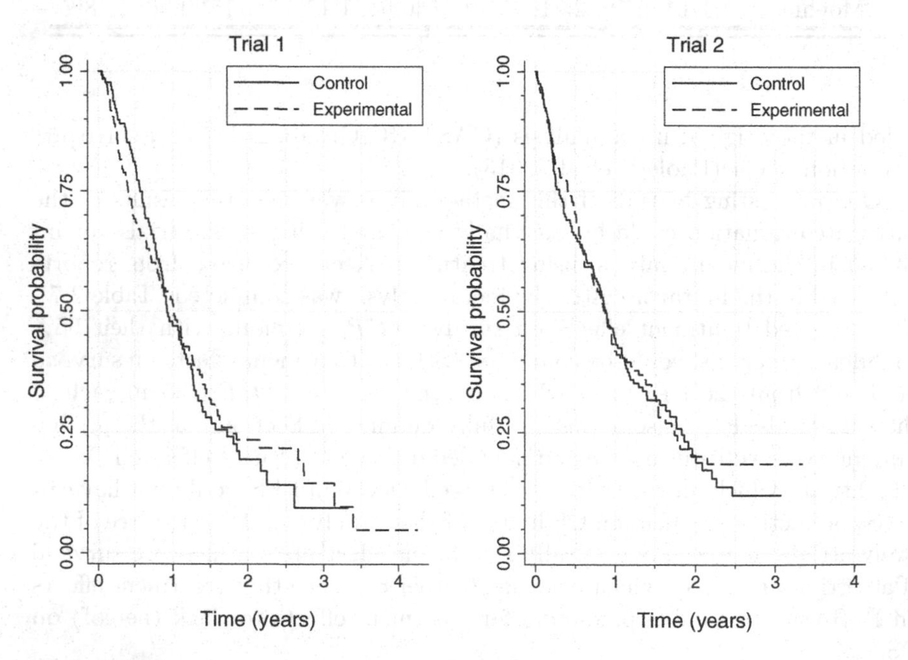

FIGURE 2.7
Advanced Prostate Cancer Trials. Survival curves by treatment arm.

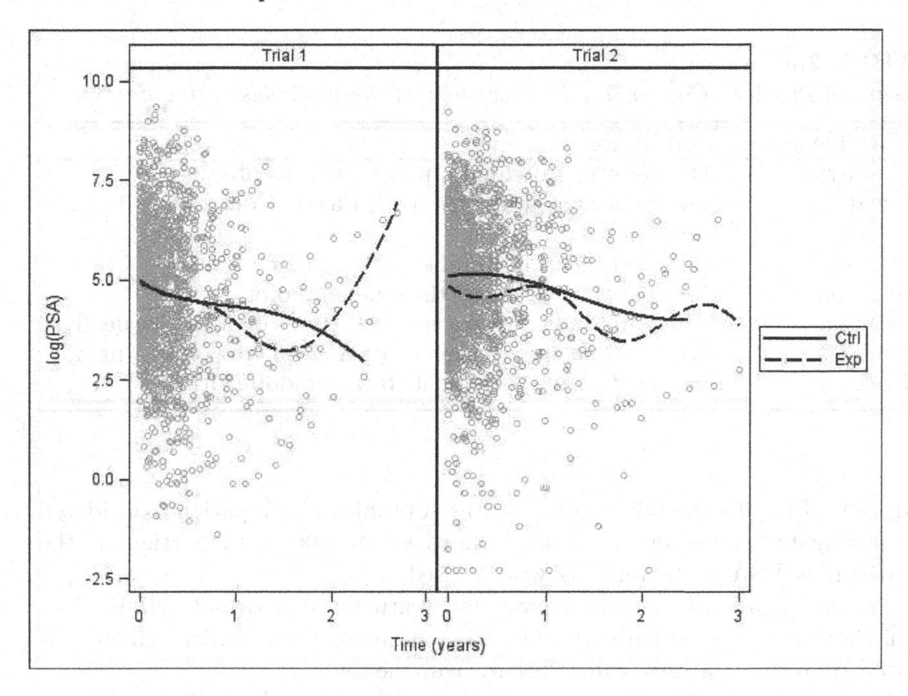

FIGURE 2.8
Advanced Prostate Cancer Trials. Mean PSA profiles by treatment arm.

2.2.7 Advanced Prostate Cancer: A Meta-Analysis of Two Trials

This dataset comprises two trials that compared oral liarozole, an experimental retinoic acid metabolism-blocking agent ($Z - 1$), with an antiandrogenic drug considered as control ($Z = 0$): cyproterone acetate in the first trial and flutamide in the second (Buyse et al., 2003). In both trials, patients were in relapse after first-line endocrine therapy. The trials accrued 312 and 284 patients, respectively. Each trial was multinational and multicentric, and the unit of analysis for the surrogacy analysis was chosen to be the country in which the patients were treated. There were 19 countries containing between 4 and 69 patients. The primary endpoint of the trials was overall survival from the start of treatment. In both trials, patients were assessed at baseline (before the start of treatment), at 2 weeks, monthly for 6 months, at 3-month intervals until the second year, and at 6-month intervals until treatment discontinuation or death. The assessments included measurement of the prostate-specific antigen (PSA) level. PSA is a glycoprotein that is found almost exclusively in normal and neoplastic prostate cells. Changes in PSA often antedate changes in bone scan, and they have been used as an indicator of response in patients with androgen-independent prostate cancer.

For the surrogacy analyses, overall survival will be considered the true

TABLE 2.9
Advanced Prostate Cancer Trials. Overview of the variables in the dataset.

Variable name	Description
Countryn	The country in which a patient was treated
Treat	The treatment indicator, coded as 0=Control and 1=Experimental
Patid	The identification number of a patient
Survtime	Survival time in days (the true endpoint)
Survind	Censoring indicator for survival time (0=alive, 1=dead)
PSA	Prostate specific androgen (PSA) measurement in ng/ml
PSAday	Day of PSA measurement (from randomization)

endpoint (T), with the full longitudinal PSA profile of each patient considered the surrogate (Buyse et al., 2003; Renard et al., 2003). In particular, the logarithm of PSA measurements will be used.

Figure 2.7 presents survival curves per treatment arm for both trials. Note that there were 18 patients without PSA measurements, which will be excluded from the analyses using PSA measurements.

Figure 2.8 presents the scatter plots of the observed log-PSA values in function of the measurement time for patients per trial. Additionally, the plots include the smoothed mean profiles for the control and treatment groups.

In the remainder of this book, this dataset will be referred to as the PSA dataset. The dataset is included in the R library Surrogate (where it can be accessed using the command data(PSA) and it can be downloaded from `http://ibiostat.be/online-resources` (file PSA.txt). Table 2.9 provides an overview of the variables that are included in the PSA dataset. The data were provided by the Janssen Research Foundation (see Buyse et al., 2003).

2.3 Acknowledgments for Use of Data

The example datasets that accompany this book can be freely downloaded from `http://ibiostat.be/online-resources`. Researchers who download and analyze the data accept the following conditions:

1. the research shall be scientifically sound and peer reviewed,
2. the data shall be used for the purpose of evaluating surrogacy,
3. the source of the data shall be acknowledged in all presentations and publications, including a reference to publication(s) by the investigator or group of investigators who generated the data,

4. the results of the analyses shall be made available to the research community, and
5. the confidentiality of individual patient data shall be protected.

3

The History of Surrogate Endpoint Evaluation: Single-Trial Methods

Ariel Alonso Abad

KU Leuven, Belgium

Wim Van der Elst

Hasselt University, and Janssen Pharmaceutica, Belgium

CONTENTS

3.1 Introduction

The seminal papers of Prentice (1989), Freedman et al. (1992), and Buyse and Molenberghs (1998) have set the scene for a large research line into surrogate marker evaluation methods. The methods that were proposed by these authors were based on the premise that information regarding the surrogate and the true endpoints is available from a single clinical trial. Hence, these methods are collectively referred to as single-trial surrogate evaluation methods. In this chapter, these methods are briefly reviewed.

It is important to emphasize that all single-trial methods are hampered by some fundamental theoretical and/or applied problems (see Sections 3.2.3–3.4.3 below). This chapter merely reviews the single-trial methods to set the scene for the statistically more informative multiple-trial surrogate evaluation methods, which assume that the data of multiple trials or other relevant clustering units are available (see Part II of this book). The use of these single-trial methods is not recommended in practice, for reasons outlined in Section 3.5.

3.2 Prentice's Approach

3.2.1 Definition

Prentice (1989) defined a surrogate endpoint as "a response variable for which a test of the null hypothesis of no relationship to the treatment groups under comparison is also a valid test of the corresponding null hypothesis based on the true endpoint" (Prentice, 1989; p. 432). This definition essentially requires that the surrogate endpoint should capture any relationship between the treatment and the true endpoint (Lin et al., 1997). Symbolically, Prentice's definition can be written as:

$$f(S \mid Z) = f(S) \Leftrightarrow f(T \mid Z) = f(T),$$

where $f(S)$ and $f(T)$ denote the probability distributions of the random variables S and T, and $f(S \mid Z)$ and $f(T \mid Z)$ denote the probability distributions of S and T conditional on the value of Z, respectively. Note that this definition involves the triplet $(T,\ S,\ Z)$, so S is a surrogate for T only with respect to the effect of some *specific* treatment Z and not (necessarily) for a different treatment (except when S is a perfect surrogate for T, i.e., except when S and T are deterministically related).

Based on his definition of a surrogate endpoint, Prentice formulated four operational criteria that should be fulfilled to validate a candidate surrogate endpoint:

$$f(S \mid Z) \neq f(S), \tag{3.1}$$

$$f(T \mid Z) \neq f(T), \tag{3.2}$$

$$f(T \mid S) \neq f(T), \tag{3.3}$$

$$f(T \mid S,\ Z) = f(T \mid S). \tag{3.4}$$

Thus, the treatment Z should have a significant effect on S (see (3.1)), the treatment Z should have a significant effect on T (see (3.2)), S should have a significant effect on T (see (3.3)), and the effect of the treatment Z on T should be fully captured by S (see (3.4)).

3.2.2 Analysis of Case Studies: The Age-Related Macular Degeneration Trial

The use of the Prentice criteria to evaluate the validity of a candidate surrogate endpoint will be illustrated here using the ARMD dataset (which was described in Section 2.2.1 of Chapter 2, starting on page 16). Recall that in the ARMD dataset, the surrogate and the true endpoints of a patient j (i.e., S_j and T_j) were the change in visual acuity at 6 and 12 months after starting the treatment, respectively. The binary indicator for the treatment of a patient j (i.e., Z_j) was coded as -1: placebo and 1: interferon-α.

In the analyses, it will be assumed that both S and T are normally distributed. In this setting, the first two Prentice criteria (see (3.1)–(3.2)) are examined by fitting the following bivariate linear regression model:

$$\begin{aligned} S_j &= \mu_S + \alpha Z_j + \varepsilon_{Sj}, && (3.5) \\ T_j &= \mu_T + \beta Z_j + \varepsilon_{Tj}, && (3.6) \end{aligned}$$

where the error terms ε_{Sj} and ε_{Tj} have a joint zero-mean normal distribution with variance-covariance matrix:

$$\Sigma = \begin{pmatrix} \sigma_{SS} & \sigma_{ST} \\ \sigma_{ST} & \sigma_{TT} \end{pmatrix}. \tag{3.7}$$

Prentice's third criterion (see (3.3)) can be examined by fitting the following univariate linear regression model (when S and T are continuous normally distributed endpoints):

$$T_j = \mu + \gamma S_j + \varepsilon_j. \tag{3.8}$$

Finally, the fourth Prentice criterion (see (3.4)) can be examined by fitting the following univariate linear regression model (when S and T are continuous normally distributed endpoints, as in (3.5)–(3.6)):

$$T_j = \widetilde{\mu}_T + \beta_S Z_j + \gamma_Z S_j + \widetilde{\varepsilon}_{Tj}, \tag{3.9}$$

where

$$\begin{aligned} \beta_S &= \beta - \sigma_{ST}\sigma_{SS}^{-1}\alpha, \\ \gamma_Z &= \sigma_{ST}\sigma_{SS}^{-1}, \end{aligned}$$

and the variance of $\widetilde{\varepsilon}_T$ equals:

$$\sigma_{TT} - \sigma_{ST}^2\sigma_{SS}^{-1}.$$

When models (3.5)–(3.6), (3.8), and (3.9) are fitted to the ARMD dataset, it is obtained that $\widehat{\alpha} = -0.8893$ (s.e. 0.9509, $p = 0.3509$), $\widehat{\beta} = -1.4562$ (s.e. 1.1771, $p = 0.2176$), $\widehat{\gamma} = 0.9256$ (s.e. 0.0617, $p < 0.0001$), and $\widehat{\beta_S} = -0.6362$ (s.e. 0.7894, $p = 0.4213$). Note that $\widehat{\alpha}$ and $\widehat{\beta}$ are negative, indicating a (albeit non-significant) negative effect of the experimental treatment on visual acuity after 24 and 52 weeks.

To be in line with Prentice's criteria, the hypotheses $H_0 : \alpha = 0$, $H_0 : \beta = 0$, and $H_0 : \gamma = 0$ in models (3.5)–(3.6) and (3.8) should be rejected, whereas the hypothesis $H_0 : \beta_S = 0$ in model (3.9) should not be rejected. Thus, in the ARMD dataset, the first and second Prentice criteria were not fulfilled (using the conventional 0.05 level of significance). Hence, based on the Prentice criteria, it is concluded that the change in visual acuity after 6 months is not a good surrogate for the change in visual acuity after 12 months.

3.2.3 An Appraisal of Prentice's Approach

The Prentice criteria are intuitively appealing and straightforward to test, but there are some fundamental problems that surround this approach.

First, the fourth Prentice criterion (3.4) requires that the statistical test for the β_S parameter is non-significant (see (3.9) for the case where both S and T are continuous normally distributed endpoints). This criterion is useful to reject a poor surrogate endpoint (i.e., a surrogate for which $\beta_S \neq 0$), but it is not suitable to validate a good surrogate (i.e., a surrogate for which $\beta_S = 0$). Indeed, validating a good surrogate in the Prentice framework would require the *acceptance* of the null hypothesis $H_0 : \beta_S = 0$, which is obviously not possible (Freedman et al., 1992). For example, the non-significant hypothesis test may always be the result of a lack of statistical power due to an insufficient number of patients in the trial.

Second, even when lack of statistical power would not be an issue, the result of the statistical test to evaluate the fourth Prentice criterion (i.e., $H_0 : \beta_S = 0$) cannot prove that the effect of the treatment Z on T is *fully* captured by S (Burzykowski, Molenberghs, and Buyse, 2005; Frangakis and Rubin, 2002). Moreover, in any practical setting, it would be more realistic to expect that a surrogate explains part of the treatment effect on the true endpoint, rather than the full effect. These considerations led Freedman et al. (1992) to the proposal that attention should be shifted from the hypothesis-testing framework of Prentice (1989), i.e., a yes/no all-or-nothing qualitative judgment of the appropriateness of a candidate S, to an estimation framework, i.e., a quantitative rating of the appropriateness of a candidate S. Their proposal (the so-called Proportion Explained) is detailed in Section 3.3.

Third, it can be shown that Prentice's operational criteria to validate a candidate S are only equivalent to his definition of a surrogate when both S and T are binary variables (in the latter case, models (3.5)–(3.6), (3.8), and

(3.9) are replaced by their logistic regression counterparts). This implies that verifying the operational criteria does not guarantee that the surrogate truly fulfills the definition, except when all members of the triplet (Z, T, S) are binary. For details, the reader is referred to Buyse and Molenberghs (1998).

Fourth, a candidate S can only be validated when the treatment Z significantly affects both S and T (see (3.1)–(3.2)). Thus, the data of a clinical trial in which the treatment has no significant effect on S and T (which was the case for the ARMD trial, see Section 3.2.2) cannot be used to validate a surrogate endpoint in Prentice's approach.

3.3 The Proportion of Treatment Effect Explained

3.3.1 Definition

In view of the problems with the Prentice criteria (see Section 3.2.3), Freedman et al. (1992) proposed to quantify surrogacy as the proportion of the effect of treatment Z on T that is explained by S (the Proportion Explained, PE):

$$PE(T, S, Z) = \frac{\beta - \beta_S}{\beta} = 1 - \frac{\beta_S}{\beta}, \tag{3.10}$$

where β is the effect of treatment on T without correction for S and β_S is the effect of the treatment on T with correction for S. The intuition behind the PE is that, if all treatment effect is mediated by S (i.e., if $\beta_S = 0$), then $PE = 1$. On the other hand, if there is no mediation at all (i.e., if $\beta = \beta_S$), then $PE = 0$ (but note that this intuitively appealing reasoning is flawed, see Section 3.3.3).

The PE is a ratio of parameters, so its confidence interval can be calculated using Fieller's theorem or the delta method (Burzykowski, Molenberghs, and Buyse, 2005). A good S should have a lower limit confidence interval value for PE that is close to 1. Note that the fourth Prentice criterion (which states that the effect of Z on T is fully captured by S, see (3.4)) is equivalent to the requirement that $PE = 1$.

3.3.2 Analysis of Case Studies: The Age-Related Macular Degeneration Trial

The use of the PE to assess surrogacy will be illustrated using the ARMD data. In the analyses, both S and T are considered to be continuous normally distributed endpoints so β and β_S can be estimated using models (3.6) and (3.9), respectively. As was found in Section 3.2.2, $\widehat{\beta} = -1.4562$ (s.e. 1.1771) and $\widehat{\beta_S} = -0.6362$ (s.e. 0.7894). Thus, $\widehat{PE} = 1 - (-0.6362/-1.4562) = 0.5631$ (95% delta method-based confidence limits $[-0.3533, 1.2271]$). The point estimate for PE thus indicates that 56.31% of the effect of Z on T can be explained by S, but notice that the 95% confidence interval covers the entire [0, 1] interval and thus no useful information is conveyed.

3.3.3 An Appraisal of the Proportion Explained

As was also the case with the Prentice criteria, there are some severe issues with the PE.

First, the intuition behind the PE is that $PE = 1$ when all treatment effect is mediated by S (i.e., if $\beta_S = 0$) and $PE = 0$ when there is no mediation (i.e., $\beta = \beta_S$). Unfortunately, this intuitively appealing reasoning is flawed because β_S is not necessarily zero when there is full mediation, and β and β_S are not necessarily equal when there is no mediation. As a result, the PE is not confined to the unit interval and it is thus *not* truly a proportion in the mathematical sense (i.e., it does not always holds that $0 \leq PE \leq 1$).

Second, to be useful in practice, a surrogate endpoint should allow for the prediction of the effect of the treatment Z on T based on the effect of Z on S (in a future clinical trial). It is not clear how such a prediction can be made within the PE framework.

Third, the confidence interval of the PE tends to be wide. This was also the case in the analysis of the ARMD dataset, where the 95% confidence interval for PE spanned the entire [0, 1] interval and thus no useful information was conveyed. Note also that Freedman (2001) found that the ratio $\widehat{\beta}/s.e.(\widehat{\beta})$ should be ≥ 5 (indicative of a very strong treatment effect on T) to achieve 80% power for a test of the hypothesis that S explains more than 50% of the effect of Z on T. Arguably, such a strong requirement makes the use of the PE infeasible in practice.

Fourth, the PE approach assumes that (3.9) is the correct model (when S and T are continuous normally distributed endpoints). If this assumption is not correct (e.g., if the association between S and T depends on Z), the PE ceases to have a simple interpretation and the validation process cannot be continued (Freedman et al., 1992).

Finally, Frangakis and Rubin (2002) strongly criticized the conceptual foundation of the PE (and the related fourth Prentice criterion), because the treatment effect on the T is obtained *after* conditioning on the post-randomization S. Consequently, it cannot be considered to be a causal effect.

3.4 The Relative Effect and Adjusted Association

3.4.1 Definition

In view of the fundamental problems with the *PE* (see Section 3.3.3), Buyse and Molenberghs (1998) proposed two new quantities to assess surrogacy, the so-called Relative Effect (*RE*) and the adjusted association (ρ_Z). In the setting where both S and T are continuous normally distributed endpoints, these quantities are:

$$RE(T,\,S,\,Z) \;=\; \frac{\beta}{\alpha}, \tag{3.11}$$

$$\rho_Z \;=\; r(S,\,T \mid Z) = \frac{\sigma_{ST}}{\sqrt{\sigma_{SS}\sigma_{TT}}}. \tag{3.12}$$

The *RE* is the ratio of the effect of Z on T and the effect of Z on S. Thus, it is a factor that allows "translating" the effect of Z on S into the effect of Z on T. Notice that, in contrast to the *PE*, the treatment effects involved in *RE* are not adjusted by post-randomization variables and thus these measures have a direct causal interpretation. Indeed, α and β are simply the average causal effects of the treatment on S and T, respectively (Alonso et al., 2014). The adjusted association ρ_Z quantifies how strongly S and T are associated at the level of the individual patients after accounting for the treatment effect. If $\rho_Z = 1$, there exists a deterministic relationship between S and T — and thus the true endpoint for an individual patient can be perfectly predicted based on his/her surrogate endpoint and the administered treatment. If $\rho_Z = 0$, knowledge of S does not improve the prediction of T in an individual patient.

The *RE* is the ratio of two parameters so its confidence interval can be computed by using the delta method or Fieller's theorem. A confidence interval for ρ_Z can be computed based on the general Fisher transformation procedure for correlations or by bootstrapping (Burzykowski, Molenberghs, and Buyse, 2005).

3.4.2 Analysis of Case Studies: The Age-Related Macular Degeneration Trial

The use of the *RE* and ρ_Z to evaluate surrogacy is again illustrated using the ARMD dataset. In the analyses, S and T are considered to be continuous normally distributed endpoints so α and β can be estimated based on model (3.5)–(3.6) and the variance-covariance matrix Σ of this model (see (3.7)) provides the estimates for σ_{ST}, σ_{SS}, and σ_{TT}.

The results in Section 3.2.2 showed that $\widehat{\alpha} = -0.8893$ (s.e. 0.9509) and $\widehat{\beta} = -1.4562$ (s.e. 1.1771), so $\widehat{RE} = -1.4562/-0.8893 = 1.6375$ (95% delta method-based confidence interval $[-0.6522, 3.9273]$). The point estimate for *RE* thus indicates that the magnitude of the treatment effect on T corresponds to about 1.6 times the magnitude of the treatment effect on S, but the confidence limits are rather wide.

For the adjusted association, it was found that $\widehat{\rho}_Z = 0.7450$ (95% confidence interval [0.6647; 0.8159]). This result is graphically illustrated in Figure

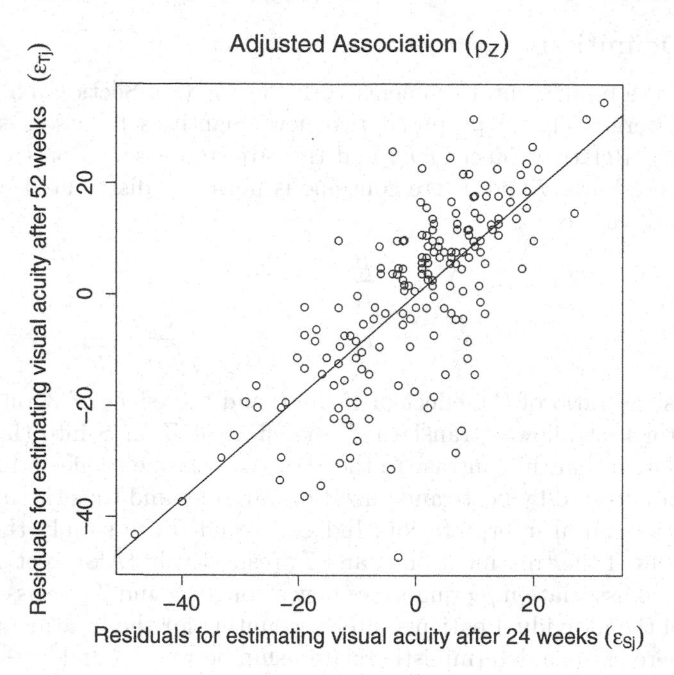

FIGURE 3.1
Age-Related Macular Degeneration (ARMD) Trial. Scatterplot of the treatment-corrected residuals of T (ε_{Tj}) against S (ε_{Sj}). The solid line results from regressing ε_{Tj} on ε_{Sj}.

3.1. In this figure, each circle depicts the treatment-corrected residuals for the S and T values of an individual patient j (i.e., $\widehat{\varepsilon}_{Sj}$ and $\widehat{\varepsilon}_{Tj}$, respectively). There is a moderately strong association between S and T at the level of an individual patient (taking the effect of treatment into account). Thus, for a given patient, the outcome on the true endpoint can be predicted using his/her outcome on the surrogate with a moderate level of accuracy.

3.4.3 An Appraisal of the Adjusted Association and the Relative Effect

3.4.3.1 Issues with the Adjusted Association

When both S and T are continuous normally distributed endpoints, there are no issues with the adjusted association (ρ_Z). Indeed, ρ_Z is simply the correlation between S and T adjusted for Z. This quantity has desirable properties, i.e., it always remains within the unit interval, it generally has a small confidence interval (because there is sufficient individual-level replication in most clinical trials), and it is straightforward to compute and interpret.

However, if we move away from the situation were both S and T are continuous normally distributed endpoints, it is no longer clear how ρ_Z, the adjusted association, should be quantified. For example, in the mixed continuous-binary setting, i.e., S is continuous and T is binary, a bivariate probit model can be used in which ρ_Z is defined as the correlation between a latent continuous variable that is assumed to underlie the observed discretized endpoint T and the continuous endpoint S. Alternatively, a bivariate Plackett-Dale model can be used in which ρ_Z is defined as the global odds ratio between S and T (Geys, 2005). A variety of other measures have been proposed to quantify ρ_Z in other settings (for details, see Burzykowski, Molenberghs, and Buyse, 2005). It would be desirable to have a single unifying approach to quantify ρ_Z across a wide variety of settings. In Chapter 10, an information-theoretic approach is introduced for this purpose.

3.4.3.2 Issues with the Relative Effect

It can be argued that a good surrogate endpoint should be able to predict the unobserved effect of Z on T in a future clinical trial $i = 0$ (i.e., $\widehat{\beta}_0$). The RE allows for such a prediction (provided that RE is sufficiently precisely estimated), but doing so requires a strong and unverifiable assumption. To illustrate this issue, consider Figure 3.2. The small circle in the figure depicts the estimated treatment effects on S and T in the ARMD trial (i.e., $\widehat{\alpha} = -0.8893$ and $\widehat{\beta} = -1.4562$; see Section 3.4.2). Obviously, based on this information alone it will not be possible to predict the effect of Z on T in a future clinical trial $i = 0$ using $\widehat{\alpha}_0$ *unless* one is willing to make an additional assumption. Indeed, an infinite number of lines can be drawn through the single point $(\widehat{\beta}, \widehat{\alpha})$ in Figure 3.2, and each of these lines would result in a different prediction of $\widehat{\beta}_0$ given a particular value of $\widehat{\alpha}_0$ (except in the trivial case when $\widehat{\alpha}_0 = \widehat{\alpha}$). Often, it is assumed that the relationship between $\widehat{\beta}$ and $\widehat{\alpha}$ is multiplicative, which comes down to a regression line through (0, 0) and $(\widehat{\beta}, \widehat{\alpha})$. In other words, it is assumed that RE remains constant *across* clinical trials. This constant RE assumption is depicted by the solid line in Figure 3.2. Based on the point estimate for RE and the constant RE assumption, the effect of Z on T can now be predicted in a straightforward way. For example, suppose that it is observed that $\widehat{\alpha}_0 = -1.1$ in a new clinical trial where the effect of interferon-α on visual acuity after 24 weeks is examined, then $\widehat{\beta}_0 = -1.8013$, i.e., $\widehat{\beta}_0 = \widehat{RE} * \widehat{\alpha}_0$, under the constant RE assumption, i.e., $\widehat{RE}_0 = \widehat{RE} = 1.6375$. Of course, the validity of the constant RE assumption cannot be verified in the single-trial setting.

Second, in contrast to ρ_Z, which has an interpretation in terms of the *strength* of the treatment-corrected association between S and T, the RE has no direct interpretation in terms of the strength of the association between β and α. This issue arises from the fact that a single clinical trial replicates patients — and thus a basis is provided for inference regarding patient-related characteristics — but not characteristics of the trial itself. Thus, even when the unverifiable constant RE assumption would not be an issue, there still is

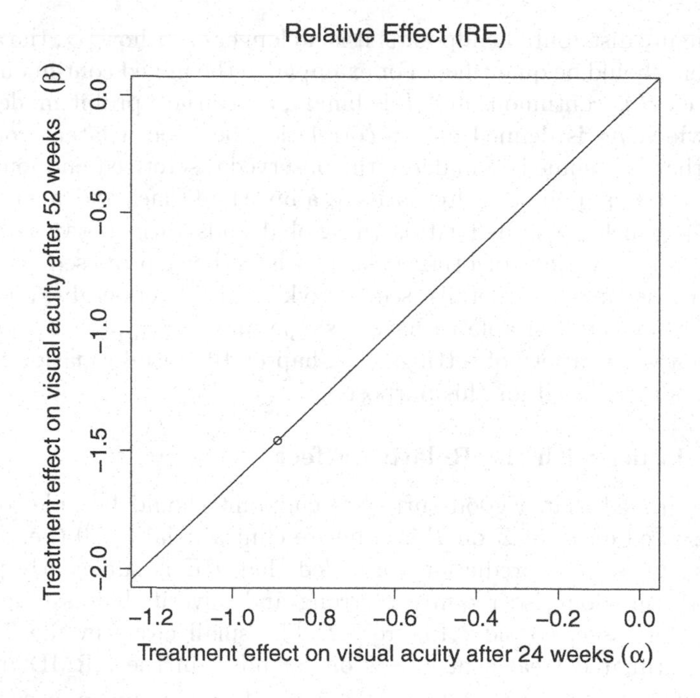

FIGURE 3.2
Age-Related Macular Degeneration (ARMD) Trial. Graphical depiction of the Relative Effect (RE). The small circle shows the estimated treatment effects on T and S, i.e., $(\widehat{\beta}, \widehat{\alpha})$ and the solid line depicts the constant RE assumption. The regression line passes through the origin $(0, 0)$.

a problem (Molenberghs et al., 2013). To see this more clearly, rewrite (3.11) as $\beta = RE * \alpha$ and include an intercept so that $\beta = \mu + RE * \alpha$ is obtained. The question is now how accurate this relationship is. To study this in proper statistical terms, a final rewrite is necessary by adding an error term ε in the previous expression: $\beta = \mu + RE * \alpha + \varepsilon$, where it is assumed that ε follows a normal distribution with mean zero and variance σ^2. Obviously, σ^2 can only be estimated when there is appropriate replication of the pair (β, α). Put differently, the data of multiple clinical trials are necessary to quantify the accuracy with which β can be predicted. Thus, the regression model can be finalized as:

$$\beta_i = \mu + RE * \alpha_i + \varepsilon_i, \tag{3.13}$$

where β_i and α_i are the treatment effects on T and S in the $i = 1, \ldots, N$ trials. If the regression model is correctly specified and σ^2 is sufficiently small, the treatment effect on T in a new trial can be accurately predicted based on the treatment effect on S in that trial.

3.5 Should the Single-Trial Methods Be Used in Practice?

As detailed in the previous sections, the earliest methodological developments to evaluate surrogate endpoints (i.e., the Prentice criteria, Freedman's proportion explained, and Buyse and Molenberghs' relative effect and adjusted association) all assumed that information regarding the surrogate (S) and the true (T) endpoints is available from a single clinical trial. Hence, these methods are collectively referred to as the single-trial surrogate evaluation methods.

These methods have the advantages (i) that the statistical analyses that are required to estimate the quantities of interest are straightforward (i.e., they merely involve the fitting of (bivariate) linear regression models, and (ii) that the data requirements are modest. Unfortunately, there are some severe issues that render the use of the single-trial methods problematic. Indeed, the Prentice approach has some fundamental flaws (i) because the validation of a good S requires the acceptance of a null hypothesis, and (ii) because it cannot be proven that the effect of the treatment (Z) on the true endpoint (T) is fully captured by the surrogate endpoint (S) (see Section 3.2.3). The proportion explained has the fundamental problem that it is actually *not* a proportion, i.e., it does not always hold that $0 \leq PE \leq 1$ (see Section 3.3.3). The adjusted association is less than ideal because it is not always clear how the correlation between S and T should be quantified if one moves away from the situation where both S and T are continuous normally distributed endpoints (see Section 3.4.3.1). The use of the relative effect (RE) is hampered by the facts (i) that it requires the unverifiable assumption that the treatment effects on S and T are multiplicative (i.e., the constant RE assumption), and (ii) that the accuracy by which β (the treatment effect on T) can be predicted based on α (the treatment effect on S) cannot be quantified (see Section 3.4.3.2).

It should be emphasized that the problems that occur with the adjusted association and the RE are of a more applied nature, whereas the Prentice approach and the proportion explained are hampered by fundamental issues. Indeed, the adjusted association has the disadvantage that it requires different computational approaches in different settings, but a way out of this problem is to use a different theoretical framework and redefine surrogacy in terms of the information content that S provides with respect to T. This framework, which is referred to as the information-theoretic approach (Alonso and Molenberghs, 2007), is detailed in Chapters 9 and 10. The problems with the RE originate in the fact that there is no trial-level replication. Indeed, when there are multiple $(\widehat{\beta}_i, \widehat{\alpha}_i)$ available rather than a single $(\widehat{\beta}_i, \widehat{\alpha}_i)$, the relation between $\widehat{\beta}_i$ and $\widehat{\alpha}_i$ (which may or may not pass through the origin, and which may or may not be linear) can be explicitly modeled and the prediction accuracy can be quantified. The latter issue clearly illustrates the need for methods in which the data of multiple clinical trials (or other relevant clustering units) are considered. The remainder of this book focuses on these so-called *multiple-trial* (or meta-analytic) methods.

Part II

Contemporary Surrogate Endpoint Evaluation Methods: Multiple-Trial Methods

4

Two Continuous Outcomes

Ariel Alonso Abad
KU Leuven, Belgium

Wim Van der Elst
Hasselt University and Janssen Pharmaceutica, Belgium

CONTENTS

4.1 Introduction

Over the years, it has become clear that the single-trial setting is too restrictive for the evaluation of surrogate endpoints (for details, see Chapter 3). Nowadays, general agreement has grown that there is a need for trial-level as well as individual-level replication. A first formal proposal along these lines used Bayesian methods (Daniels and Hughes, 1997). These ideas were subsequently extended using the theory of linear mixed-effects models (Buyse et al., 2000) and generalized estimating equations (Gail et al., 2000). This chapter focuses on the approach proposed in (Buyse et al., 2000). The methodology assumes that both endpoints are normally distributed random variables that are measured cross-sectionally. In Chapters 5–11, non-normally distributed endpoints (e.g., categorical, time-to-event, etc.) and longitudinally measured continuous endpoints will be considered.

4.2 The Meta-Analytic Framework

Assume that data from $i = 1, \ldots, N$ trials are available, in the ith in which $j = 1, \ldots, n_i$ subjects are enrolled. Further, denote by T_{ij} and S_{ij} the true and surrogate endpoints for patient j in trial i, respectively, and by Z_{ij} the indicator variable for the new treatment.

Buyse et al. (2000) proposed to evaluate surrogacy based on the following mixed-effects model:

$$\begin{cases} S_{ij} = \mu_S + m_{Si} + (\alpha + a_i) Z_{ij} + \varepsilon_{Sij}, \\ T_{ij} = \mu_T + m_{Ti} + (\beta + b_i) Z_{ij} + \varepsilon_{Tij}, \end{cases} \tag{4.1}$$

where μ_S, μ_T are the fixed intercepts for S and T, m_{Si}, m_{Ti} are the corresponding trial-specific random intercepts, α, β are the fixed treatment effects for S and T, and a_i, b_i are the corresponding random treatment effects. The vector of the random effects $(m_{Si}, m_{Ti}, a_i, b_i)$ is assumed to be mean-zero normally distributed with variance-covariance matrix D:

$$D = \begin{pmatrix} d_{SS} & d_{ST} & d_{Sa} & d_{Sb} \\ & d_{TT} & d_{Ta} & d_{Tb} \\ & & d_{aa} & d_{ab} \\ & & & d_{bb} \end{pmatrix}. \tag{4.2}$$

The error terms ε_{Sij} and ε_{Tij} in (4.1) are assumed to be mean-zero normally distributed with variance-covariance matrix Σ:

$$\Sigma = \begin{pmatrix} \sigma_{SS} & \sigma_{ST} \\ & \sigma_{TT} \end{pmatrix}. \tag{4.3}$$

In the meta-analytic framework, surrogacy is quantified based on two metrics, i.e., the trial- and individual-level coefficients of determination. These two metrics are detailed in the next sections.

4.2.1 Trial-Level Surrogacy

The trial-level coefficient of determination quantifies the strength of the association between the treatment effects on T ($\beta_i = \beta + b_i$) and the treatment effects on S ($\alpha_i = \alpha + a_i$) in the N different trials:

$$R^2_{\text{trial(f)}} = R_{b_i|m_{Si},\, a_i} = \frac{\begin{pmatrix} d_{Sb} \\ d_{ab} \end{pmatrix}^T \begin{pmatrix} d_{SS} & d_{Sa} \\ d_{Sa} & d_{aa} \end{pmatrix}^{-1} \begin{pmatrix} d_{Sb} \\ d_{ab} \end{pmatrix}}{d_{bb}}. \quad (4.4)$$

All quantities in (4.4) are based on the D matrix (4.2). The $R^2_{\text{trial(f)}}$ value is unitless and lies within the unit interval when the D matrix is positive definite. A 95% confidence interval around $R^2_{\text{trial(f)}}$ can be computed as

$$R^2_{\text{trial(f)}} \pm 1.96 \sqrt{\frac{4\, R^2_{\text{trial(f)}} \left(1 - R^2_{\text{trial(f)}}\right)^2}{N-3}}, \quad (4.5)$$

where the variance of $R^2_{\text{trial(f)}}$ is estimated using the delta method (Buyse et al., 2000; Burzykowski, Molenberghs, and Buyse, 2005). For a derivation of (4.5), we refer to Cortiñas, Shkedy, and Molenberghs (2008).

An $R^2_{\text{trial(f)}}$ that is close to 1 indicates that there is a strong association between the treatment effects on S and T in the N different trials. A surrogate is called trial-level valid when this is the case. The term "trial-level" surrogacy refers to the fact that the treatment effects on S and T, i.e., $\left(\widehat{\alpha}_i,\, \widehat{\beta}_i\right)$, are observed at the level of the clinical trial. Notice that the (f) indicator in the $R^2_{\text{trial(f)}}$ subscript is used to indicate that a so-called "full model" is used to evaluate surrogacy — as opposed to the situation where a reduced model is used (see Section 4.3.2 below).

The key motivation to evaluate a surrogate endpoint is to be able to predict the expected treatment effect on T based on the treatment effect on S in a new trial $i = 0$. To this end, observe that $\left(\beta + b_0 \mid m_{S0},\, a_0\right)$ follows a normal distribution with mean and variance:

$$E\left(\beta + b_0 \mid m_{S0},\, a_0\right) = \beta + \begin{pmatrix} d_{Sb} \\ d_{ab} \end{pmatrix}^T \begin{pmatrix} d_{SS} & d_{Sa} \\ d_{Sa} & d_{aa} \end{pmatrix}^{-1} \begin{pmatrix} \mu_{S0} - \mu_S \\ \alpha_0 - \alpha \end{pmatrix}, \quad (4.6)$$

$$\text{Var}\left(\beta + b_0 \mid m_{S0},\, a_0\right) = d_{bb} - \begin{pmatrix} d_{Sb} \\ d_{ab} \end{pmatrix}^T \begin{pmatrix} d_{SS} & d_{Sa} \\ d_{Sa} & d_{aa} \end{pmatrix}^{-1} \begin{pmatrix} d_{Sb} \\ d_{ab} \end{pmatrix}, \quad (4.7)$$

where $m_{S0} = \mu_{S0} - \mu_S$ and $a_0 = \alpha_0 - \alpha$. Estimates for μ_S and α are obtained from fitting Model (4.1), and estimates for μ_{S0} and α_0 are obtained by fitting the following univariate linear regression model to the data of the new clinical trial $i = 0$ (in which data are available for S but not for T):

$$S_{0j} = \mu_{S0} + \alpha_0 Z_{0j} + \varepsilon_{S0j}. \quad (4.8)$$

4.2.2 Individual-Level Surrogacy

Similar to the adjusted association defined in Section 3.4, the individual-level coefficient of determination quantifies the strength of the association between S and T after adjustment for both the trial and treatment effects:

$$R^2_{\text{indiv}} = R^2_{\varepsilon_{Tij}|\varepsilon_{Sij}} = \frac{\sigma^2_{ST}}{\sigma_{SS}\sigma_{TT}}, \tag{4.9}$$

where the quantities in (4.9) are based on the Σ matrix (4.3). A 95% confidence interval around R^2_{indiv} can be obtained as

$$R^2_{\text{indiv}} \pm 1.96\sqrt{\frac{4\,R^2_{\text{indiv}}\,\left(1 - R^2_{\text{indiv}}\right)^2}{N_{total} - 3}},$$

where the variance of R^2_{indiv} is estimated using the delta method and N_{total} refers to the total number of patients in the study. An R^2_{indiv} close to 1 indicates that there is a strong association between S and T at the level of the individual patients, after adjusting for treatment and trial effects. A surrogate is called individual-level valid when this is the case. The term "individual-level" refers to the fact that S and T are observed at the level of the individual patients.

Apart from estimating the treatment effect on T based on the treatment effect on S in a new trial $i = 0$ (see Section 4.2.1), one may also be interested in making a prediction of the expected T based on S and Z in an individual patient. This prediction (and its accuracy) can also be made based on Model (4.1):

$$\begin{aligned}
E\left(T_{ij} \mid S_{ij}, Z_{ij}\right) &= \mu_T + m_{Ti} - \frac{\sigma_{TS}}{\sigma_{SS}}\left(\mu_S + m_{Si}\right) \\
&\quad + \left[\beta + b_i - \frac{\sigma_{TS}}{\sigma_{SS}}\left(\alpha + a_i\right)\right] Z_{ij} + \frac{\sigma_{TS}}{\sigma_{SS}} S_{ij}, \\
\text{Var}\left(\varepsilon_{Tij} \mid \varepsilon_{Sij}\right) &= \sigma_{TT} - \frac{\sigma^2_{TS}}{\sigma_{SS}}.
\end{aligned}$$

4.3 Simplified Model-Fitting Strategies

The mixed-effects (hierarchical) modeling approach of Buyse et al. (2000) poses considerable computational challenges. Indeed, fitting a linear mixed-effects model is typically done using Newton-Raphson or quasi-Newton-based procedures (Lindstrom and Bates, 1988; Verbeke and Molenberghs, 2000). Based on some starting values for the parameters of interest, these procedures iteratively update the parameter estimates until convergence is achieved. Unfortunately, non-converging iteration processes may occur when complex linear mixed-effects models are considered. This means that the iterative process does not converge at all, or that it converges to values that are close to or outside the boundary of the parameter space (i.e., variances that are close to zero or even negative). Simulation studies have shown that such problems mainly occur (i) when the number of clustering (trial-level) units is small, (ii) when the size of the between-cluster variability (i.e., the components in the D matrix (4.2)) is small relative to the size of the residual variability (i.e., the components in the Σ matrix (4.3)), and (iii) when the number of patients in each of the trials is strongly unbalanced (Burzykowski, Molenberghs, and Buyse, 2005; Buyse et al., 2000; Renard et al., 2002; Van der Elst et al., 2015).

Unfortunately, the conditions described in (i)–(iii) are often encountered in real-life surrogate evaluation settings and thus convergence problems tend to be prevalent. Buyse et al. (2000) and Tibaldi et al. (2003) proposed a number of simplified model-fitting strategies that can be used when model convergence problems occur. In particular, Model (4.1) can be simplified along four dimensions. The simplified model-fitting strategies are discussed in more detail in the subsequent sections, and an overview that summarizes the different strategies is provided in Table 4.1. Alternatively, the multiple-imputation-based strategy, described in Chapter 15, can be used to improve convergence.

4.3.1 The Trial Dimension: Fixed- versus Random-Effects Models

To avoid the computational problems that arise in the estimation of the variance components of Model (4.1), the mixed-effects model representation can be replaced by its fixed-effects, two-stage, counterpart (Buyse et al., 2000; Tibaldi et al., 2003). When the fixed-effects approach is used, either a single bivariate or two univariate linear regression models are fitted to the data of each of the i trials separately. The choice for a bivariate or a univariate approach is determined by the assumptions that are made regarding the association structure of the errors (see Section 4.3.3). Thus, in Stage 1, the following (bi- or univariate) fixed-effects model is fitted:

$$\begin{aligned} S_{ij} &= \mu_{Si} + \alpha_i Z_{ij} + \varepsilon_{Sij}, \\ T_{ij} &= \mu_{Ti} + \beta_i Z_{ij} + \varepsilon_{Tij}, \end{aligned} \tag{4.10}$$

where μ_{Si}, μ_{Ti} are the trial-specific intercepts and α_i, β_i are the trial-specific treatment effects. The error terms ε_{Sij}, ε_{Tij} are assumed to be mean-zero normally distributed with variance-covariance matrix Σ (4.3) when a bivariate regression model is fitted, or they are assumed to be independent when two univariate models are fitted (see Section 4.3.3 below). The parameter estimates for β_i, μ_{Si}, and α_i that are obtained by fitting Model (4.10) are subsequently used in Stage 2 of the analysis, where the following univariate regression model

TABLE 4.1
Summary of the different models that can be fitted to evaluate surrogacy when both S and T are normally distributed endpoints. For the stage 2 models, it is recommended to use weighted regression (with the trial sizes as weights) to account for the heterogeneity in information content in the trial-specific estimated parameters (see Section 4.3.4).

	Full	Reduced
	Mixed-effects approach	
Bivariate	$\begin{cases} S_{ij} = \mu_S + m_{Si} + (\alpha + a_i) Z_{ij} + \varepsilon_{Sij} \\ T_{ij} = \mu_T + m_{Ti} + (\beta + b_i) Z_{ij} + \varepsilon_{Tij} \end{cases}$	$\begin{cases} S_{ij} = \mu_S + (\alpha + a_i) Z_{ij} + \varepsilon_{Sij} \\ T_{ij} = \mu_T + (\beta + b_i) Z_{ij} + \varepsilon_{Tij} \end{cases}$
Univariate	Stage 1: $S_{ij} = \mu_S + m_{Si} + (\alpha + a_i) Z_{ij} + \varepsilon_{Sij}$; $T_{ij} = \mu_T + m_{Ti} + (\beta + b_i) Z_{ij} + \varepsilon_{Tij}$ Stage 2: $(\beta + b_i) = \lambda_0 + \lambda_1 (\mu_S + m_{Si}) + \lambda_2 (\alpha + a_i) + \varepsilon_i$	Stage 1: $S_{ij} = \mu_S + (\alpha + a_i) Z_{ij} + \varepsilon_{Sij}$; $T_{ij} = \mu_T + (\beta + b_i) Z_{ij} + \varepsilon_{Tij}$ Stage 2: $(\beta + b_i) = \lambda_0 + \lambda_1 (\alpha + a_i) + \varepsilon_i$
	Fixed-effects approach	
Bivariate	Stage 1: $\begin{cases} S_{ij} = \mu_{Si} + \alpha_i Z_{ij} + \varepsilon_{Sij} \\ T_{ij} = \mu_{Ti} + \beta_i Z_{ij} + \varepsilon_{Tij} \end{cases}$ Stage 2: $\beta_i = \lambda_0 + \lambda_1 \mu_{Si} + \lambda_2 \alpha_i + \varepsilon_i$	Stage 1: $\begin{cases} S_{ij} = \mu_S + \alpha_i Z_{ij} + \varepsilon_{Sij} \\ T_{ij} = \mu_T + \beta_i Z_{ij} + \varepsilon_{Tij} \end{cases}$ Stage 2: $\beta_i = \lambda_0 + \lambda_1 \alpha_i + \varepsilon_i$
Univariate	Stage 1: $S_{ij} = \mu_{Si} + \alpha_i Z_{ij} + \varepsilon_{Sij}$; $T_{ij} = \mu_{Ti} + \beta_i Z_{ij} + \varepsilon_{Tij}$ Stage 2: $\beta_i = \lambda_0 + \lambda_1 \mu_{Si} + \lambda_2 \alpha_i + \varepsilon_i$	Stage 1: $S_{ij} = \mu_S + \alpha_i Z_{ij} + \varepsilon_{Sij}$; $T_{ij} = \mu_T + \beta_i Z_{ij} + \varepsilon_{Tij}$ Stage 2: $\beta_i = \lambda_0 + \lambda_1 \alpha_i + \varepsilon_i$

is fitted:

$$\widehat{\beta}_i = \lambda_0 + \lambda_1 \widehat{\mu}_{Si} + \lambda_2 \widehat{\alpha}_i + \varepsilon_i. \tag{4.11}$$

The classical coefficient of determination that is obtained by fitting Model (4.11) provides an estimate for $R^2_{\text{trial(f)}}$. Similar to when the mixed-effects approach is used to estimate trial-level surrogacy, the (f) indicator in the $R^2_{\text{trial(f)}}$ subscript indicates that a "full model" is used. Alternatively, trial-level surrogacy can be estimated based on a reduced fixed-effects modeling approach (see Section (4.3.2)).

4.3.2 The Model Dimension: Full versus Reduced Models

Model (4.1) is referred to as the *full* mixed-effects model, i.e., the model that contains random intercepts for S and T as well as random treatment effects for S and T. Similarly, Model (4.10) is referred to as the full (bi- or univariate) fixed-effects model, i.e., the model that contains both trial-specific intercepts for S and T as well as trial-specific treatment effects for S and T.

The random-effects structure of the full mixed-effects model can be simplified by assuming that there is no heterogeneity in the random intercepts for S and T:

$$\begin{cases} S_{ij} = \mu_S + (\alpha + a_i)\, Z_{ij} + \varepsilon_{Sij}. \\ T_{ij} = \mu_T + (\beta + b_i)\, Z_{ij} + \varepsilon_{Tij}. \end{cases} \tag{4.12}$$

Thus, the trial-specific intercepts for S and T in Model (4.1) are replaced by common intercepts for S and T, and consequently the D matrix reduces to

$$D = \begin{pmatrix} d_{aa} & d_{ab} \\ & d_{bb} \end{pmatrix}. \tag{4.13}$$

Further, the computation of the trial-level coefficient of determination simplifies to:

$$R^2_{\text{trial(r)}} = R_{b_i|a_i} = \frac{d^2_{ab}}{d_{aa} d_{bb}}, \tag{4.14}$$

where the (r) indicator in the $R^2_{\text{trial(r)}}$ subscript now indicates that a reduced mixed-effects model is used. When a reduced modeling approach is used, the prediction of the treatment effect on T in a new trial $i = 0$ based on the treatment effect on S also simplifies, i.e., (4.6) and (4.7) become where the (r) indicator in the $R^2_{\text{trial(r)}}$ subscript now indicates that a reduced mixed-effects model is used. When a reduced modeling approach is used, the prediction of the treatment effect on T in a new trial $i = 0$ based on the treatment effect on S also simplifies, i.e., (4.6) and (4.7) become where the (r) indicator in the $R^2_{\text{trial(r)}}$ subscript now indicates that a reduced mixed-effects model is used. When a reduced modeling approach is used, the prediction of the treatment effect on T in a new trial $i = 0$ based on the treatment effect on S also simplifies, i.e., (4.6) and (4.7) become where the (r) indicator in the $R^2_{\text{trial(r)}}$ subscript now indicates that a reduced mixed-effects model is used. When a reduced modeling approach is used, the prediction of the treatment effect on T in a new trial $i = 0$ based on the treatment effect on S also simplifies, i.e., (4.6) and (4.7) become

$$E\left(\beta + b_0 \mid a_0\right) = \beta + \frac{d_{ab}}{d_{aa}}\left(\alpha_0 - \alpha\right), \tag{4.15}$$

$$\text{Var}\left(\beta + b_0 \mid a_0\right) = d_{bb} - \frac{d_{ab}^2}{d_{aa}}. \tag{4.16}$$

When the fixed-effects approach is used, Model (4.10) can be simplified by assuming common intercepts for S and T in Stage 1 of the analysis. Thus, μ_{Si} and μ_{Ti} in Model (4.10) are replaced by μ_S and μ_T. Further, in Stage 2, the $\lambda_1\widehat{\mu}_{Si}$ component is dropped from Model (4.11).

4.3.3 The Endpoint Dimension: Univariate versus Bivariate Models

The error terms for S and T may be assumed to be independent rather than dependent by fitting univariate instead of bivariate (mixed- or fixed-effects) models. This consideration seems odd at first sight, because it is natural to assume that S and T are correlated in a surrogate marker evaluation context. Nonetheless, making the simplifying assumption that the error terms are uncorrelated is not necessarily a problem. Indeed, the explicit consideration of the bivariate nature of the endpoints is mainly of importance to obtain the Σ matrix, which is mainly of interest to estimate R^2_{indiv}, and often the focus of the analysis is on trial-level surrogacy rather than on individual-level surrogacy. It has been shown that the R^2_{trial} values that are obtained by using mixed-effects univariate and mixed-effects bivariate models are similar (Tibaldi et al., 2003), and the R^2_{trial} values that are obtained by using fixed-effects univariate and fixed-effects bivariate models are identical (Johnson and Wichern, 2007). Moreover, if interest is also in R^2_{indiv}, this quantity can always be estimated by computing the squared correlation of the residuals of the fitted univariate models (Molenberghs et al., 2010), or by using the information-theoretic approach (see Chapter 9 and 10).

4.3.4 The Measurement Error Dimension: Weighted versus Unweighted Models

When the bivariate mixed-effects model is not used, one is confronted with measurement error because the treatment effects on S and T in the different trials are affected by sampling variability. The magnitude of this error likely depends on the trial size. Therefore, a straightforward approach to address this issue is to use weighted regression with trial sizes as the weights in the Stage 2 model (Burzykowski, Molenberghs, and Buyse, 2005; Tibaldi et al., 2003). Notice that the measurement error dimension is not relevant when a bivariate mixed-effects model is used, because it is automatically accounted for and therefore explicit corrections are not needed.

4.4 General Considerations in the Multiple-Trial Setting

The choice of trial-level units

An important issue that arises in the multiple-trial surrogate evaluation setting pertains to the choice of the cluster-level unit of the analysis (Molenberghs et al., 2010). Viable choices are clinical trial, treating physician, country, or hospital (Burzykowski, Molenberghs, and Buyse, 2005; Cortiñas et al., 2004).

As a general paradigm, clinical trial is taken as the level of replication (hence the terminology "trial-level surrogacy" and the R^2_{trial} notation), but this is not always possible or sensible. For example, it may occur that only a few clinical trials are available (see also Chapter 15). When the number of clustering units is too small, convergence problems tend to occur when mixed-effects models are fitted to the data. The use of a simplified two-stage modeling strategy (see Section 4.3.1) provides no viable alternative in this situation, because Model (4.11) that is fitted in the second stage of the analysis would then be based on only a few data points. This could result in an overestimation of the trial-level surrogacy.

The other extreme situation, where the number of clusters is high and the number of participants per cluster is low, is also not ideal. Indeed, this situation is convenient to explain the between-cluster variability but not the within-cluster variability. The use of a simplified two-stage approach is again not an ideal alternative, because the estimation of the fixed cluster-specific treatment effects for S and T would be based on relatively few observations per cluster, which impacts the precision of these estimates. This problem can be remedied to some extent by using a weighted regression procedure at the second stage of the analysis (see Section 4.3.4), but some other issues still remain. For example, when the number of participants per cluster is low, it may occur that only one type of treatment is administered within certain clusters. The cluster-specific treatment effects cannot be estimated in such clusters, and thus data are lost from the analyses.

In general, the choice for a particular clustering unit will depend on several considerations, such as the information that is available in the dataset, experts' opinion regarding the most suitable clustering unit, and the number of patients per clustering unit. Importantly, simulation studies have shown that the impact of shifting between (hierarchical) clustering units, e.g., using hospital instead of trial, on the estimated R^2_{trial} is small when the magnitude of the variability in the treatment effects at the different levels (trial, hospital) is roughly similar. However, when there are large differences in the magnitude of this variability, the impact of shifting between clustering units on the estimated R^2_{trial} can be substantial and thus caution is needed (Cortiñas et al., 2004).

The coding of the treatment effect

In the single-trial setting (see Chapter 3), the coding of the treatment effect (using e.g., $-1/1$, $1/0$ or any other coding scheme) is essentially irrelevant. The same holds in the multiple-trial setting when models are considered in which treatment occurs as a fixed effect only. Indeed, in these scenarios, all treatment coding choices lead to an equivalent model fit and the parameters are connected by simple linear transformations.

In contrast, the choice for a $0/1$ or $-1/1$ coding for treatment is relevant and impacts the results when mixed-effects models are used. Indeed, a $1/0$ coding, for a positive-definite D matrix, forces the variability in the experimental arm to be greater than or equal to the variability in the control arm. A $-1/1$ coding on the other hand ensures that the same components of variability operate in both treatment arms (Burzykowski, Molenberghs, and Buyse, 2005; Molenberghs et al., 2010). In practice, both situations may be relevant and it is of importance to illicit views from the study investigators regarding the appropriate treatment coding scheme.

A "good" surrogate

A "good" candidate surrogate endpoint should ideally have high levels of both individual- and trial-level surrogacy. It is important to emphasize that there is *not* necessarily a relationship between both metrics, except in the trivial case where S and T are deterministically related. Indeed, an endpoint can have excellent individual-level properties but poor trial-level properties, or vice versa.

When R^2_{indiv} and R^2_{trial} equal 1, surrogacy is perfect at the individual and at the trial level (Buyse et al., 2000). In practice, both coefficients will be below 1 and thus the question arises how large these metrics should be in order to conclude that the candidate S is an appropriate surrogate for T (given the treatment that was considered). In this respect, it may be useful to consider the confidence intervals of R^2_{indiv} and R^2_{trial} as well as expert opinion. For example, a candidate S that has high trial- and individual-level coefficients of surrogacy (e.g., lower bound trial- and individual-level surrogacy confidence intervals that are ≥ 0.80) may nonetheless not be useful in practice, because the gain of using the candidate S instead of T itself, in terms of the time needed to conduct the trial, the cost of the measurement, or the burden to the patients enrolled in the trial, may be considered too small by substantive experts. On the other hand, an endpoint that has substantially lower coefficients of trial- and individual-level surrogacy may be considered a useful surrogate when it can be measured much earlier or cheaper than T, or when it involves a substantial reduction in the burden to the patients. An alternative way to evaluate *goodness* of a candidate surrogate endpoint is to use the surrogacy measure that is described in the next section.

4.5 Prediction of Treatment Effect: Surrogate Threshold Effect (STE)

The key motivation for validating a surrogate endpoint is the ability to predict the effect of treatment on the true endpoint based on the observed effect of treatment on the surrogate endpoint. Suppose that we have fitted the mixed-effects model (4.1) to data from a meta-analysis of N trials. Suppose further that a new trial is considered for which data are available on the surrogate endpoint but not on the true endpoint. It is essential to explore the quality of the prediction of the effect of Z on T in the new trial $i = 0$, based on the information contained in the trials $i = 1, \ldots, N$ used in the evaluation process, and the estimate of the effect of Z on S in the new trial. We can fit the following linear model to the surrogate outcomes S_{0j}:

$$S_{0j} = \mu_{S0} + \alpha_0 Z_{0j} + \varepsilon_{S0j}. \tag{4.17}$$

We are interested in an estimate of the effect $\beta + b_0$ of Z on T, given the effect of Z on S. To this end, one can observe that $(\beta + b_0|m_{S0}, a_0)$, where m_{S0} and a_0 are, respectively, the surrogate-specific random intercept and treatment effect in the new trial, follows a normal distribution with mean linear in μ_{S0}, μ_S, α_0, and α, and variance

$$\text{Var}(\beta + b_0|m_{S0}, a_0) \quad = \quad (1 - R^2_{\text{trial}})\text{Var}(b_0). \tag{4.18}$$

Here, $\text{Var}(b_0)$ denotes the unconditional variance of the trial-specific random effect of Z on T. The smaller the conditional variance given by (4.18), the better the precision of the prediction. Denote ϑ to group the fixed-effects parameters and variance components related to the mixed-effects model (4.1), with $\widehat{\vartheta}$ denoting the corresponding estimates. Fitting the linear model (4.17) to data on the surrogate endpoint from the new trial provides estimates for m_{S0} and a_0. The prediction variance can be written as:

$$\begin{aligned} \text{Var}(\beta + b_0|\mu_{S0}, \alpha_0, \vartheta) \quad &\approx \quad f\{\text{Var}(\widehat{\mu}_{S0}, \widehat{\alpha}_0)\} + f\{\text{Var}(\widehat{\vartheta})\} \\ &\quad + (1 - R^2_{\text{trial}})\text{Var}(b_0), \end{aligned} \tag{4.19}$$

where $f\{\text{Var}(\widehat{\mu}_{S0}, \widehat{\alpha}_0)\}$ and $f\{\text{Var}(\widehat{\vartheta})\}$ are functions of the asymptotic variance-covariance matrices of $(\widehat{\mu}_{S0}, \widehat{\alpha}_0)^T$ and $\widehat{\vartheta}$, respectively. The third term on the right-hand side of (4.19), which is equivalent to (4.18), describes the prediction's variability if μ_{S0}, α_0, and ϑ were known. The first two terms describe the contributions to the variability due to the use of the estimates of these parameters, respectively, in the new trial (estimation of μ_{S0} and of α_0) and in the meta-analysis (estimation of ϑ).

In reality, the parameters of models (4.1) and (4.17) all have to be estimated, in which case the prediction variance is given by the three terms on the right-hand side of (4.19). It is useful, however, to consider two theoretical situations:

1. **No estimation error.** If the parameters of models (4.1) and (4.17) were known, the prediction variance for $\beta + b_0$ would only contain the last term on the right-hand side of (4.19). Thus, the variance would be reduced to (4.18) and the precision of the prediction would be driven entirely by the value R^2_{trial}. While this situation is of theoretical relevance only, as it would require an infinite number of trials and infinite sample sizes for the estimation in the meta-analysis and in the new trial, it provides important insights about the intrinsic quality of the surrogate, and shows that R^2_{trial} measures the "potential" validity of a surrogate endpoint at the trial level.
2. **Estimation error only in the meta-analysis.** This scenario is again possible only in theory, as it would require an infinite sample size in the new trial. In that case, the parameters of the single-trial regression model (4.17) would be known and the first term on the right-hand side of (4.19) would vanish:

$$\text{Var}(\beta + b_0|\alpha_0, \vartheta) \approx f\{\text{Var}(\widehat{\vartheta})\} + (1 - R^2_{\text{trial(r)}})\text{Var}(b_0). \quad (4.20)$$

In this case, equation (4.19) would provide the minimum variance of the prediction of $\beta + b_0$ that is achievable when the size of the meta-analysis is finite. Gail et al. (2000) used this fact to point out that the use of a surrogate validated through a meta-analytic approach will always be less efficient than the direct use of the true endpoint. Even so, a surrogate can be of great use in terms of reduced sample size, shortened trial duration, or both.

Using the aforementioned considerations, Burzykowski and Buyse (2006) have proposed a useful measure of surrogacy, alternative to $R^2_{\text{trial(r)}}$. In particular, assume that the prediction of $\beta + b_0$ can be made independently of μ_{S0}. Under this assumption, the conditional mean of $\beta + b_0$ is a linear function of α_0, the treatment effect on the surrogate. Assume further that α_0 is estimated without error. Then the conditional variance of $\beta + b_0$ can be expressed as in (4.20) and it can be shown that it is approximately a quadratic function of α_0.

Consider a $(1 - \gamma)100\%$ prediction interval for $\beta + b_0$:

$$E(\beta + b_0|\alpha_0, \vartheta) \pm \sqrt{\text{Var}(\beta + b_0|\alpha_0, \vartheta)}, \quad (4.21)$$

where $z_{1-\gamma/2}$ is the $(1-\gamma/2)$ quantile of the standard normal distribution. The limits of the interval (4.21) are functions of α_0. Define the lower and upper prediction limit functions of α_0 as

$$l(\alpha_0), u(\alpha_0) \equiv E(\beta + b_0|\alpha_0, \vartheta) \pm \sqrt{\text{Var}(\beta + b_0|\alpha_0, \vartheta)}. \tag{4.22}$$

One can then compute a value of α_0 such that

$$l(\alpha_0) = 0. \tag{4.23}$$

This value is called the *surrogate threshold effect* (STE). The STE is the smallest treatment effect on the surrogate necessary to be observed to predict a treatment effect on the true endpoint that is statistically significantly different from zero. The STE depends on the variance of the prediction. The larger the variance, the larger the absolute value of the STE. In practical terms, one would hope to get a value of STE that can realistically be achieved, given the range of treatment effects on surrogates observed in previous clinical trials. If the STE were too large to be achievable, the surrogate would not be useful for the purposes of predicting a treatment effect on the true endpoint. In such a case, the use of the surrogate would not be reasonable, even if the surrogate were "potentially" valid, i.e., with $R^2_{\text{trial(r)}} \simeq 1$. The STE thus provides important information about the usefulness of a surrogate in practice.

4.6 Case Study: The Age-Related Macular Degeneration Trial

The methodology that was detailed in the earlier sections of the current chapter is illustrated based on the data of the ARMD trial. The results of the case study are discussed without reference to the software tools that can be used to conduct the analyses. In Sections 12.3, 13.2.1, and 14.2, it is detailed how the analyses can be conducted in R, R Shiny, and SAS, respectively.

The ARMD study is a multi-center clinical trial in which the efficacy of interferon-α to treat age-related macular degeneration (ARMD) was evaluated (for details, see Section 2.2.1). Obviously, since the ARMD dataset consists of a single clinical trial, it is not possible to use trial as the clustering unit. Instead, center is used as the clustering unit in the analysis. A total of $N = 36$ such centers were available.

Analyses

The hierarchical modeling approach and the different simplifying model-fitting strategies (detailed in Sections 4.2 and 4.3) were applied to the data of the ARMD study. Table 4.2 summarizes the results. As can be seen, no trial- and

TABLE 4.2
Age-Related Macular Degeneration (ARMD) Trial. Trial- and individual-level surrogacy estimates and their 95% confidence intervals.
Note. – *: model did not converge.*

		Full		Reduced	
		Unweighted	Weighted	Unweighted	Weighted
		Mixed-effects approach			
Bivariate	$\widehat{R}^2_{\text{trial}}$	—	—	—	—
	$\widehat{R}^2_{\text{indiv}}$	—	—	—	—
Univariate	$\widehat{R}^2_{\text{trial}}$	0.6772 [0.4959; 0.8584]	0.8126 [0.6973; 0.9279]	0.6888 [0.5125; 0.8650]	0.8151 [0.7012; 0.9290]
	$\widehat{R}^2_{\text{indiv}}$	0.5387 [0.3772; 0.7001]	0.5387 [0.3772; 0.7001]	0.5469 [0.4172; 0.6765]	0.5469 [0.4172; 0.6765]
		Fixed-effects approach			
Bivariate	$\widehat{R}^2_{\text{trial}}$	0.6968 [0.5240; 0.8695]	0.7031 [0.5333; 0.8730]	0.6423 [0.4466; 0.8379]	0.6585 [0.4695; 0.8476]
	$\widehat{R}^2_{\text{indiv}}$	0.4866 [0.3814; 0.5919]	0.4866 [0.3814; 0.5919]	0.5318 [0.4315; 0.6321]	0.5318 [0.4315; 0.6321]
Univariate	$\widehat{R}^2_{\text{trial}}$	0.6968 [0.5240; 0.8695]	0.7031 [0.5333; 0.8730]	0.6423 [0.4466; 0.8379]	0.6585 [0.4695; 0.8476]
	$\widehat{R}^2_{\text{indiv}}$	0.4866 [0.2941; 0.6792]	0.4866 [0.2941; 0.6792]	0.5318 [0.3876; 0.6761]	0.5318 [0.3876; 0.6761]

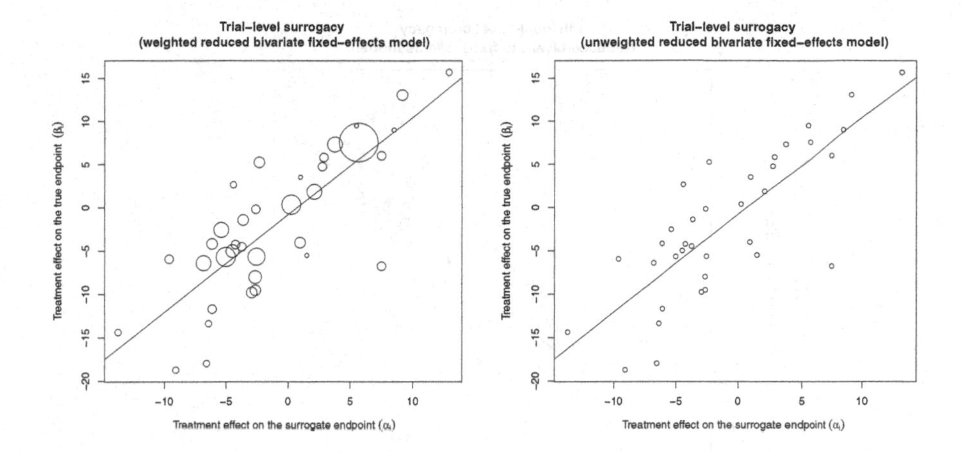

FIGURE 4.1

Age-Related Macular Degeneration Trial. Scatter plot of the estimated β_i (the treatment effect on the true endpoint, i.e., visual acuity after 52 weeks) against α_i (the treatment effect on the surrogate endpoint, i.e., visual acuity after 24 weeks) based on the weighted and unweighted full bivariate fixed-effects model (left and right figures, respectively).

individual-level surrogacy estimates are provided for the (full and reduced) bivariate mixed-effects (hierarchical) models. The reason for this is that these models did not converge, a problem that often occurs in real-life datasets.

Trial-level surrogacy

The point estimates of $\widehat{R}^2_{\text{trial}}$ that were obtained using the different models ranged between 0.6423 and 0.8151, and their 95% confidence intervals largely overlapped (see Table 4.2). It can thus be concluded that the accuracy by which $\widehat{\beta}_i$ (i.e., the treatment effect on T = visual acuity after 52 weeks in center i) can be predicted based on $\widehat{\alpha}_i$ (i.e., the treatment effect on S = visual acuity after 24 weeks in center i) is moderate.

Trial-level surrogacy can be visualized using a scatter plot that shows the estimated treatment effects on T = visual acuity after 52 weeks (i.e., $\widehat{\beta}_i$) against the estimated treatment effects on S = visual acuity after 24 weeks (i.e., $\widehat{\alpha}_i$) in the N = 36 different centers. Such a plot can be made for each of the different models shown in Table 4.1. By way of illustration, Figure 4.1 shows the results based on the reduced bivariate fixed-effects model, with and without weighting for cluster size in Stage 2 of the analysis (left and right figures, respectively). Note that the sizes of the circles in the left figure are proportional to the number of patients in the particular center. These plots

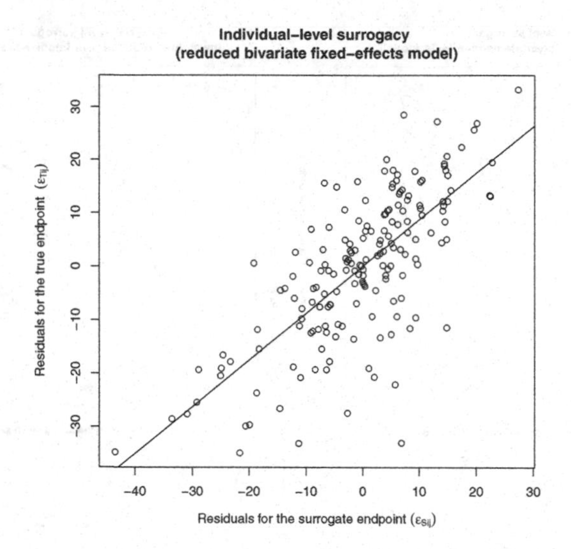

FIGURE 4.2
Age-Related Macular Degeneration Trial. Scatter plot of the estimated residuals for T (the treatment effect on the true endpoint, i.e., visual acuity after 52 weeks) against the estimated residuals for S (the treatment effect on the surrogate endpoint, i.e., visual acuity after 24 weeks) based on a (weighted or unweighted) reduced bivariate fixed-effects model.

confirm the earlier conclusion about the prediction accuracy. The plots also suggest that the relationship between $\widehat{\beta}_i$ and $\widehat{\alpha}_i$ is approximately linear (when this is not the case, a quadratic or cubic model may be considered in Stage 2 of the analysis), and that the constant RE assumption (see Section 3.4.3.2) appears to be reasonable in the ARMD trial (i.e., the regression lines approximately pass through zero).

Individual-level surrogacy

As shown in Table 4.2, the point estimates of R^2_{indiv} that were obtained in the different models ranged between 0.4866 and 0.5469, and their 95% confidence intervals largely overlapped. Notice that the point estimates for R^2_{indiv} are identical in the weighted and unweighted scenarios for all models (see Table 4.2). This result is expected, because the choice for a weighted versus unweighted model only affects the Stage 2 models (upon which the estimation of R^2_{trial} is based) but not the Stage 1 models (upon which the estimation of R^2_{indiv} is based). Overall, the results indicate that $S =$ visual acuity after 24 weeks is a moderate surrogate for $T =$ visual acuity after 52 weeks at the level of individual patients.

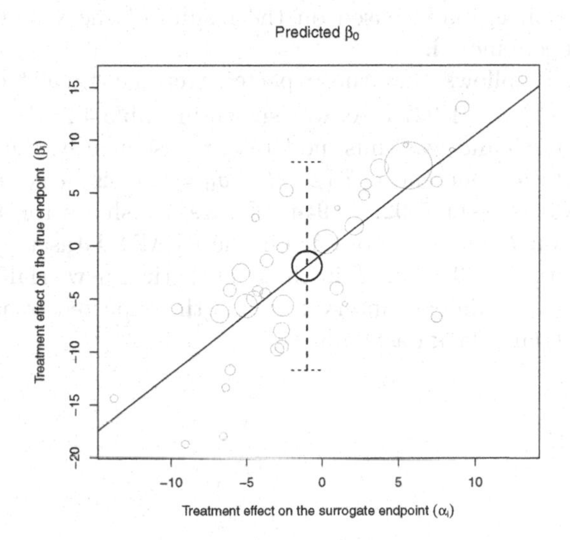

FIGURE 4.3
Age-Related Macular Degeneration Trial. Scatter plot of the treatment effects on the true endpoint against the treatment effects on the surrogate endpoint in the ARMD data (gray circles), the expected treatment effect on T in a new trial where $\widehat{\alpha}_0 = -1$ (black circle), and the 95% confidence interval around the expected treatment effect in the new trial (dashed black line).

Individual-level surrogacy can be graphically illustrated based on a scatter plot that depicts the treatment- and trial-corrected residuals for T (i.e., ε_{Tij}) against the treatment- and trial-corrected residuals for S (i.e., ε_{Sij}) for the $N_{total} = 181$ patients. By means of illustration, Figure 4.2 provides such a plot using the (weighted or unweighted) reduced bivariate fixed-effects model. This plot is in line with the earlier conclusion that the accuracy by which T can be predicted based on S (taking treatment and trial into account) is moderate (i.e., there remains substantial variability in ε_{Tij} for a given value of ε_{Sij}).

The expected treatment effect on T in a new trial

The main motivation to evaluate a surrogate endpoint is to be able to predict the treatment effect on T based on the treatment effect on S in a new trial $i = 0$. For example, suppose that a new clinical trial was conducted that is similar to the ARMD study in which only S (and not T) is measured. Figure 4.3 presents a scenario in which in the new trial it is found that $\widehat{\alpha}_0 = -1$, i.e., the estimated treatment effect on visual acuity measured after 24 weeks equals -1. Interest is in the prediction of the expected treatment effect after 52 weeks.

Here, the prediction is made based on the results of the weighted reduced bivariate fixed-effects model.

Using (4.15), it follows that the expected treatment effect on T equals $E\left(\beta + b_0 \mid a_0 = -1\right) = -1.9324$. As was shown in Table 4.2, the $\widehat{R}^2_{\text{trial}}$ of the model equaled 0.6585 and was thus moderate. Consequently, the uncertainty in the expected treatment effect $E\left(\beta + b_0 \mid a_0 = -1\right)$ is large, i.e., its 95% confidence interval is $[-11.7592; 7.8944]$. Figure 4.3 shows the trial-specific treatment effects on T and S as obtained in the ARMD dataset (gray circles), the expected treatment effect on T in the hypothetical new trial $i = 0$ (black circle), and the 95% confidence interval around the expected treatment effect on T in the new trial (black dashed line).

5

Two Failure-Time Endpoints

Tomasz Burzykowski

Hasselt University, Belgium and IDDI, Belgium

CONTENTS

5.1 Introduction

In this chapter, we focus on the case when both the surrogate and the true endpoint are failure-time endpoints. We mainly follow the two-stage approach proposed by Burzykowski et al. (2001).

5.2 Theoretical Background

Assume now that S_{ij} and T_{ij} are failure-time endpoints. Similar to the case with two normally distributed endpoints, the two-stage approach can be applied. In particular, model (4.10) is replaced by a model for two correlated failure-time random variables. Burzykowski et al. (2001) used single-parameter copulas toward this end (Clayton, 1978; Dale, 1986; Hougaard, 1986). In particular, the joint survivor function of (S_{ij}, T_{ij}) is expressed as

$$F(s, t) = P(S_{ij} \geq s, T_{ij} \geq t) = C_\theta\{F_{Sij}(s), F_{Tij}(t)\}, \qquad s, t \geq 0, \qquad (5.1)$$

where (F_{Sij}, F_{Tij}) denote marginal survivor functions and C_θ is a copula, i.e., a distribution function on $[0, 1]^2$ with $\theta \in R^1$. The marginal survivor functions can be specified by using, e.g., the proportional hazard model:

$$F_{Sij}(s) = \exp\left\{-\int_0^s \lambda_{Si}(x)\exp(\alpha_i Z_{ij})dx\right\}, \quad (5.2)$$

$$F_{Tij}(t) = \exp\left\{-\int_0^t \lambda_{Ti}(x)\exp(\beta_i Z_{ij})dx\right\}, \quad (5.3)$$

where $\lambda_{Si}(t)$ and $\lambda_{Ti}(t)$ are trial-specific marginal baseline hazard functions and α_i and β_i are trial-specific effects of treatment Z on S and T, respectively, in trial i. The hazard functions can be specified parametrically or can be left unspecified as in the classical formulation of the model proposed by Cox (1972).

When the hazard functions are specified, estimates of the parameters of the model defined by (5.1)–(5.3) can be obtained by using maximum likelihood. Alternately, as suggested by Shih and Louis (1995), the marginal models (5.2)–(5.3) can be fitted first, and then the copula parameter θ can be estimated from a profile-likelihood.

Note that different copulas may be used in (5.1), depending on assumptions made about the nature of the association between the surrogate and the true endpoint; such assumptions are generally unavailable, in which case the best fitting copula may be chosen. We will consider three particular copulas:

The Clayton copula The copula function (Clayton, 1978) has the following form:

$$C_\theta(u, v) = (u^{1-\theta} + v^{1-\theta} - 1)^{\frac{1}{1-\theta}}, \quad \theta > 1. \quad (5.4)$$

It implies a positive, "late" dependence, i.e., mainly for large failure-times. The strength of the association decreases with decreasing θ and reaches independence when $\theta \to 1$.

The Hougaard copula The copula function (Hougaard, 1986) is given by

$$C_\theta(u, v) = \exp[-\{(-\ln u)^{\frac{1}{\theta}} + (-\ln v)^{\frac{1}{\theta}}\}^\theta], \quad 0 < \theta < 1. \quad (5.5)$$

It induces a positive, "early" dependence, i.e., mainly for early failure-times. The strength of the association decreases with increasing θ and reaches independence when $\theta \to 1$.

The Plackett copula The copula function (Dale, 1986) is defined as follows:

$$C_\theta(u,v) = \begin{cases} \dfrac{1 + (u+v)(\theta-1) - H_\theta(u,v)}{2(\theta-1)} & \text{if } \theta \neq 1 \\ uv & \text{otherwise,} \end{cases} \quad (5.6)$$

where

$$H_\theta(u, v) = \sqrt{\left[1 + (\theta - 1)(u + v)\right]^2 + 4\theta(1 - \theta)uv} \tag{5.7}$$

and $\theta \in [0, +\infty]$. Parameter θ has an interesting interpretation as the constant global cross-ratio (Dale, 1986). The value of $\theta = 1$ corresponds to independence.

Individual-level surrogacy

To assess the quality of the surrogate at the individual level, a measure of association between S_{ij} and T_{ij}, calculated while adjusting the marginal distributions of the two endpoints for both the trial and treatment effects, is needed. In the copula model (5.1), the strength of the association depends on the copula parameter θ. Hence, θ could be used as the individual-level surrogacy measure. However, the value of the parameter is generally hard to interpret. Instead, one can use Kendall's concordance-coefficient τ, which can be obtained from θ by the following transformation (Nelsen, 2006):

$$\tau = 4 \int_0^1 \int_0^1 C_\theta(u, v) C_\theta(du, dv) - 1. \tag{5.8}$$

Alternately, one can use Spearman's rank-correlation coefficient ρ (Nelsen, 2006):

$$\rho = 12 \int_0^1 \int_0^1 C_\theta(u, v) du dv - 3. \tag{5.9}$$

The relationship (5.8) is especially simple for the Clayton and Hougaard copulas, defined in (5.4) and (5.5), respectively. In particular, for the former,

$$\tau = \frac{\theta - 1}{\theta + 1}, \tag{5.10}$$

whereas for the latter

$$\tau = 1 - \theta. \tag{5.11}$$

On the other hand, for the Plackett copula (5.6)–(5.7), the relationship (5.9) between θ and ρ is explicit:

$$\rho = \frac{\theta + 1}{\theta - 1} - \frac{2\theta}{(\theta - 1)^2} \ln \theta. \tag{5.12}$$

Trial-level surrogacy

The quality of the surrogate at the trial level can be evaluated by considering the correlation coefficient between the treatment effects α_i and β_i. The coefficient can be estimated by using the estimates $\widehat{\alpha}_i$ and $\widehat{\beta}_i$ of the treatment effects obtained from (5.2)–(5.3). Note that, in this step, the adjustment for the estimation error, present in $\widehat{\alpha}_i$ and $\widehat{\beta}_i$, should be made. Toward this aim, as suggested by Burzykowski and Cortiñas Abrahantes (2005), assume that the estimated treatment effects $\widehat{\alpha}_i$ and $\widehat{\beta}_i$ follow the model

$$\begin{pmatrix} \widehat{\alpha}_i \\ \widehat{\beta}_i \end{pmatrix} = \begin{pmatrix} \alpha_i \\ \beta_i \end{pmatrix} + \begin{pmatrix} \varepsilon_{ai} \\ \varepsilon_{bi} \end{pmatrix}, \tag{5.13}$$

where the estimation errors ε_{ai} and ε_{bi} are normally distributed with mean zero and variance-covariance matrix

$$\Omega_i = \begin{pmatrix} \omega_{aa,i} & \omega_{ab,i} \\ \omega_{ab,i} & \omega_{bb,i} \end{pmatrix}, \tag{5.14}$$

and $(\alpha_i, \beta_i)^T$ follows a bivariate-normal distribution with mean $(\alpha, \beta)^T$ and variance-covariance matrix D given by (4.13). Consequently, $(\widehat{\alpha}_i, \widehat{\beta}_i)^T$ follows a normal distribution with mean $(\alpha, \beta)^T$ and variance-covariance matrix $D + \Omega_i$. One can then fit model (5.13)–(5.14) while fixing matrices Ω_i at their values estimated in the first-stage model, and obtain an estimate of D.

If the individual-level association is not of immediate interest, one may base analysis on the marginal models (5.2)–(5.3) without specifying the baseline hazards. When fitting the models, it is important to use the "robust" estimator of the variance-covariance matrix of the estimated treatment effects $\widehat{\alpha}_i$ and $\widehat{\beta}_i$ (see, e.g., Lin, 1994). This is because the estimator takes into account the correlation between the surrogate and true endpoints and provides a correct estimate of the variance-covariance matrix. The latter can then be used to adjust the estimation of the correlation coefficient of α_i and β_i for the estimation error present in $\widehat{\alpha}_i$ and $\widehat{\beta}_i$.

5.3 Analysis of Case Studies

In this section, we illustrate the application of the methods, mentioned in the previous section, by using data from the individual-patient-data meta-analysis of patients with advanced or recurrent gastric cancer (Section 2.2.6). The analysis includes individual data on 4,069 patients with documented OS and PFS who were randomized in 20 trials (Paoletti et al., 2013). The goal of the analysis is to evaluate PFS as a surrogate for OS.

5.3.1 Using SAS

5.3.1.1 Copula-Based Models

We first conduct the analysis applying the two-stage approach with a copula model (5.1) used in the first stage. In particular, we consider models defined by using the Clayton (5.4), Hougaard (5.5), and Plackett (5.6)–(5.7) copulas. The marginal models (5.2)–(5.3) are specified by assuming the Weibull hazard functions.

We fit the three models with the help of the SAS macros (`%COPULA`, Section 12.3.4). The obtained maximum log-likelihood values are equal to −2989.5, −2438.8, and −2549.4 for the Clayton, Hougaard, and Plackett copula, respectively. Given that all models include the same number of parameters (121), we can select as the best fitting model the one with the largest maximum-likelihood value, i.e., the model based on the Hougaard copula.

For this model, the estimated value of the copula parameter θ is equal to 0.328 (95% CI: [0.317, 0.339]). From (5.11) it follows that the value of τ can be estimated to be equal to 0.672 (95% CI: [0.661, 0.683]). Spearman's rank correlation coefficient, computed from (5.9) by numerical integration, is equal to 0.853 (95% CI: [0.842, 0.865]). It indicates substantial correlation between PFS and OS at the individual-patient level.

Figure 5.1 presents the estimated trial-specific treatment effects, i.e., logarithms of hazard ratios, on PFS and on OS; each trial is represented by a circle, the size of which is proportional to the trial sample size. The association between the effects is only moderate. A simple linear regression model, fitted without any adjustment for the estimation error present in the estimated treatment effects, yields the following regression equation:

$$\ln(HR_{OS}) = 0.043 + 0.747 \times \ln(HR_{PFS}), \tag{5.15}$$

with the standard errors of the intercept and slope estimated to be equal to 0.050 and 0.138, respectively. The corresponding value of $R^2_{\text{trial(r)}}$ is equal to 0.621 (95% CI: [0.359, 0.883]). The value is based on the following estimate of the variance-covariance matrix D of the (random) treatment effects:

$$\begin{pmatrix} 0.0477 & 0.0396 \\ 0.0396 & 0.0531 \end{pmatrix}, \tag{5.16}$$

for which the condition number (the ratio of the largest to the smallest eigenvalue) is equal to 8.5. This value is small enough to regard the obtained estimate as numerically stable.

To adjust the analysis for the estimation of treatment effects by using model (5.13)–(5.14), we need data in the "long" format, with two records per trial, one providing the estimate of effect for PFS, and the other for OS. An illustration of a few first records in a such dataset is:

```
trial        effect     endp
    1      -0.09382     MAIN
    1      -0.46722     SURR
    2       0.03852     MAIN
    2      -0.16112     SURR
```

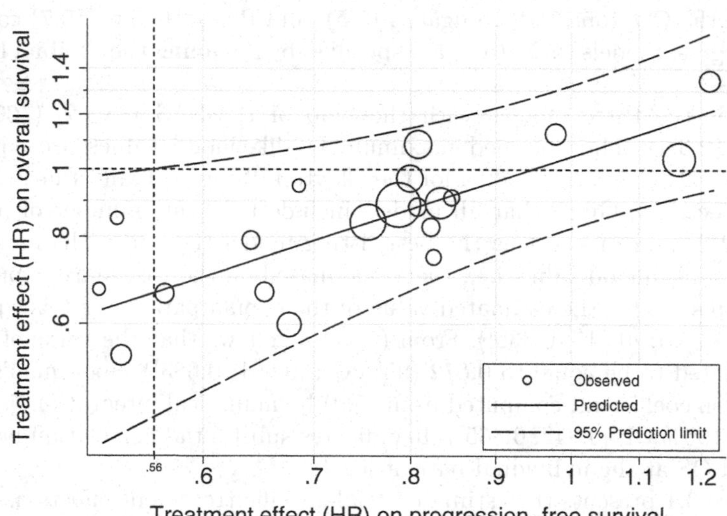

FIGURE 5.1
Advanced Gastric Cancer Data. Trial-level association between copula-model-based treatment effects on PFS and OS (both axes are on a log scale). The circle surfaces are proportional to trial size.

```
     3          -0.32230      MAIN
     3          -0.29295      SURR
...
```

To fit model (5.13)–(5.14), we can use `PROC MIXED`:

```
PROC MIXED data=both order=data method=reml covtest asycov;
 MODEL effect=surr main/s covb noint;
 RANDOM surr main/subject=trial type=un;
 REPEATED /subject=trial group=trial type=un;
 PARMS /parmsdata=parms eqcons=4 to \&nobs;
RUN;
```

Note the use of the `PARMS` statement. It uses the dataset indicated in the `parmsdata` option to provide the starting values for the variance-covariance parameters of the model. In particular, the values starting from the fourth one are fixed, as indicated by the `eqcons=4 to &nobs` option, where `&nobs` is a SAS macro variable indicating the number of observations in the `parmsdata` dataset. The macro variable has to be created and initialized or replaced by the concrete number for the data at hand, which is the $3 \times (\#\text{trials} + 1)$. The first three values in the `parmsdata` dataset become the starting values for the estimation of matrix D.

Thus, the `parmsdata` dataset should include just one variable called `Est` containing the elements of matrices D and the estimated variance-covariance matrices Ω_i for all trials. The first three values should be the starting values for the elements of D, given in the order d_{bb}, d_{ab}, and d_{aa}. The fourth and subsequent values should be the values of $\omega_{bb,i}$, $\omega_{ab,i}$, and $\omega_{aa,i}$ (see equation (5.14)) for all trials, estimated by using the first-stage model. Note that the selection of the starting values for D is very important, as it may influence the convergence of the optimization algorithm. However, even with reasonable starting values, the optimization algorithm is not guaranteed to converge, especially if the magnitude of the estimation error (elements of Ω_i) is considerable as compared to the between-trial variability (elements of D).

Note that alternative variance-covariance parameterizations could be used in the `type` option of the `RANDOM` statement. In particular, one can use `type=unr` or `type=fa0(2)` options. The former has the advantage of providing directly the estimate of $R_{\text{trial(r)}} = \sqrt{R^2_{\text{trial(r)}}}$ with its standard error, while the latter explicitly constraints the estimates of D to be positive-definite.

After adjusting for the estimation error by using model (5.13)–(5.14) fitted with the `PROC MIXED` code described above, $R^2_{\text{trial(r)}}$ is estimated to be equal to 0.606 (95% CI: [0.041, 1.170]). The value is based on the following estimate of the variance-covariance matrix D of the (random) treatment effects:

$$\begin{pmatrix} 0.0226 & 0.0176 \\ 0.0176 & 0.0227 \end{pmatrix}, \qquad (5.17)$$

for which the condition number is equal to 8.0. It is worth noting that the elements of matrix (5.17) are about twice smaller than the elements of matrix (5.16). This is due to the fact that (5.16) is obtained by considering the total variability of the estimated treatment-effects as due to the between-trial variability, whereas (5.17) is obtained after removing from the total variability the part due to the estimation of treatment effects.

Note that the CI for the "adjusted" $R^2_{\text{trial(r)}}$ is much wider than the CI obtained for the "naïve" regression model (5.15). Thus, after accounting for the fact that we analyze estimated, and not the true random, treatment effects, our uncertainty regarding the true value of $R^2_{\text{trial(r)}}$ increases.

The linear regression model obtained with an adjustment for estimation errors is

$$\ln(HR_{OS}) = 0.042 + 0.779 \times \ln(HR_{PFS}), \qquad (5.18)$$

with the standard errors of the intercept and slope estimated to be equal to 0.079 and 0.295, respectively. There is only a slight difference between the estimated values of the intercept and slope as compared to the "naïve" regression (5.15); this is not always the case. The standard errors of the coefficients of the equation (5.18) are larger than the corresponding estimates for (5.15).

Regression line (5.18) is labeled "predicted" in Figure 5.1. The 95% prediction limits, presented in the plot, indicate the range of effects on OS that can be expected for a given effect on PFS.

The moderate correlation at the trial level is reflected by a surrogate threshold effect (STE; Section 4.5) equal to 0.56 (indicated by the vertical dashed line in Figure 5.1). Hence, one should observe an HR_{PFS} smaller than 0.56 in order to predict, with 95% confidence, an HR_{OS} significantly smaller than 1.

5.3.1.2 Marginal Models

If we focus on the trial-level surrogacy, we can conduct an analysis based solely on the marginal models (5.2)–(5.3) specified without assuming any particular form for the baseline hazards. Toward this aim, we can use `PROC PHREG`. In particular, the data have to be transformed to the "long" format, with two records per patient, one providing the time and censoring indicator for PFS, and the other the time and censoring indicator for OS. An illustration of the first few records in such a dataset is:

```
treat   idpat   endp       time   status
    1     219      1    2.35729        1
    1     219      2    0.75838        1
    0     220      1    1.79877        1
    0     220      2    0.39151        1
    1     221      1    0.71458        1
    1     221      2    0.71458        1
...
```

Then, for each trial, treatment effects on PFS and OS can be estimated by the following SAS syntax:

```
PROC PHREG data=joined covs(aggregate) covout outest=outests;
   MODEL time*status(0)=treat1 treat2 / ties=efron;
   STRATA endp;
   ID idpat;
   treat1 = treat * (endp=1);
   treat2 = treat * (endp=2);
RUN;
```

Note the use of the `covs(aggregate)` option and the `ID idpat` statement that allow estimating the variance-covariance of the estimated treatment effects by using the "robust" estimator, which takes into account the association between PFS and OS. Variables `treat1` and `treat2` define treatment indicators specific for, respectively, the surrogate and true endpoints.

Figure 5.2 presents the estimated log-hazard ratios. As was the case in the copula-based estimates (see Figure 5.1), the association between the treatment effects is only moderate. A simple linear regression model, fitted without any adjustment for the estimation error present in the estimated treatment effects, yields the value of $R^2_{\text{trial(r)}}$ equal to 0.452 (95% CI: [0.130, 0.775]), somewhat smaller than the estimate obtained from the copula model with Weibull marginal hazards. The value is based on the following estimate of matrix D:

$$\begin{pmatrix} 0.0343 & 0.0279 \\ 0.0279 & 0.0504 \end{pmatrix}, \tag{5.19}$$

for which the condition number is equal to 5.4. The resulting regression equation is

$$\ln(HR_{OS}) = -0.022 + 0.555 \times \ln(HR_{PFS}), \tag{5.20}$$

with the standard errors of the intercept and slope estimated to be equal to 0.052 and 0.144, respectively. The slope is markedly smaller than it was in the case of the "naïve" regression model (5.15) corresponding to the copula model. with the standard errors of the intercept and slope estimated to be equal to 0.052 and 0.144, respectively. The slope is markedly smaller than it was in the case of the "naïve" regression model (5.15) corresponding to the copula model.

After adjusting for the estimation error, $R^2_{\text{trial(r)}}$ is estimated to be equal to 0.224 (95% CI: [-0.638, 1.085]), based on the following estimate of the variance-covariance matrix D:

$$\begin{pmatrix} 0.0218 & 0.0065 \\ 0.0065 & 0.0088 \end{pmatrix}, \tag{5.21}$$

for which the condition number is equal to 4.0. The estimated value of $R^2_{\text{trial(r)}}$ is much smaller than the estimates obtained for the copula model or for the "naïve" regression model (5.15). However, the CI for the adjusted $R^2_{\text{trial(r)}}$ is very wide; it essentially covers the entire admissible range [0,1]. In fact, it extends beyond the range; this is due to the fact that the CI was obtained as $(\widehat{R}_{\text{trial(r)}})^2 \pm 1.96 \times \widehat{SE}\{(\widehat{R}_{\text{trial(r)}})^2\}$, where $\widehat{SE}\{(\widehat{R}_{\text{trial(r)}})^2\}$ was computed by applying the delta method to the standard error of $\widehat{R}_{\text{trial(r)}}$, i.e.,

$$\widehat{SE}\{(\widehat{R}_{\text{trial(r)}})^2\} \approx 2 \times |\widehat{R}_{\text{trial(r)}}| \times \widehat{SE}\{(\widehat{R}_{\text{trial(r)}})\}.$$

The linear regression model obtained with an adjustment for estimation errors is

$$\ln(HR_{OS}) = -0.076 + 0.300 \times \ln(HR_{PFS}), \tag{5.22}$$

with the standard errors of the intercept and slope estimated to be equal to 0.101 and 0.379, respectively. There is a marked difference between the estimated values of the intercept and slope as compared to the "naïve" regression (5.20); however, given the (im)precision of the estimates, the difference is not significant. The standard errors of the coefficients of the equation (5.22) are larger than the corresponding estimates for (5.20).

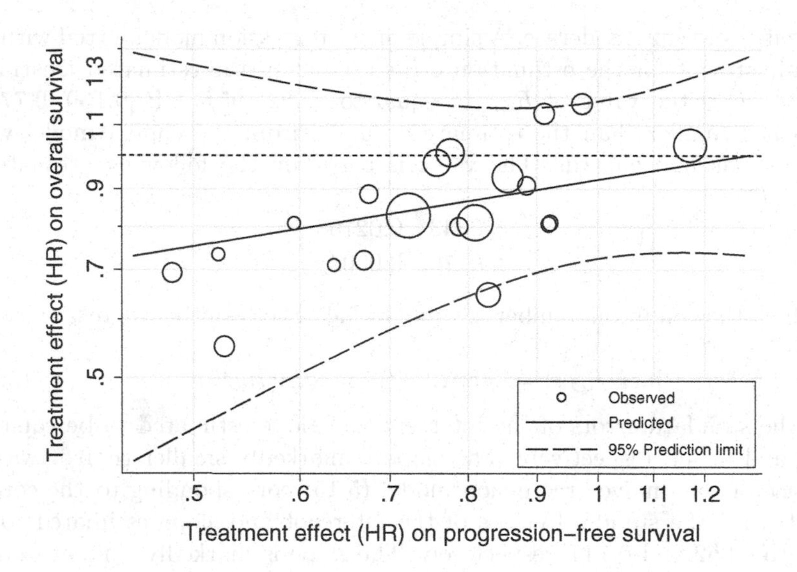

FIGURE 5.2
Advanced Gastric Cancer Data. Trial-level association between marginal-PH-model-based treatment effects on PFS and OS (both axes are on a log scale). The circle surfaces are proportional to trial size.

Regression line (5.22) is labeled "predicted" in Figure 5.2. The 95% prediction limits, presented in the plot, indicate the range of effects on OS that can be expected for a given effect on PFS. Note that the limits do not cross the horizontal line corresponding to $HR = 1$. Hence, it is not possible to estimate the surrogate threshold effect STE.

5.3.2 Using R

Currently, there are no specific tools in R aimed at evaluation of a failure-time surrogate for a failure-time true endpoint. Using the existing packages it is possible to conduct an analysis based on the marginal proportional hazard models (5.2)–(5.3). Toward this aim, the *survival* package can be used. In particular, function `coxph` can be used to fit the marginal models while using the "robust" estimator of the variance-covariance matrix of the estimated treatment effects.

More specifically, assume that the data frame, `long` say, contains the data for the two endpoints for a particular trial in the "long" format, with two records per patient, as described in the previous section in the context of the use of `PROC PHREG`. Then the following R command fits the required marginal

TABLE 5.1

Prostate Data. Studies of potential failure-time surrogate endpoints for a failure-time true endpoint in cancer. (Abbreviations: endpoint, DFS = Disease-free Survival, LFS = Leukemia-free Survival, OS = Overall Survival, PFS = Progression-free Survival, RFS = Relapse-free Survival, TTPP = Time to Prostate-specific-antigen Progression).

Tumor	Surrogate	True	References
Acute myeloid leukemia	LFS	OS	Buyse et al. (2011)
Resectable colorectal cancer	DFS	OS	Sargent et al. (2005)
Resectable gastric cancer	DFS	OS	Oba et al. (2013)
Locally advanced head and neck cancer	RFS/EFS	OS	Michiels et al. (2009)
Advanced colorectal cancer	PFS	OS	Burzykowski et al. (2001)
			Buyse et al. (2007)
Advanced ovarian cancer	PFS	OS	Burzykowski et al. (2001)
Advanced breast cancer	PFS	OS	Burzykowski et al. (2008)
Advanced gastric cancer	PFS	OS	Paoletti et al. (2013)
Advanced lung cancer	PFS	OS	Laporte et al. (2013)
			Foster et al. (2015)
Advanced prostate cancer	TTPP	OS	Buyse et al. (2003)
			Collette et al. (2005)

models with the robust estimator of the variance-covariance matrix of the estimated treatment effects:

```
coxph(Surv(time, status, type='right') ~
    treat1 + treat2 + strata(endp) + cluster(idpat), data=long)
```

The command can be used to estimate treatment effects for each trial. The estimates can then be collected and subsequently analyzed to provide an estimate of $R^2_{\text{trial(r)}}$. In particular, assume that the estimates are collected in data frame `ph.long` with the following structure:

```
trial          est    endp
    1   -0.309128428     1
    1   -0.649782310     2
    2   -0.212360463     1
    2   -0.520637024     2
    3   -0.094950157     1
```

```
    3    -0.123028658        2
...
```

where `est` is the estimated effect for endpoint `endp`. Then function `gls` from the *nlme* package can be used to estimate $R^2_{\text{trial(r)}}$ and its CI (without adjusting for the estimation error in the estimated treatment effects). In particular, the following syntax can be applied:

```
gls.fit <- gls(est ~ factor(endp) -1,
weights=varIdent(form = ~1 | endp),
correlation = corCompSymm(form = ~ 1 | trial), data=ph.long)
intervals(gls.fit,which = "var-cov")$corStruct ^ 2
```

The `intervals`-function call provides the squared values of the correlation coefficient of the estimated treatment effects and its 95% CI, which can be taken as an estimate of $R^2_{\text{trial(r)}}$ and its 95% CI. In particular, for the estimated marginal log-hazard ratios, the presented R code yields $R^2_{\text{trial(r)}}$ equal to 0.453 with the 95% CI equal to [0.123, 0.727]. The CI is similar to the one ([0.130, 0.775]) reported for the corresponding marginal analysis using SAS tools.

One could consider using function `lme` from the *nlme* package to adjust the analysis for the estimation error present in the estimated treatment effects by using model (5.13)–(5.14). However, unlike `PROC PHREG` in SAS, function `lme` does not allow for fixing the residual scale parameter, which prohibits specifying the desired form of the model.

5.4 Concluding Remarks

The approach to evaluation of a failure-time surrogate for a failure-time true endpoint, presented in the current chapter, has already been applied multiple times in oncology. Table 5.1 provides details of several applications.

The results of the analysis, presented in the current chapter, suggest that PFS does not seem to be a useful surrogate for OS in advanced gastric cancer, although, given the imprecision of the estimation of $R^2_{\text{trial(r)}}$, this statement may need to be treated with caution. These findings parallel those in advanced breast cancer (Burzykowski et al., 2008). They are at variance with those in advanced colorectal cancer and advanced ovarian cancer, where PFS seemed a good surrogate for OS (Burzykowski et al., 2001; Buyse et al., 2007). In advanced lung cancer, the value of PFS as a surrogate for OS is questionable (Laporte et al., 2013). It seems difficult to draw general conclusions about the surrogacy of PFS as a surrogate for OS in advanced forms of cancer.

The choice of the copula in model (5.1) requires some attention, as misspecification of the shape of the association between S and T may lead to bias (Renfro, Shang, and Sargent, 2015). Renfro, Shang, and Sargent (2015) provide some recommendations in that respect. It should be noted that copulas (5.1) treat both endpoints symmetrically. However, if the true endpoint is, e.g., the overall survival time, there is a natural restriction that $S \leq T$. Obviously, in that case, the copula model is misspecified and it may lead to, e.g., a biased estimate of the individual-level association. A possible solution to this issue is an accelerated failure-time model that takes into account the ordering of the two endpoints as proposed by Ghosh, Taylor, and Sargent (2012).

6

A Categorical (Ordinal) and a Failure-Time Endpoint

Tomasz Burzykowski
Hasselt University, Belgium and IDDI, Belgium

CONTENTS

6.1 Introduction

In this chapter, we focus on the case when the surrogate is a categorical ordinal (or binary) endpoint and the true endpoint is a failure-time endpoint. Note that the described approach is applicable also in the reverse case, i.e., with a failure-time surrogate and an ordinal true endpoint. We mainly follow the two-stage approach proposed by Burzykowski, Molenberghs, and Buyse (2004).

6.2 Theoretical Background

Assume that the true endpoint T is a failure-time random variable and the surrogate S is a categorical variable with K ordered categories, i.e., an ordinal variable. For each of $j = 1, \ldots, n_i$ patients from trial i ($i = 1, \ldots, N$) we thus have quadruplets $(X_{ij}, \Delta_{ij}, S_{ij}, Z_{ij})$, where X_{ij} is a possibly censored version of survival time T_{ij} and Δ_{ij} is the censoring indicator assuming a value of 1 for observed failures and 0 otherwise.

Model (4.10) is replaced by a copula-based model (see, e.g., Section 5.2) for the true endpoint T_{ij} and a latent continuous variable $\tilde{S}_{ij}$ underlying the surrogate endpoint S_{ij} (Burzykowski, Molenberghs, and Buyse, 2004). In particular, Burzykowski, Molenberghs, and Buyse (2004) used the Plackett copula (Hougaard, 1986) (see also (5.6)–(5.7)). The marginal model for S_{ij} is the proportional odds model:

$$\text{logit}\{P(S_{ij} \leq k \mid Z_{ij})\} = \gamma_{ik} + \alpha_i Z_{ij}. \tag{6.1}$$

The model can be interpreted as assuming a logistic distribution for the latent variable $\tilde{S}_{ij}$. Note that, in the case of a binary surrogate S_{ij}, model (6.1) is equivalent to logistic regression.

It is worth re-parameterizing model (6.1) as follows:

$$\text{logit}\{P(S_{ij} \leq k \mid Z_{ij})\} = \eta_k^0 + \eta_i + \eta_{i,k} + \alpha_i Z_{ij}, \tag{6.2}$$

where, for identifiability purposes, one might specify that, for example,

$$\eta_1 = \eta_{1,1} = \ldots = \eta_{1,K-1} = 0.$$

If, for a particular trial, i_0 say, not all levels of S are observed, one can use model (6.2) with some of the terms $\eta_{i_0,1}, \ldots, \eta_{i_0,K-1}$, corresponding to the unobserved levels, constrained to 0. As a special case, the following model might be considered:

$$\text{logit}\{P(S_{ij} \leq k \mid Z_{ij})\} = \eta_k^0 + \eta_i + \alpha_i Z_{ij}. \tag{6.3}$$

The model assumes a fixed set of cut-points $\eta_1^0, \ldots, \eta_{K-1}^0$, but allows for trial-specific shifts η_i of the set.

For T_{ij}, the proportional hazard model is used:

$$\lambda_{ij}(t \mid Z_{ij}) = \lambda_i(t) \exp(\beta_i Z_{ij}), \tag{6.4}$$

where β_i are trial-specific effects of treatment Z and $\lambda_i(t)$ is a trial-specific baseline hazard function. Burzykowski, Molenberghs, and Buyse (2004) used a Weibull-distribution-based baseline hazard.

Using the joint distribution function defined by the copula and the marginal models (6.1) and (6.4), it is possible to construct the likelihood function for the observed data ($X_{ij} = x_{ij}, \Delta_{ij} = \delta_{ij}, S_{ij} = s_{ij}, Z_{ij} = z_{ij}$) and obtain estimates of the treatment effects α_i and β_i.

If, as proposed by Burzykowski, Molenberghs, and Buyse (2004), the Plackett copula is used in the construction of the joint model for T_{ij} and $\widetilde{S}_{ij}$, the quality of the surrogate at the individual level can be evaluated by using the copula parameter θ. This is because, for the Plackett copula, θ takes the form of a (constant) global odds ratio. Specifically, in the current setting (for $k = 1, \ldots, K-1$ and $t > 0$):

$$\begin{aligned} \theta &= \frac{P(T_{ij} > t,\, S_{ij} > k)\, P(T_{ij} \leq t, S_{ij} \leq k)}{P(T_{ij} > t,\, S_{ij} \leq k)\, P(T_{ij} \leq t,\, S_{ij} > k)} \\ &= \frac{P(T_{ij} > t \mid S_{ij} > k)}{P(T_{ij} \leq t \mid S_{ij} > k)} \left\{ \frac{P(T_{ij} > t \mid S_{ij} \leq k)}{P(T_{ij} \leq t \mid S_{ij} \leq k)} \right\}^{-1}. \end{aligned} \quad (6.5)$$

Thus, θ is naturally interpreted as the (constant) ratio of the odds of surviving beyond time t given response higher than k to the odds of surviving beyond time t given response at most k. For a binary surrogate, it is just the odds ratio for responders *versus* non-responders (assuming that $k = 2$ indicates response).

The quality of the surrogate at the trial level can be evaluated by considering the correlation coefficient between the estimated treatment effects α_i and β_i. Note that, in this step, the adjustment for the estimation error, present in $\widehat{\alpha}_i$ and $\widehat{\beta}_i$, should be made. Toward this aim, model (5.13)–(5.14) (see Section 5.2) can be used.

If the individual-level association is not of immediate interest, one may base analysis on the marginal models (6.1) and (6.4), without specifying the baseline hazards in the latter. When fitting the models, it is worth estimating the variance-covariance matrix of the estimated treatment effects $\widehat{\alpha}_i$ and $\widehat{\beta}_i$ while taking into account the association between S and T. Toward this aim, an estimator based on a combination of the results obtained by Liang and Zeger (1986), Lin and Wei (1989), Lin (1994), and Lipsitz, Kim, and Zhao (1994) can be used (see Appendix 6.5).

6.3 Analysis of a Case Study

In this section, we illustrate the application of the methods, mentioned in the previous section, by using data from the individual-patient-data meta-analysis of patients with advanced colorectal cancer (see Section 2.2.4). The data were analyzed before by Burzykowski, Molenberghs, and Buyse (2004). The goal of the analysis is to evaluate tumor response as a surrogate for overall survival (OS). In particular, we consider two forms of the response:

the four-category (complete response, CR; partial response, PR; stable disease, SD; progressive disease, PD) and the binary (complete/partial versus stable disease/progression) ones.

6.3.1 Using SAS

6.3.1.1 Four-Category Tumor Response

We first conduct the analysis of the four-category response using the Plackett-copula model with the marginal models (6.3) and (6.4); the latter is specified by assuming the Weibull hazard functions. Note that, as the response, we use the best response observed across the entire observation period for a patient.

We fit the model with the help of the SAS macro (see Section 12.5.4). For this model, the estimated value of the copula parameter θ is equal to 6.52 (95% CI: [5.79, 7.25]). It indicates a substantial association between response and OS at the individual-patient level: the odds for surviving beyond time t given a higher (for instance, complete) response are about 6.5 times higher than the odds of surviving beyond time t given any lower response (partial response, stable disease, or progression). Note that the estimated value differs slightly from the value of 6.78 reported by Burzykowski, Molenberghs, and Buyse (2004). This is due to the fact that these authors used the marginal model (6.2) with some of the terms $\eta_{i_0,1}, \ldots, \eta_{i_0,K-1}$ constrained to 0 for trials with missing response categories.

It should be noted that θ involves a comparison of survival times of patients classified according to tumor response. It is well known that such a comparison is likely to be length-biased, because a response to treatment is not observed instantaneously. As a result, patients who enjoy long survival times are more likely to be responders than non-responders, and therefore the survival of responders is likely to be biased upward compared with that of non-responders. One method of correcting for length bias in such a comparison is a landmark analysis (Anderson et al., 1983). We do not attempt to conduct such an analysis here; it was considered by Burzykowski, Molenberghs, and Buyse (2004).

Figure 6.1 presents the estimated trial-specific treatment effects, i.e., logarithms of hazard ratios on OS and log-odds ratios for tumor response; each trial is represented by a circle of the size proportional to the trial sample size. In the dataset, higher response categories (PD, SD, PR, CR) were coded with higher scores (1, 2, 3, 4). Hence, according to the parameterization used in model (6.3), α_i is the logarithm of the ratio of the odds of observing a lower tumor-response category for the experimental treatment to the odds for the control treatment. On the other hand, following (6.4), β_i is the logarithm of the ratio of the hazard of death for the experimental treatment to the hazard for the control treatment. Thus, Figure 6.1 indicates that the larger experimental-treatment-induced reduction of the odds of a "worse" response (OR<1), the larger the corresponding reduction in the hazard of death (HR<1). However,

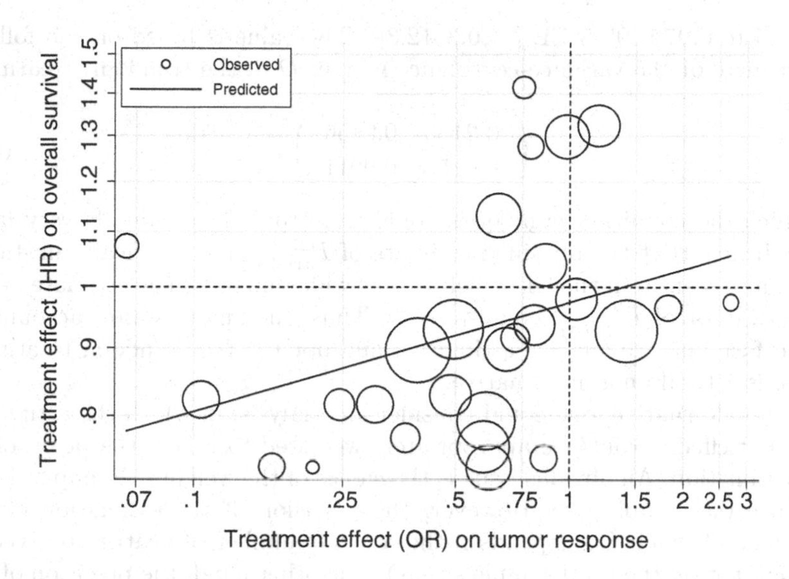

FIGURE 6.1
Advanced Colorectal Cancer. Trial-level association between copula-model-based treatment effects on four-category tumor response and OS (both axes on a log scale). The circle surfaces are proportional to trial size.

the association between the effects appears weak. A simple linear regression model, fitted without any adjustment for the estimation error present in the estimated treatment effects, yields the following regression equation:

$$\ln(HR_{OS}) = -0.027 + 0.082 \times \ln(OR_{\mathbf{response}}), \tag{6.6}$$

with the standard errors of the intercept and slope estimated to be equal to 0.044 and 0.043, respectively. The corresponding value of $R^2_{\text{trial(r)}}$ is equal to 0.125 (95% CI: [-0.108, 0.358]); the negative lower limit of the CI is due to the use of the normal approximation to the distribution of $(\widehat{R}_{\text{trial(r)}})^2$ (see Section 5.3.1.1). The value is based on the following estimate of the variance-covariance matrix D of the (random) treatment effects:

$$\begin{pmatrix} 0.0363 & 0.0551 \\ 0.0551 & 0.6707 \end{pmatrix}, \tag{6.7}$$

for which the condition number (the ratio of the largest to the smallest eigenvalue) is equal to 21.4. This value is small enough to regard the obtained estimate as numerically stable.

After adjusting for the estimation error by using model (5.13)–(5.14) fitted with the `PROC MIXED` code described in Section 5.3.1, $R^2_{\text{trial(r)}}$ is estimated to be equal to 0.979 (95% CI: $[-10.3, 12.3]$). The value is based on the following estimate of the variance-covariance matrix D of the (random) treatment effects:

$$\begin{pmatrix} 0.2183 & 0.0156 \\ 0.0156 & 0.0011 \end{pmatrix}, \tag{6.8}$$

for which the condition number is equal to 9216.7. This value is very large and indicates that the obtained estimate of $R^2_{\text{trial(r)}}$ is numerically unstable. This is also seen from the CI, which is very wide due to a huge estimate of the standard error of $\widehat{R}^2_{\text{trial(r)}}$, equal to 5.77. Thus, the analysis after accounting for the fact that we analyze estimated, and not the true random, treatment effects, is actually non-informative.

As an alternative, one could consider an analysis, in which the estimated treatment effects would be appropriately weighted to reflect the precision of their estimation. An obvious issue is the choice of the weights. A simple choice is to use the sample size. However, the precision of the estimation of the treatment effect on OS depends rather on the number of deaths observed in the trial, not on the total sample size. On the other hand, the precision of the estimation of the treatment effect on tumor response depends on the observed numbers of different types of responses. Hence, it is not clear to what extent the analysis weighted by the trial sample size can correct for the estimation error and provide a correct estimate of $R^2_{\text{trial(r)}}$.

If the weighted estimate of $R^2_{\text{trial(r)}}$ is desired, it can be obtained by using any procedure providing the coefficient of determination for a simple linear regression model, e.g., `PROC REG`. However, an important issue is the estimation of the precision of the obtained estimate. Toward this aim, `PROC MIXED` can be used. In particular, we need data in the "long" format, with two records per trial, one providing the estimate of effect for OS, and the other one for tumor response. An illustration of a few first records in a such dataset is:

```
trial      effect    ssize      endp
    1    -0.23164      306      MAIN
    1    -0.50734      306      SURR
    2    -0.27657      249      MAIN
    2    -0.52413      249      SURR
    3     0.03843      164      MAIN
    3    -0.14893      164      SURR
...
```

Then we fit a (weighted) linear model with the help of the following SAS syntax:

```
PROC MIXED data=ests;
   CLASS trial endp;
   WEIGHT ssize;
```

```
   MODEL effect=endp / noint;
   REPEATED endp / subject=trial type=unr;
RUN;
```

Note the use of the WEIGHT statement, which applies the sample sizes, contained in the variable ssize, as weights. Moreover, the type=unr option in the REPEATED statement provides directly an estimate of the correlation coefficient between the treatment effects, $\widehat{R}_{\text{trial(r)}}$, and its estimated variance. Subsequently, we can obtain the estimate of $R^2_{\text{trial(r)}}$ as $\widehat{R}^2_{\text{trial(r)}}$, with an estimate of its variance computed by using the delta method, i.e., $\text{Var}(\widehat{R}^2_{\text{trial(r)}}) \approx 4 \times \widehat{R}^2_{\text{trial(r)}} \times \text{Var}(\widehat{R}_{\text{trial(r)}})$.

The aforementioned approach is applied to the treatment-effect estimates obtained from the copula model by using a dedicated SAS macro (see Section 12.5.4). It yields an estimate of $R^2_{\text{trial(r)}}$ equal to 0.144 (95% CI: $[-0.106, 0.394]$). The underlying weighted linear regression model is

$$\ln(HR_{OS}) = -0.033 + 0.100 \times \ln(OR_{\text{response}}), \tag{6.9}$$

with the standard errors of the intercept and slope estimated to be equal to 0.039 and 0.048, respectively. This is the line indicated in Figure 6.1 as "predicted." The "weighted" estimates are based on the following estimate of the variance-covariance matrix D of the (random) treatment effects:

$$\begin{pmatrix} 62.5 & 6.2 \\ 6.2 & 4.3 \end{pmatrix}, \tag{6.10}$$

for which the condition number is equal to 17.3.

The "weighted" results are quite similar to those obtained based on the unweighted, "naïve" linear regression model (6.6). It is worth mentioning that the use of PROC REG yields the same estimates of $R^2_{\text{trial(r)}}$ and linear-regression coefficients, but with somewhat larger standard errors for the intercept (0.04) and slope (0.049) of equation (6.9). This is due to the fact that the PROC MIXED estimates are based on the (restricted) likelihood based on a normal distribution, whereas the PROC REG estimates are obtained by using the weighted least-squares method.

If we focus on the trial-level surrogacy, we can conduct an analysis based solely on the marginal models (6.2) and (6.4), with the latter specified without assuming any particular form of the baseline hazards. Toward this aim, model (6.2) can be fitted by using PROC LOGISTIC and (6.4) by using PROC PHREG. In particular, the call to PROC LOGISTIC can be as follows:

```
PROC LOGISTIC data=dataset;
   CLASS trial treat(ref=first) / param=glm;
   MODEL response=trial treat(trial);
RUN;
```

Variable `trial` is the trial identifier, `treat` is the treatment indicator (with 0 for the control group and 1 for the experimental one), and `response` is the response. Of interest are the trial-specific treatment-effect estimates, provided by the nested effect `treat(trial)`.

On the other hand, (6.4) can be fitted by using `PROC PHREG`, with a call as follows:

```
PROC PHREG data=dataset;
    CLASS trial treat(ref=first) / param=glm;
    MODEL surv*survind(0)=treat(trial);
    STRATA trial;
RUN;
```

Variable `surv` is the observed survival time, while `survind` is the event indicator (with 0 for censored times and 1 for event times).

After fitting the models, the variance-covariance of the estimated coefficients of the models can be estimated while taking into account the association between the response and OS. Toward this aim, a dedicated SAS macro can be used (see Section 12.5.4).

Figure 6.2 presents the estimated log-odds ratios and log-hazard ratios. As was the case in the copula-based estimates (see Figure 6.1), the association between the treatment effects is only moderate. A simple linear regression model, fitted without any adjustment for the estimation error present in the estimated treatment effects, yields the value of $R^2_{\text{trial(r)}}$ equal to 0.145 (95% CI: $[-0.105, 0.395]$), somewhat smaller than the estimate obtained from the copula model with Weibull marginal hazards. The value is based on the following estimate of matrix D:

$$\begin{pmatrix} 0.0308 & 0.0541 \\ 0.0541 & 0.0658 \end{pmatrix}, \tag{6.11}$$

for which the condition number is equal to 25.3. The resulting regression equation is

$$\ln(HR_{OS}) = -0.023 + 0.082 \times \ln(OR_{PFS}), \tag{6.12}$$

with the standard errors of the intercept and slope estimated to be equal to 0.052 and 0.144, respectively. The regression equation is very similar to (6.6) obtained for the model based on the Plackett copula.

Analysis adjusted for the estimation error leads to an estimate of variance-covariance matrix D which is singular. The analysis weighted by the trial sample size, conducted with the help of the dedicated SAS macro (see Section 12.5), yields the following estimate of the variance-covariance matrix D of the (random) treatment effects:

$$\begin{pmatrix} 64.2 & 5.7 \\ 5.7 & 3.5 \end{pmatrix}, \tag{6.13}$$

for which the condition number is equal to 22.0. The corresponding estimate of

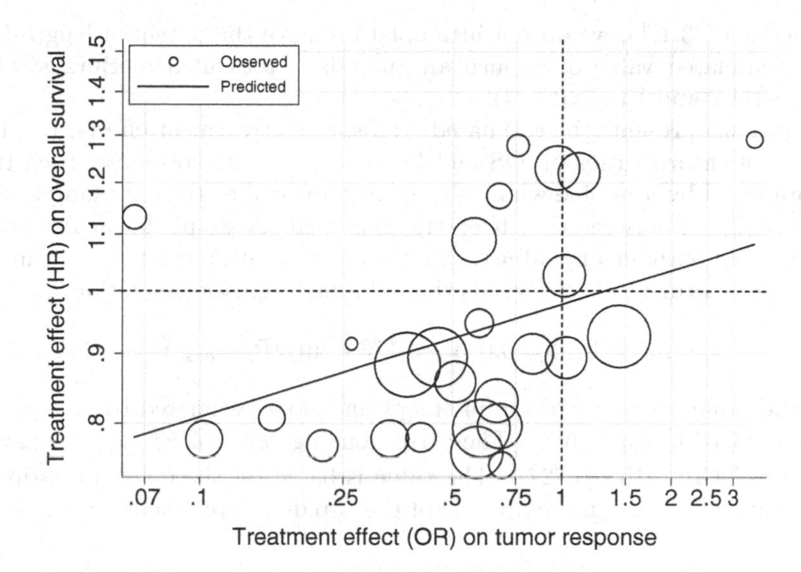

FIGURE 6.2
Advanced Colorectal Cancer. Trial-level association between the marginal-model-based treatment effects on OS and four-category tumor response (both axes on a log scale). The circle surfaces are proportional to trial size.

$R^2_{\text{trial(r)}}$ is equal to 0.144 (95% CI: $[-0.111, 0.399]$), with the linear regression equation

$$\ln(HR_{OS}) = -0.054 + 0.088 \times \ln(OR_{\text{response}}) \tag{6.14}$$

and standard errors of the intercept and slope estimated equal to 0.036 and 0.043, respectively. The line corresponding to equation (6.14) is indicated in Figure 6.2 as "predicted."

6.3.1.2 Binary Tumor Response

We now conduct the analysis of the binary tumor response (complete/partial *vs.* stable disease/progression) using the two-stage approach. Note that in the analysis, one of the trials (no. 6) is excluded due to the fact that there were no complete nor partial responses in one of the treatment groups.

For the Plackett copula with the marginal models (6.3) and (6.4), the estimated value of the copula parameter θ is equal to 4.91 (95% CI: [4.16, 5.66]). It indicates a substantial association between response and OS at the individual-patient level: the odds for surviving beyond time t for responders are about 5 times higher than the odds of surviving beyond time t for non-responders. The same result was reported by Burzykowski, Molenberghs, and Buyse (2004). As was the case in the analysis of the four-category response (see Section 6.3.1.1), we do not attempt to remove the potential length-bias in the estimated value of θ; such an analysis is presented in Burzykowski, Molenberghs, and Buyse (2004).

Figure 6.3 presents the estimated trial-specific treatment effects, i.e., logarithms of hazard ratios on OS and log-odds for tumor response; each trial is represented by a bubble whose size is proportional to the trial sample size. The association between the effects appears weak. A simple linear regression model, fitted without any adjustment for the estimation error present in the estimated treatment effects, yields the following regression equation:

$$\ln(HR_{OS}) = 0.073 + 0.173 \times \ln(OR_{\text{response}}), \tag{6.15}$$

with the standard errors of the intercept and slope estimated to be equal to 0.046 and 0.040, respectively. The corresponding value of $R^2_{\text{trial(r)}}$ is equal to 0.442 (95% CI: [0.156, 0.727]). The value is based on the following estimate of the variance-covariance matrix D of the (random) treatment effects:

$$\begin{pmatrix} 0.0365 & 0.0931 \\ 0.0931 & 0.5377 \end{pmatrix}, \tag{6.16}$$

for which the condition number (the ratio of the largest to the smallest eigenvalue) is equal to 28.0. This value is small enough to regard the obtained estimate as numerically stable.

Attempts to adjust the analysis for the estimation error by using model (5.13)–(5.14) fail due to the fact that the estimated variance-covariance matrix D is not positive-definite. The analysis weighed by the sample size yields the following estimate of the variance-covariance matrix D of the (random) treatment effects:

$$\begin{pmatrix} 69.1 & 11.2 \\ 11.2 & 4.7 \end{pmatrix}, \tag{6.17}$$

for which the condition number is equal to 25.5. The resulting estimate of $R^2_{\text{trial(r)}}$ is equal to 0.390 (95% CI: [0.092, 0.689]) and the weighted linear regression model is

$$\ln(HR_{OS}) = 0.030 + 0.163 \times \ln(OR_{\text{response}}), \tag{6.18}$$

with the standard errors of the intercept and slope estimated to be equal to 0.042 and 0.041, respectively. This is the line indicated in Figure 6.3 as "predicted." The results are similar to those obtained for the "naïve," unweighted linear regression.

Implementation of the models can be performed as explained on page 87. Figure 6.4 presents the estimated log-odds ratios and log-hazard ratios. The association between the treatment effects is only moderate. A simple linear regression model, fitted without any adjustment for the estimation error present in the estimated treatment effects, yields the value of $R^2_{\text{trial(r)}}$ equal to 0.398

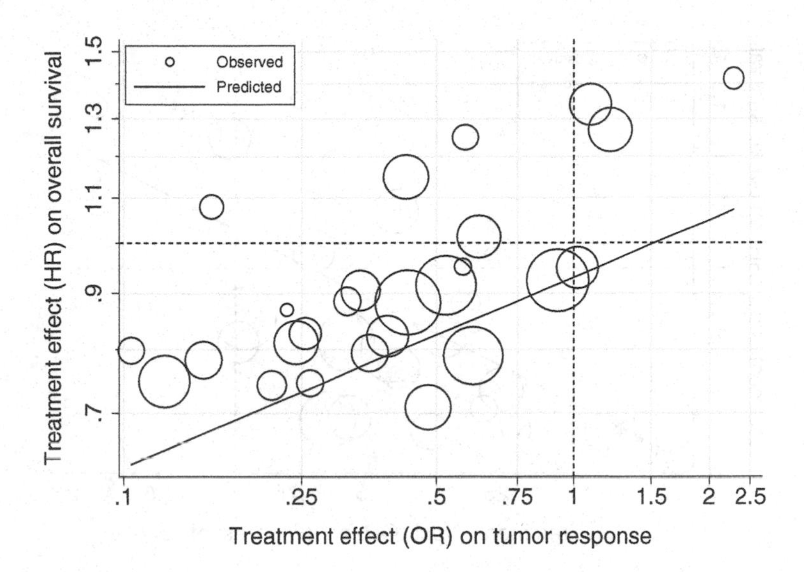

FIGURE 6.3
Advanced Colorectal Cancer. Trial-level association between copula-model-based treatment effects on binary tumor response and OS (both axes on a log scale). The circle surfaces are proportional to trial size.

(95% CI: [0.106, 0.690]). The value is based on the following estimate of matrix D:

$$\begin{pmatrix} 0.0308 & 0.0825 \\ 0.0825 & 0.5553 \end{pmatrix}, \tag{6.19}$$

for which the condition number is equal to 31.3. The resulting regression equation is

$$\ln(HR_{OS}) = 0.058 + 0.149 \times \ln(OR_{\text{response}}), \tag{6.20}$$

with the standard errors of the intercept and slope estimated to be equal to 0.043 and 0.037, respectively.

Analysis adjusted for the estimation error leads to an estimate of variance-covariance matrix D which is singular. The analysis weighed by the sample size yields the estimate of $R^2_{\text{trial(r)}}$ equal to 0.371 (95% CI: [0.070, 0.671]), based on the estimated variance-covariance matrix D of the (random) treatment effects:

$$\begin{pmatrix} 71.5 & 9.6 \\ 9.6 & 3.5 \end{pmatrix}, \tag{6.21}$$

with the condition number equal to 34.0. The weighted linear regression model is

$$\ln(HR_{OS}) = 0.005 + 0.1341 \times \ln(OR_{response}), \tag{6.22}$$

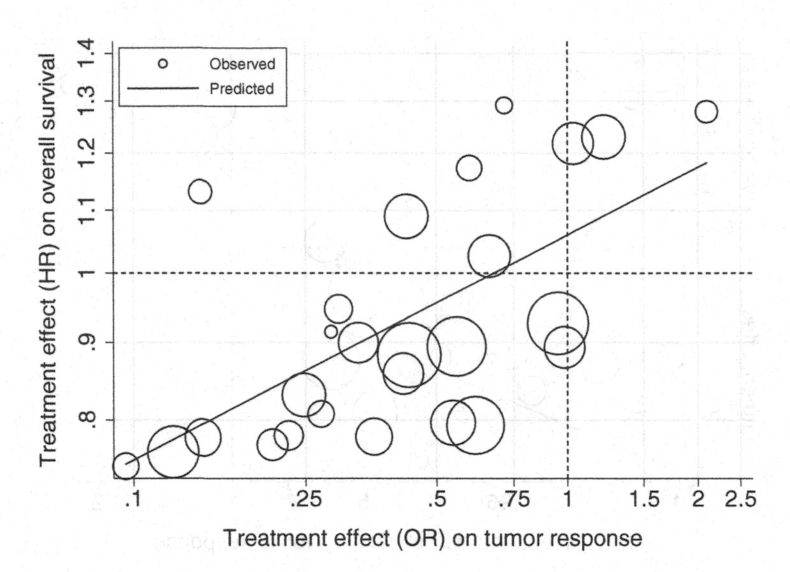

FIGURE 6.4
Advanced Colorectal Cancer. Trial-level association between the marginal-model-based treatment effects on OS and binary tumor response (both axes on a log scale). The circle surfaces are proportional to trial size.

with the estimated standard errors of the intercept and slope equal to 0.036 and 0.035, respectively. This is the line indicated in Figure 6.4 as "predicted."

6.3.2 Using R

Currently, there are no specific tools aimed at evaluation of an ordinal surrogate for a failure-time true endpoint, or for the reverse.

6.4 Concluding Remarks

The results of the analysis, presented in the current chapter, suggest that tumor response is substantially associated with OS in patients with advanced colorectal cancer. The survival odds ratio, estimated by using the Plackett copula, is equal to 6.5 and 4.9 for the four-category and binary response, respectively. Thus, tumor response could be regarded as a valid surrogate at the individual level. However, it is not a valid surrogate at the trial level:

for the four-category response, the estimated values of $R^2_{\text{trial(r)}}$ were around 0.15, while for the binary response, they were oscillating around 0.40. The estimated confidence intervals were relatively wide, but were excluding values larger than 0.75. Note that, given the small estimated values of $R^2_{\text{trial(r)}}$, no attempts to estimate the surrogate threshold effects (STE; Section 4.5) were made.

Unsatisfactory performance of tumor response as a surrogate for OS in advanced colorectal cancer was reported by Burzykowski, Molenberghs, and Buyse (2004) and Buyse et al. (2000). A similar conclusion was made by Burzykowski et al. (2008) regarding the validity of binary tumor response as a surrogate for OS in metastatic breast cancer.

The analyses presented in the current chapter illustrate problems that one can encounter when trying to properly adjust the analysis for the presence of the estimation error in the observed trial-specific treatment effects. The analysis weighted by the sample size offers a solution in this regard. However, its validity may be questioned, as outlined in Section 6.3.1.1. Another alternative is to consider the Bayesian approach for the "adjusted" analysis, proposed by Renfro et al. (2012).

6.5 Appendix

We will first summarize the results obtained by Lin and Wei (1989) and Lin (1994) for failure times. For each of $j = 1, 2, \ldots, n$ patients, define $Y_j(t) = I(X_j \geq t)$, where $I(\cdot)$ is the indicator function and X_j is the observed failure-time with failure indicator Δ_j. Consider a proportional hazard model:

$$\lambda_j(t) = \lambda_0(t) \exp(\boldsymbol{z}_{T,j}\boldsymbol{\eta}_T'), \tag{6.23}$$

where $\boldsymbol{z}_{T,j}$ is a (general) $p-$dimensional vector of covariates and $\boldsymbol{\eta}_T$ is a corresponding $p-$dimensional vector of coefficients. The score function for $\boldsymbol{\eta}_T$ equals

$$U_T(\boldsymbol{\eta}_T) = \sum_{j=1}^{n} \Delta_j \left\{ \boldsymbol{z}_{T,j} - \frac{S^{(1)}(\boldsymbol{\eta}_T, X_j)}{S^{(0)}(\boldsymbol{\eta}_T, X_j)} \right\}, \tag{6.24}$$

where Δ_j is the censoring indicator, $S^{(0)}(\boldsymbol{\eta}_T, t) = \sum_{j=1}^{n} Y_j(t) \exp(\boldsymbol{z}_{T,j}\boldsymbol{\eta}_T')$ and $S^{(1)}(\boldsymbol{\eta}_T, t) = \sum_{j=1}^{n} Y_j(t) \exp(\boldsymbol{z}_{T,j}\boldsymbol{\eta}_T')\boldsymbol{z}_{T,j}$. Denote by $\widehat{\boldsymbol{\eta}}_T$ the solution of $U_T(\boldsymbol{\eta}_T) = 0$.

Lin and Wei (1989) showed that $n^{1/2}(\widehat{\boldsymbol{\eta}}_T - \boldsymbol{\eta}_T)$ has, asymptotically, a normal distribution with zero mean and variance-covariance matrix that can be estimated by

$$A_T^{-1}(\widehat{\boldsymbol{\eta}}_T)\left\{\sum_{j=1}^{n} W_{T,j}(\boldsymbol{\eta}_T)W'_{T,j}(\widehat{\boldsymbol{\eta}}_T)\right\}A_T^{-1}(\widehat{\boldsymbol{\eta}}_T),$$

where

$$\begin{aligned} W_{T,j}(\boldsymbol{\eta}_T) &= \Delta_j\left\{\boldsymbol{z}_{T,j}-\frac{S^{(1)}(\boldsymbol{\eta}_T,X_j)}{S^{(0)}(\boldsymbol{\eta}_T,X_j)}\right\} \\ &- \sum_{k=1}^{n}\frac{\Delta_k Y_j(X_k)e^{\boldsymbol{z}_{T,j}\boldsymbol{\eta}'_T}}{S^{(0)}(\boldsymbol{\eta}_T,X_k)}\left\{\boldsymbol{z}_{T,j}-\frac{S^{(1)}(\boldsymbol{\eta}_T,X_k)}{S^{(0)}(\boldsymbol{\eta}_T,X_k)}\right\}, \quad (6.25) \\ A_T(\boldsymbol{\eta}_T) &= \sum_{j=1}^{n}\Delta_j\left\{\frac{S^{(2)}(\boldsymbol{\eta}_T,X_j)}{S^{(0)}(\boldsymbol{\eta}_T,X_j)}\right. \\ &\left. -\frac{S^{(1)}(\boldsymbol{\eta}_T,X_j)S^{(1)}(\boldsymbol{\eta}_T,X_j)'}{\left\{S^{(0)}(\boldsymbol{\eta}_T,X_j)\right\}^2}\right\}, \quad (6.26) \\ S^{(2)}(\boldsymbol{\eta}_T,t) &= \sum_{j=1}^{n}Y_j(t)\exp(\boldsymbol{z}_{T,j}\boldsymbol{\eta}'_T)\boldsymbol{z}_{T,j}(\boldsymbol{z}_{T,j})'. \quad (6.27) \end{aligned}$$

For a categorical ordinal response S_j ($S_j = 1,\ldots,K$), consider a proportional odds model (for $k = 1,\ldots K-1$):

$$\text{logit}\{P(S_j \le k \mid \boldsymbol{z}_{S,j})\} = \eta_k^0 + \boldsymbol{z}_{S,j}\boldsymbol{\theta}'_S\,, \quad (6.28)$$

where $\boldsymbol{z}_{S,j}$ is a (general) $q-$dimensional vector of covariates and $\boldsymbol{\eta}_S$ is a corresponding $q-$dimensional vector of coefficients. Hence,

$$\pi_{j,k} = P(S_j = k) = \frac{e^{\eta_k^0+\boldsymbol{z}_{S,j}\boldsymbol{\theta}'_S}}{1+e^{\eta_k^0+\boldsymbol{z}_{S,j}\boldsymbol{\theta}'_S}} - I(k>1)\frac{e^{\eta_{k-1}^0+\boldsymbol{z}_{S,j}\boldsymbol{\theta}'_S}}{1+e^{\eta_{k-1}^0+\boldsymbol{z}_{S,j}\boldsymbol{\theta}'_S}}.$$

Put $\boldsymbol{\eta}_S = (\eta_1^0,\ldots,\eta_{K-1}^0,\boldsymbol{\theta}'_S)'$.

Let $\tilde{S}_j = (\tilde{S}_{j,1},\ldots,\tilde{S}_{j,K-1})'$, where $\tilde{S}_{j,k} = I(S_j = k)$, and $\boldsymbol{\pi}_j = (\pi_{j,1},\ldots,\pi_{j,K-1})'$. The estimating equations for $\boldsymbol{\eta}_S$ can then be expressed as follows (Lipsitz, Kim, and Zhao, 1994):

$$U_S(\boldsymbol{\eta}_S) = \sum_{j=1}^{n} D_{S,j}\boldsymbol{V}_{S,j}^{-1}(\tilde{S}_j - \boldsymbol{\pi}_j) = \sum_{j=1}^{n} U_{S,j}(\boldsymbol{\eta}_S)\,, \quad (6.29)$$

where $D_{S,j} = \partial\boldsymbol{\pi}_j/\partial\boldsymbol{\eta}'_S$ and $\boldsymbol{V}_{S,j} = \text{diag}(\boldsymbol{\pi}_j) - \boldsymbol{\pi}_j\boldsymbol{\pi}'_j$, where $\text{diag}(\boldsymbol{\pi}_j)$ is a diagonal matrix with the elements of $\boldsymbol{\pi}_j$ on the diagonal. Define

$$A_S(\boldsymbol{\eta}_S) = \sum_{j=1}^{n} D_{S,j}\boldsymbol{V}_{S,j}^{-1}D'_{S,j}\,.$$

It can be shown (Lipsitz, Kim, and Zhao, 1994) that $n^{1/2}(\widehat{\boldsymbol{\eta}}_S - \boldsymbol{\eta}_S)$ has, asymptotically, a normal distribution with mean 0 and variance-covariance matrix that can be estimated by

$$A_S^{-1}(\widehat{\boldsymbol{\eta}}_S)\left\{\sum_{j=1}^{n} U_{S,j}(\widehat{\boldsymbol{\eta}}_S)U_S'(\widehat{\boldsymbol{\eta}}_S)\right\} A_S^{-1}(\widehat{\boldsymbol{\eta}}_S).$$

Consider now a bivariate random variable (T_j, S_j). Let models (6.23) and (6.28) be marginal models for T_j and S_j, respectively. The estimating equations for the coefficient vector $(\boldsymbol{\eta}_T', \boldsymbol{\eta}_S')'$ are

$$\begin{cases} U_T(\boldsymbol{\eta}_T) = 0, \\ U_S(\boldsymbol{\eta}_S) = 0. \end{cases} \tag{6.30}$$

These equations can be seen as arising under "independence working assumptions" (Liang and Zeger, 1986). Denote the solution to (7.12) by $(\widehat{\boldsymbol{\eta}}_T', \widehat{\boldsymbol{\eta}}_S')'$. Let

$$W_{TS,j}(\boldsymbol{\eta}_T, \boldsymbol{\eta}_S) = (W_{T,j}(\boldsymbol{\eta}_T)', U_{S,j}(\boldsymbol{\eta}_S)')'.$$

Define $A_{ST}(\boldsymbol{\eta}_T, \boldsymbol{\eta}_S)$ to be a block-diagonal matrix with $A_T(\boldsymbol{\eta}_T)$ and $A_S(\boldsymbol{\eta}_S)$ on the diagonal and zeros elsewhere. Then it follows from the developments by Liang and Zeger (1986) that $(\widehat{\boldsymbol{\eta}}_T', \widehat{\boldsymbol{\eta}}_S')'$ is asymptotically normal with mean $(\boldsymbol{\eta}_T', \boldsymbol{\eta}_S')'$ and the variance-covariance matrix that can be estimated by

$$\begin{aligned} &C_{ST}(\widehat{\boldsymbol{\eta}}_T, \widehat{\boldsymbol{\eta}}_S) \\ &= A_{ST}^{-1}(\widehat{\boldsymbol{\eta}}_T, \widehat{\boldsymbol{\eta}}_S)\left\{\textstyle\sum_{j=1}^{n} W_{TS,j}(\widehat{\boldsymbol{\eta}}_T, \widehat{\boldsymbol{\eta}}_S)W_{TS,j}(\widehat{\boldsymbol{\eta}}_T, \widehat{\boldsymbol{\eta}}_S)'\right\} A_{ST}^{-1}(\widehat{\boldsymbol{\eta}}_T, \widehat{\boldsymbol{\eta}}_S)\,. \end{aligned}$$

In particular, the covariance between $\widehat{\boldsymbol{\eta}}_T$ and $\widehat{\boldsymbol{\eta}}_S$ can be estimated by

$$A_T^{-1}(\widehat{\boldsymbol{\eta}}_T)\left\{\sum_{j=1}^{n} W_{T,j}(\widehat{\boldsymbol{\eta}}_T)U_{S,j}(\widehat{\boldsymbol{\eta}}_S)'\right\} A_S^{-1}(\widehat{\boldsymbol{\eta}}_S)\,.$$

7

A Continuous (Normally-Distributed) and a Failure-Time Endpoint

Tomasz Burzykowski

Hasselt University, Belgium, and IDDI, Belgium

CONTENTS

7.1 Introduction

In this chapter, we focus on the case when the surrogate is a continuous, normally distributed endpoint and the true endpoint is a failure-time endpoint. Note that the described approach is applicable also in the reverse case, i.e., with a failure-time surrogate and a continuous true endpoint.

7.2 Theoretical Background

Assume that the true endpoint T is a failure-time random variable and the surrogate S is a normally distributed, continuous variable. For each of $j = 1, \ldots, n_i$ patients from trial i $(i = 1, \ldots, N)$ we thus have quadruplets

$(X_{ij}, \Delta_{ij}, S_{ij}, Z_{ij})$, where X_{ij} is a possibly censored version of survival time T_{ij} and Δ_{ij} is the censoring indicator assuming a value of 1 for observed failures and 0 otherwise.

As in Chapter 4, we consider the two-stage approach with model (4.10) replaced by a copula-based model (see, e.g., Section 5.2) for the true endpoint T_{ij} and the continuous variable S_{ij}. Toward this aim, various copula functions can be used (see Section 5.2).

The marginal model for S_{ij} is the classical linear regression model:

$$S_{ij} = \alpha_{0,i} + \alpha_i Z_{ij} + \varepsilon_{ij}, \tag{7.1}$$

where ε_{ij} is normally distributed with mean zero and variance σ_i^2.

For T_{ij}, the proportional hazard model is used:

$$\lambda_{ij}(t \mid Z_{ij}) = \lambda_i(t) \exp(\beta_i Z_{ij}), \tag{7.2}$$

where β_i are trial-specific effects of treatment Z and $\lambda_i(t)$ is a trial-specific baseline hazard function.

If a parametric (e.g., Weibull-distribution-based) baseline hazard is used in (7.2), the joint distribution function defined by the copula and the marginal models (7.1) and (7.2) allows constructing the likelihood function for the observed data $(X_{ij} = x_{ij}, \Delta_{ij} = \delta_{ij}, S_{ij} = s_{ij}, Z_{ij} = z_{ij})$ and obtaining estimates of the treatment effects α_i and β_i.

The quality of the surrogate at the individual level can be evaluated by using Kendall's τ or Spearman's ρ (see Section 5.2). The quality at the trial level can be evaluated by considering the correlation coefficient between the estimated treatment effects α_i and β_i. Note that, in this step, the adjustment for the estimation error, present in $\widehat{\alpha}_i$ and $\widehat{\beta}_i$, should be made. Toward this aim, model (5.13)–(5.14) (see Section 5.2) can be used.

If the individual-level association is not of immediate interest, one may base analysis on the marginal models (7.1) and (7.2), without specifying the baseline hazards in the latter. When fitting the models, it is worth estimating the variance-covariance matrix of the estimated treatment effects $\widehat{\alpha}_i$ and $\widehat{\beta}_i$ while taking into account the association between S and T. Toward this aim, an estimator similar to the one proposed in Appendix 6.5 can be used (see also Appendix 7.5).

7.3 Analysis of a Case Study

In this section, we illustrate the application of the methods, mentioned in the previous section, by the individual-patient-data meta-analysis of patients with advanced (metastatic) prostate cancer (see Section 2.2.7). The goal of the analysis is to evaluate the logarithm of PSA, measured at about 28 days, as a

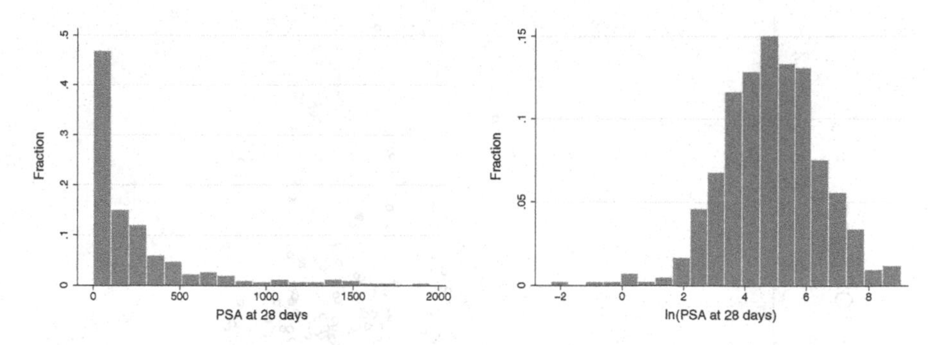

FIGURE 7.1
Histograms of PSA and log-PSA at 28 days.

surrogate for overall survival (OS). The data were analyzed before by Buyse et al. (2003), but without considering the value of PSA at a particular time point as a candidate surrogate for OS. For analysis purposes, patients were grouped by trial and by country. Treatment with flutamide or cyproterone acetate is considered the control treatment, while liarozole is regarded as the experimental treatment.

7.3.1 Using SAS

7.3.1.1 Copula-Based Models

Among the 596 patients included in the dataset, 421 had a PSA measurement obtained at about 28 days (±6 days). There are 19 trial-by-country groups containing between two and 55 patients per group. Two groups (one with two and one with seven patients) have to be eliminated from the analysis, because at least one of the treatment arms within the group does not contain any deaths. Consequently, the analysis includes 412 patients spread across 17 groups.

Figure 7.1 presents histograms of PSA (left-hand-side panel) and log-PSA values for the 412 patients. Note that, for legibility purposes, the histogram of PSA has been obtained for PSA values smaller than 2000 ng/mL. The histogram on the right-hand side of Figure 7.1 shows that the logarithmic transformation makes the distribution of the data more symmetric.

Figure 7.2 presents the scatter plot of log-PSA at 28 days and OS. Note that we ignore censoring in the latter variable. The scatter plot indicates a negative association between the two variables. Given that Clayton and Hougaard copula models assume a positive association (see Section 5.2), in what follows we will consider the negative of log-PSA as a surrogate.

We first conduct a two-stage analysis using the Clayton, Hougaard, and Plackett copula with the marginal models (7.1) and (7.2); the latter is speci-

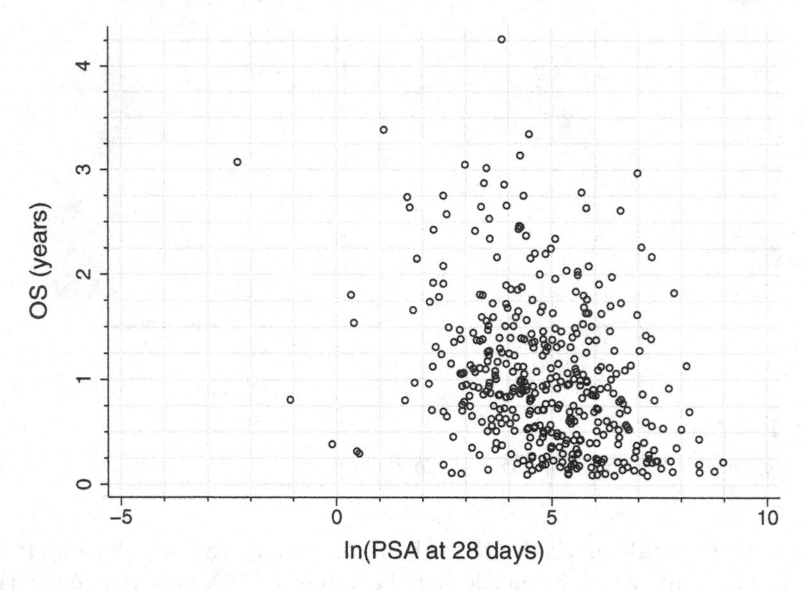

FIGURE 7.2
Scatter plot of overall survival and logarithmic PSA at 28 days.

fied by assuming the Weibull hazard functions. Toward this aim, we use the dedicated SAS macros (see Section 12.4.1). We use the copula-based likelihood function to estimate the copula parameter and all the coefficients of the marginal models.

The estimated value of the copula parameter θ for the Clayton copula is equal to 1.61 (95% CI: [1.40, 1.83]). Given the relationship (5.10), the value of τ is estimated to be equal to 0.235 (95% CI: [0.171, 0.298]). Spearman's rank-correlation coefficient ρ, computed from (5.9) by numerical integration, is equal to 0.344 (95% CI: [0.255, 0.433]).

For the Hougaard copula, the estimated value of θ is equal to 0.724 (95% CI: [0.662, 0.790]). Following (5.11), the estimated value of τ is equal to 0.276 (95% CI: [0.212, 0.340]). Spearman's ρ, computed by numerical integration, is equal to 0.400 (95% CI: [0.305, 0.495]).

Finally, for the Plackett copula, the estimated value of θ is equal to 3.56 (95% CI: [2.49, 4.64]). Note that it can interpreted in the following way (see Sections 5.2 and 6.2): the odds of surviving beyond time t given a value of negative-log-PSA at 28 days larger than x, say, are about 3.6 times higher than the odds of surviving beyond time t given a value of negative-log-PSA smaller than or equal to x. As $-\ln(PSA) > x \equiv PSA < e^{-x}$, we can equivalently conclude that the odds of surviving beyond time t given a lower value of PSA at 28 days are about 3.6 times higher than the odds of surviving beyond time t given a higher value of PSA. From (5.12) it follows that the estimated value

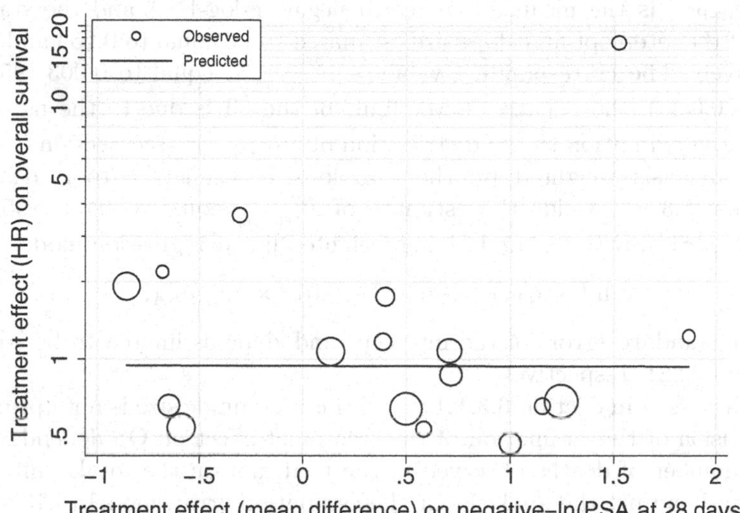

FIGURE 7.3

Trial-level association between the marginal treatment effects on negative-log-PSA and OS in advanced prostate cancer (vertical axis on a log scale).

of ρ is equal to 0.402 (95% CI: [0.317, 0.488]). Kendall's τ, computed from (5.8) by numerical integration, is equal to 0.276 (95% CI: [0.214, 0.339]).

Thus, all three copula models suggest a weak association between the negative-log-PSA at 28 days and OS at the individual-patient level. It is worth noting that the value of the maximum log-likelihood for the Clayton, Hougaard, and Plackett copulas are equal to −1047.8, −1042.2, and −1043.6, respectively. Thus, one could conclude that the Hougaard-copula-based model offers the best fit to the data.

Figure 7.3 presents the estimated trial-specific treatment effects, i.e., logarithms of the Weibull-model-based hazard ratios for OS and mean differences for negative-log-PSA, obtained by using the Hougaard-copula-based model; each trial is represented by a circle of the size proportional to the group sample size.

The figure indicates almost no association between the treatment effects. It seems to suggest that the larger the mean difference in negative-log-PSA (the larger mean reduction of PSA for the experimental treatment), the smaller corresponding log-hazard ratio for OS (the larger reduction in hazard of death for the experimental treatment). A simple linear regression model, fitted without any adjustment for the estimation error present in the estimated treatment effects, yields the following regression equation:

$$\ln(HR_{OS}) = 0.142 + 0.057 \times \delta_{-lnPSA}, \tag{7.3}$$

where $\delta_{\text{ln-PSA}}$ is the mean difference in negative-log-PSA and the standard errors of the intercept and slope are estimated to be equal to 0.253 and 0.282, respectively. The corresponding value of $R^2_{\text{trial(r)}}$ is equal to 0.003 (95% CI: $[-0.046, 0.052]$); the negative lower limit of the CI is due to the use of the normal approximation to the distribution of $(\widehat{R}_{\text{trial(r)}})^2$ (see Section 5.3.1.1).

The analysis weighted by the sample size, using the tools described in Section 6.3.1.1, yields the estimate of $R^2_{\text{trial(r)}}$ equal to 0.007 (95% CI: $[-0.072, 0.086]$), with the underlying weighted linear regression model

$$\ln(HR_{OS}) = -0.022 - 0.072 \times \delta_{-lnPSA}, \tag{7.4}$$

with the standard errors of the intercept and slope estimated to be equal to 0.183 and 0.221, respectively.

As discussed in Section 6.3.1.1, weighting by sample size is not optimal, as the precision of the estimation of the treatment effect on OS depends rather on the number of deaths observed in the trial, not on the total sample size. To properly adjust the analysis for the estimation error, model (5.13)–(5.14) can be used. Applying it, using `PROC MIXED` code described in Section 5.3.1, yields the estimate of $R^2_{\text{trial(r)}}$ equal to 0.0001 (95% CI: $[-0.054, 0.055]$). The value is based on the following estimate of the variance-covariance matrix D of the (random) treatment effects:

$$\begin{pmatrix} 0.2758 & -0.0011 \\ -0.0011 & 0.0286 \end{pmatrix}, \tag{7.5}$$

for which the condition number is equal to 9.6. Thus, the obtained estimate of $R^2_{\text{trial(r)}}$ can be regarded as numerically stable. The underlying linear regression model for the treatment effect is

$$\ln(HR_{OS}) = -0.061 - 0.004 \times \delta_{-lnPSA}, \tag{7.6}$$

with the standard errors of the intercept and slope estimated to be equal to 0.202 and 0.372, respectively. This is the line indicated in Figure 7.3 as "predicted."

7.3.1.2 Marginal Models

If we focus on the trial-level surrogacy, we can conduct an analysis based solely on the marginal models (7.1) and (7.2), with the latter specified without assuming any particular form of the baseline hazards. Toward this aim, model (7.1) can be fitted by using `PROC MIXED` and (7.2) by using `PROC PHREG`. In particular, a possible call to `PROC MIXED` is:

```
PROC MIXED data=dataset;
   CLASS trial;
   MODEL contsurr = trial treat(trial) / noint;
   REPEATED / group = trial;
RUN;
```

Variable `trial` is the trial identifier (trial-by-country group in our example), while `treat` is the treatment indicator (with 0 for the control group and 1 for the experimental one). The response variable `contsurr` is the logarithm of PSA at day 28. Of interest are the trial-specific treatment-effect estimates, provided by the nested effect `treat(trial)`. The `REPEATED` statement includes the `group=trial` option, which implies the use of trial-specific residual variances.

On the other hand, (7.2) can be fitted by using `PROC PHREG`, as described in Section 6.3.1.1.

After fitting the models, the variance-covariance of the estimated coefficients of the models can be estimated while taking into account the association between the negative-log-PSA and OS (see Appendix 7.5). Toward this aim, a dedicated SAS macro can be used (see Section 12.6.3).

Figure 7.4 presents the estimated mean differences and log-hazard-ratios. As was the case in the copula-based estimates (see Figure 7.3), the association between the treatment effects is weak. A simple linear regression model yields the value of $R^2_{\text{trial(r)}}$ equal to 0.0007 (95% CI: $[-0.025, 0.026]$). The resulting regression equation is

$$\ln(HR_{OS}) = 0.166 - 0.024 \times \delta_{-lnPSA}, \tag{7.7}$$

with the standard errors of the intercept and slope estimated to be equal to 0.212 and 0.229, respectively.

Analysis adjusted for the estimation error leads to an estimate of the variance-covariance matrix D that is singular. The analysis weighted by the group sample size, conducted with the help of the dedicated SAS macro (see Section 12.6.3), yields the following estimate of the variance-covariance matrix D of the (random) treatment effects:

$$\begin{pmatrix} 15.4 & -1.5 \\ -1.5 & 8.6 \end{pmatrix}, \tag{7.8}$$

for which the condition number is equal to 1.9. The corresponding estimate of $R^2_{\text{trial(r)}}$ is equal to 0.017 (95% CI: $[-0.108, 0.141]$), with the linear regression equation given by

$$\ln(HR_{OS}) = 0.012 - 0.091 \times \delta_{-lnPSA} \tag{7.9}$$

and standard errors of the intercept and slope estimated equal to 0.155 and 0.185, respectively. The line corresponding to equation (7.9) is indicated in Figure 7.4 as "predicted."

7.3.2 Using R

Currently, there are no specific tools aimed at evaluation of a continuous (normally distributed) surrogate for a failure-time true endpoint.

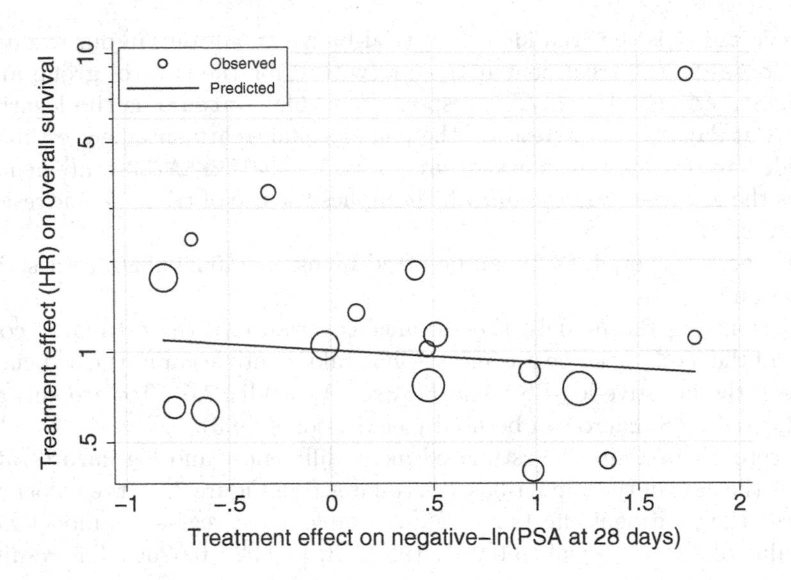

FIGURE 7.4
Trial-level association between the marginal treatment effects on negative-log-PSA and OS in advanced prostate cancer (vertical axis on a log scale).

7.4 Concluding Remarks

The results of the analysis presented in the current chapter suggest that (the logarithm of) PSA at 28 days is very weekly associated with OS in patients with advanced prostate cancer. Also, the association between treatment effects on (the logarithm of) PSA and OS is very weak. Thus, PSA is not a valid surrogate at the individual or at the trial level. Note that, given the small estimated values of $R^2_{\mathrm{trial(r)}}$, no attempts to estimate the surrogate threshold effects (STE; Section 4.5) were made.

Unsatisfactory performance of PSA as a surrogate for OS in advanced prostate cancer was reported, among others, by Buyse et al. (2003) and Collette et al. (2005).

The analyses presented in the current chapter illustrate problems that one can encounter when trying to evaluate a surrogate when using a limited dataset. In such a situation, the "natural" grouping of patients by trial may not be feasible due to an insufficient number of trials. Considering other grouping, e.g., by countries (as in our example) or centers, may be possible, but raises several issues (Cortiñas et al., 2004; Renfro et al., 2014). One of them is related to the smaller sample size of the groups, which, in turn, implies a larger estimation error in the estimated group-specific treatment effects. In such a situation, an analysis adjusted for the estimation error is of special importance. Yet, it is often difficult to conduct, as it requires a considerable between-group variability of the treatment effects for the association between the true random treatment effects to become estimable. The analysis weighted by the sample size offers a solution in this regard. However, its validity may be questioned, as outlined in Section 6.3.1.1. An alternative is to consider the Bayesian approach, proposed by Renfro et al. (2012).

7.5 Appendix

Consider a continuous variable S_j and the linear model

$$S_j = \boldsymbol{\eta}_S' \boldsymbol{z}_{S,j} + \varepsilon_j, \tag{7.10}$$

where $\boldsymbol{z}_{S,j}$ is a (general) $q-$dimensional vector of covariates (including the intercept), $\boldsymbol{\eta}_S$ is a corresponding $q-$dimensional vector of coefficients, and $\varepsilon_j \sim N(0, \sigma^2)$. The estimating equations for $\boldsymbol{\eta}_S$ can then be expressed as follows (Molenberghs and Verbeke, 2005):

$$U_S(\boldsymbol{\eta}_S) = \sum_{j=1}^{n} \boldsymbol{z}_{S,j}'(S_j - \boldsymbol{\eta}_S' \boldsymbol{z}_{S,j})/\sigma^2 = \sum_{j=1}^{n} U_{S,j}(\boldsymbol{\eta}_S). \tag{7.11}$$

Define

$$A_S(\boldsymbol{\eta}_S) = \sum_{j-1}^{n} \boldsymbol{z}_{S,j}' \boldsymbol{z}_{S,j}/\sigma^2 .$$

It can be shown (Molenberghs and Verbeke, 2005) that $n^{1/2}(\hat{\boldsymbol{\eta}}_S - \boldsymbol{\eta}_S)$ has, asymptotically, a normal distribution with mean 0 and variance-covariance matrix that can be estimated by

$$A_S^{-1}(\widehat{\boldsymbol{\eta}}_S) \left\{ \sum_{j=1}^{n} U_{S,j}(\widehat{\boldsymbol{\eta}}_S) U_S'(\widehat{\boldsymbol{\eta}}_S) \right\} A_S^{-1}(\widehat{\boldsymbol{\eta}}_S).$$

For the failure-time variable T_j, consider the proportional hazard model (7.2) with coefficients $\boldsymbol{\eta}_T$.

Consider now a bivariate random variable (T_j, S_j). Let models (7.2) and (7.10) be marginal models for T_j and S_j, respectively. The estimating equations for the coefficient vector $(\boldsymbol{\eta}_T', \boldsymbol{\eta}_S')'$ are

$$\begin{cases} U_T(\boldsymbol{\eta}_T) &= 0, \\ U_S(\boldsymbol{\eta}_S) &= 0. \end{cases} \tag{7.12}$$

These equations can be seen as arising under "independence working assumptions" (Liang and Zeger, 1986). Denote the solution to (7.12) by $(\hat{\boldsymbol{\eta}}_T', \hat{\boldsymbol{\eta}}_S')'$. Let

$$W_{TS,j}(\boldsymbol{\eta}_T, \boldsymbol{\eta}_S) = (W_{T,j}(\boldsymbol{\eta}_T)', U_{S,j}(\boldsymbol{\eta}_S)')',$$

with $W_{T,j}(\boldsymbol{\eta}_T)$ was defined in (6.25). Define $A_{ST}(\boldsymbol{\eta}_T, \boldsymbol{\eta}_S)$ to be a block-diagonal matrix with $A_T(\boldsymbol{\eta}_T)$, defined in (6.26), and $A_S(\boldsymbol{\eta}_S)$ on the diagonal and zeros elsewhere. Then it follows (see Appendix 6.5) that $(\hat{\boldsymbol{\eta}}_T', \hat{\boldsymbol{\eta}}_S')'$ is asymptotically normal with mean $(\boldsymbol{\eta}_T', \boldsymbol{\eta}_S')'$ and the variance-covariance matrix that can be estimated by

$$\begin{aligned} & C_{ST}(\hat{\boldsymbol{\eta}}_T, \hat{\boldsymbol{\eta}}_S) \\ = \; & A_{ST}^{-1}(\hat{\boldsymbol{\eta}}_T, \hat{\boldsymbol{\eta}}_S) \left\{ \sum_{j=1}^{n} W_{TS,j}(\hat{\boldsymbol{\eta}}_T, \hat{\boldsymbol{\eta}}_S) W_{TS,j}(\hat{\boldsymbol{\eta}}_T, \hat{\boldsymbol{\eta}}_S)' \right\} A_{ST}^{-1}(\hat{\boldsymbol{\eta}}_T, \hat{\boldsymbol{\eta}}_S) \,. \end{aligned}$$

In particular, the covariance between $\hat{\boldsymbol{\eta}}_T$ and $\hat{\boldsymbol{\eta}}_S$ can be estimated by

$$A_T^{-1}(\hat{\boldsymbol{\eta}}_T) \left\{ \sum_{j=1}^{n} W_{T,j}(\hat{\boldsymbol{\eta}}_T) U_{S,j}(\hat{\boldsymbol{\eta}}_S)' \right\} A_S^{-1}(\hat{\boldsymbol{\eta}}_S) \,.$$

8

A Longitudinal (Normally Distributed) and a Failure-Time Endpoint

Tomasz Burzykowski
Hasselt University, Belgium, and IDDI, Belgium

CONTENTS

8.1 Introduction

In this chapter, we focus on the case when the surrogate is a continuous, normally-distributed endpoint measured repeatedly over time and the true endpoint is a failure-time endpoint. Technically, the evaluation of the candidate surrogate requires a joint model for longitudinal measurements and failure-time data. Methodology for such joint modeling has been considerably developed in recent years (see, e.g., the recent monograph by Rizopoulos, 2012). The proposed joint models couple the failure-time model, which is usually of primary interest, with a suitable model for the longitudinal measurements of a covariate. We follow the meta-analytic approach developed by Renard et al. (2003), which uses the joint model proposed by Henderson, Diggle, and Dobson (2000).

8.2 Theoretical Background

Assume that the true endpoint T is a failure-time random variable and the surrogate S is a normally distributed, continuous variable that is repeatedly measured over time. In particular, for each of $j = 1, \ldots, n_i$ patients from trial i $(i = 1, \ldots, N)$ we have measurements s_{ijk} $(k = 1, \ldots, n_{ij})$ made at times τ_{ijk}. Let $\boldsymbol{s}_{ij} = (s_{ij1}, \ldots, s_{ijn_i})'$ and $\boldsymbol{\tau}_{ij} = (\tau_{ij1}, \ldots, \tau_{ijn_i})'$. Thus, for each patient we have a vector of data $(X_{ij}, \Delta_{ij}, \boldsymbol{s}'_{ij}, \boldsymbol{\tau}'_{ij}, Z_{ij})$, where X_{ij} is a possibly censored version of survival time T_{ij}, Δ_{ij} is the censoring indicator, assuming value of 1 for observed failures and 0 otherwise, and Z_{ij} is the treatment indicator.

To evaluate a longitudinal surrogate S, Renard et al. (2003) applied the joint model proposed by Henderson, Diggle, and Dobson (2000). In what follows, we briefly describe the model.

A central feature of the model is an unobserved (latent) zero-mean bivariate Gaussian process, $W_{ij}(\tau) = \{W_{1,ij}(\tau), W_{2,ij}(\tau)\}$ used to induce the association between the longitudinal measurement and event processes. The measurement and intensity models are linked as follows:

(1) The sequence of measurements $\{s_{ijk} : k = 1, \ldots, n_{ij}\}$ of a subject is modeled using a standard linear mixed-effects model (LMM), possibly allowing for a serially correlated component:

$$S_{ijk} = \mu_{ij}(\tau_{ijk}; \boldsymbol{\alpha}_i) + W_{1,ij}(\tau_{ijk}) + \varepsilon_{ijk}, \tag{8.1}$$

where $\mu_{ij}(\tau_{ijk})$ describes the mean profile and

$$\varepsilon_{ijk} \sim N(0, \sigma_e^2)$$

is a sequence of mutually independent measurement errors. In (8.1) we have explicitly indicated the dependence of the mean response profile μ_{ij} on $\boldsymbol{\alpha}_i$, which is a vector of parameters for the trial-specific treatment effects used in modeling the mean response profile. We will discuss the composition of $\boldsymbol{\alpha}_i$ in what follows.

(2) The event intensity process is modeled by using a semi-parametric proportional-hazards (PH) model:

$$\lambda_{ij}(\tau) = Y_{ij}(\tau)\lambda_0(\tau)\exp\{\beta_{0,i} + \beta_i Z_{ij} + W_{2,ij}(\tau)\}, \tag{8.2}$$

where the form of $\lambda_0(\tau)$ is left unspecified and $Y_{ij}(\tau)$ is a binary indicator of whether a subject is at risk of experiencing an event at time τ. The parameters $\beta_{0,i}$ and β_i represent, respectively, trial-specific overall effects and treatment effects on the hazard function.

$W_{1,ij}$ and $W_{2,ij}$ can be specified in various forms. For example, suppressing the indices for notational simplicity, we can assume:

$$W_1(\tau) = U_1 + U_2\tau, \tag{8.3}$$

with (U_1, U_2) being normally distributed with mean zero and variance-covariance matrix G. This implies the use of a model with random intercepts and slopes for the longitudinal surrogate. Then, $W_2(\tau)$ can be defined by including distinct elements of $W_1(\tau)$ and/or its entire current value. For instance, we can specify that:

$$W_2(\tau) = \gamma_1 U_1 + \gamma_2 U_2 + \gamma_3(U_1 + U_2\tau) = U_1(\gamma_1 + \gamma_3) + U_2(\gamma_2 + \gamma_3\tau). \quad (8.4)$$

The model can be estimated by using the EM algorithm (Henderson, Diggle, and Dobson, 2000; Renard et al., 2003).

In the meta-analytic approach proposed by Renard et al. (2003), model (8.1)–(8.2) is fitted to data from all trials, providing estimates of $\boldsymbol{\alpha}_i$ and β_i. The quality of the surrogate at the trial level is evaluated by the coefficient $R^2_{\text{trial(r)}}$, the reduced value based on not using a trial-specific intercept, obtained from a linear model associating $\widehat{\beta}_i$ and $\widehat{\boldsymbol{\alpha}}_i$. Note that the structure of $\boldsymbol{\alpha}_i$ depends on the chosen form of the mean profile over time in (8.1). For practical purposes, the mean trajectory of the surrogate within each treatment group is specified parsimoniously by using, e.g., a low-order polynomial or fractional polynomials. For the sake of illustration, suppose that the profile is quadratic; then $\mu_{ij}(\tau_{ijk})$ can be defined as follows:

$$\mu_{ij}(\tau_{ijk}; \boldsymbol{\alpha}_i) = \mu_{0,i} + \mu_{1,i}\tau_{ijk} + \mu_{2,i}\tau^2_{ijk} + \alpha_{0,i}Z_{ij} + \alpha_{1,i}Z_{ij}\tau_{ijk} + \alpha_{2,i}Z_{ij}\tau^2_{ijk},$$

with $\boldsymbol{\alpha}_i \equiv (\alpha_{0,i}, \alpha_{1,i}, \alpha_{2,i})'$. Subsequently, $R^2_{\text{trial(f)}}$ can be calculated as the coefficient of determination from the regression model:

$$\widehat{\beta}_i = \lambda_0 + \lambda_1\widehat{\alpha}_{0,i} + \lambda_2\widehat{\alpha}_{1,i} + \lambda_3\widehat{\alpha}_{2,i} + \varepsilon_i. \quad (8.5)$$

Note that, in this step, the adjustment for the estimation error present in $\widehat{\beta}_i$ and $\widehat{\boldsymbol{\alpha}}_i$ should ideally be considered (see Section 5.2).

At the individual level, Renard et al. (2003) proposed to consider the strength of the association between W_1 and W_2 and estimate R^2_{indiv} as the square of the correlation coefficient of the pair (W_1, W_2). Note that, in that case, R^2_{indiv} will not refer to the direct association between the two endpoints, but rather to the association between the two latent processes governing the longitudinal and event processes. Moreover, as W_1 and W_2 can be functions of time, it may no longer be possible to summarize the strength of the association by a single number. To illustrate the point, assume that W_1 and W_2 are defined by (8.3) and (8.4), respectively. Thus, given that $(U_1, U_2)' \sim N(0, G)$, we have:

$$\begin{aligned}
\text{Var}\{W_1(\tau_1)\} &= G_{11} + 2G_{12}\tau_1 + G_{22}\tau_1^2, && (8.6)\\
\text{Var}\{W_2(\tau_2)\} &= (\gamma_1 + \gamma_3)^2 G_{11} + 2(\gamma_1 + \gamma_3)(\gamma_2 + \gamma_3\tau_2)G_{12} \\
&\quad +(\gamma_2 + \gamma_3\tau_2)^2 G_{22}, && (8.7)\\
\text{Cov}\{W_1(\tau_1), W_2(\tau_2)\} &= (\gamma_1 + \gamma_2)G_{11} + \{(\gamma_1 + \gamma_2)\tau_1 \\
&\quad +(\gamma_2 + \gamma_3)\tau_2)\}G_{12} + \tau_1(\gamma_2 + \gamma_3\tau_2)G_{22}, && (8.8)
\end{aligned}$$

where G_{11}, G_{12}, and G_{22} are the elements of the variance-covariance matrix G. From (8.6)–(8.8) it is clear that the correlation between W_1 and W_2, or its squared value R^2_{indiv}, is a function of time. In fact, (8.6)–(8.8) defines a two-dimensional surface, $R^2_{\text{indiv}}(\tau_1, \tau_2)$, which can be estimated by using the estimates for γ_1, γ_2, γ_3, and G.

Note that the form of the correlation function very much depends on the assumed form of W_1 and W_2. For instance, if we assume that $W_2(\tau) = \gamma W_1(\tau)$, then, necessarily, $R^2_{\text{indiv}} \equiv 1$. Hence, Renard et al. (2003) recommended including a sufficiently large number of association parameters $\{\gamma_k\}$ in (8.4) to avoid undue constraints on R^2_{indiv}.

8.3 Analysis of a Case Study

In this section, we illustrate the application of the methods, mentioned in the previous section, by the individual-patient-data meta-analysis of patients with advanced (metastatic) prostate cancer (see Section 2.2.7). The goal of the analysis is to evaluate the repeated measurements of (the logarithm of) PSA as a surrogate for overall survival (OS). The data were analyzed before by Renard et al. (2003) and Buyse et al. (2003). For analysis purposes, patients were grouped by trial and by country (see also Section 7.3). Treatment with flutamide or cyproterone acetate is considered as the control treatment, while liarozole is regarded as the experimental treatment.

8.3.1 Using SAS

The dataset includes PSA measurements for 596 patients. There are 19 trial-by-country groups containing between four and 69 patients per group. Two groups (one with four and one with eight patients) have to be eliminated from the analysis, because at least one of the treatment arms within the group does not contain any deaths. Consequently, the analysis includes 567 patients spread across 17 groups (see Table 8.1).

Figure 2.8 presents the scatter plots of the observed log-PSA values as a function of the measurement time for patients per trial. Additionally, the plots include the smoothed profiles for the control and treatment groups. It can be seen that most of the patients had their PSA measurements taken within the first few months after randomization. Also, it is worth noting that the smoothed profiles are not fully informative about the change in the log-PSA levels over time due to drop-out. In particular, patients who experienced a PSA progression, i.e., an increase in the PSA level, left the study. Hence, the smoothed profiles, especially at the later points in time, do not include those patients. A more informative way of looking at log-PSA levels over time is to consider cohorts of patients defined by the time they leave the study (for

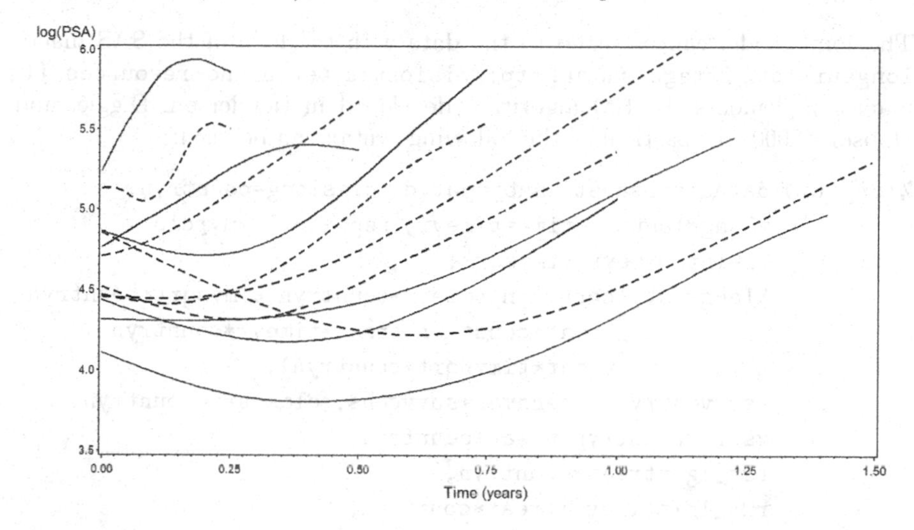

FIGURE 8.1
Prostate Cancer. Smoothed mean log-PSA profiles for cohorts of patients with similar follow-up times. Solid line for the control treatment, dashed line for the experimental one.

any reason). Smoothed profiles for such cohorts (with observation time in the interval of (0, 0.25], (0.25, 0.5], (0.5, 0.75], (0.75, 1], (1, 1.25], and (1.25, 1.5] years) are shown in Figure 8.1. Note that the plot does not include profiles of patients with follow-up longer than 1.5 years, as there were too few such patients. The smoothed profiles in Figure 8.1 indicate the tendency of PSA to go down initially (PSA response) and then increase again (PSA progression).

8.3.1.1 Joint-Model-Based Analysis

Based on the shape of the profiles presented in Figure 8.1, Renard et al. (2003) applied the following LMM to describe the dependence of the logarithm of PSA on time τ and treatment Z:

$$\begin{aligned} S_{ijk} &= \mu_{0,i} + \mu_{1,i}\tau_{ijk} + \mu_{2,i}\sqrt{\tau_{ijk}} + \alpha_{0,i}Z_{ij} + \alpha_{1,i}Z_{ij}\tau_{ijk} \\ &\quad + \alpha_{2,i}Z_{ij}\sqrt{\tau_{ijk}} + W_{1,ij}(\tau_{ijk}) + \varepsilon_{ijk}, \end{aligned} \tag{8.9}$$

with

$$W_{1,ij}(\tau) = U_{1,ij} + U_{2,ij}\tau + U_{3,ij}\sqrt{\tau}, \tag{8.10}$$

where $\varepsilon_{ijk} \overset{iid}{\sim} N(0, \sigma_e^2)$ and $(U_{1,ij}, U_{2,ij}, U_{3,ij})' \overset{iid}{\sim} N(0, G)$. For the survival data, they applied model (8.2) with

$$W_{2,ij}(\tau) = \gamma_1 U_{1,ij} + \gamma_2 U_{2,ij} + \gamma_3 U_{3,ij} + \gamma_4 W_{1,ij}(\tau). \tag{8.11}$$

The joint model can be fitted to the data with the help of the SAS macro `longsurvtst2_2stage.sas` at `http://ibiostat.be/online-resources`. The macro implements the EM algorithm developed in Henderson, Diggle, and Dobson (2000). In particular, the following syntax can be used:

```
%longsurv(dataset=psadat, subj=patid, claslong=countryn,
          ylong=logpsa, time=timeyr, repeated=timyrcls,
          W1=int timeyr timysqrt,
          Xlong=%str(countryn timeyr*countryn timysqrt*countryn
                     treat*countryn treat*timeyr*countryn
                     treat*timysqrt*countryn),
          ysurv=survyr, censvar=survcens, classurv=countryn,
          xsurv=countryn treat*countryn,
          r2t_lg0=treat*countryn,
          r2t_lg1=timeyr*treat*countryn,
          r2t_lg2=timysqrt*treat*countryn,
          r2t_sv=treat*countryn,
          noint=1, niter=500, label=psa45asqrt, tbeg=0, tend=9,
          step=0.05);
```

Argument `dataset=psadat` indicates the name of the dataset. The dataset is in the "long" format, i.e., it contains as many records per patient as there are PSA measurements for the patient. An illustration of a few first records is presented below:

patid	countryn	treat	survyr	survcens	timeyr	timysqrt	logpsa	timyrcls
1	7	1	2.30527	0	0.00274	0.05232	3.83081	0.00274
2	7	1	0.65708	1	0.00000	0.00000	2.63189	0.00000
2	7	1	0.65708	1	0.04107	0.20265	2.46810	0.04107
2	7	1	0.65708	1	0.09309	0.30510	3.14415	0.09309
2	7	1	0.65708	1	0.16701	0.40867	3.15274	0.16701
2	7	1	0.65708	1	0.34771	0.58967	2.99072	0.34771
3	7	1	1.55784	1	0.00274	0.05232	3.69138	0.00274
...	...	...	...	...	...	...	...	...

Variable `patid` is the patient identifier, `countryn` is a numerical code for the trial-by-country group, while `treat` is the treatment indicator (equals 0 for the control and 1 for the experimental treatment). Survival time (in years) and survival status of the patient (0 for alive and 1 for death) are provided in the variables `survyr` and `survcens`, respectively. Variable `timeyr` indicates the time (in years from randomization) at which the log-PSA value `logpsa` was obtained. Variable `timysqrt` provides the square root of `timeyr`, while `timyrcls` is a copy of `timeyr` that will be used as a factor, not as a numeric variable.

Argument `subj=patid` indicates the variable containing patient identifiers, while `claslong=countryn` specifies that variable `countryn` is the factor (class-variable) defining the grouping of patients. The longitudinal surrogate endpoint (log-PSA) is identified by `ylong=logpsa` and `time=timeyr` indicates the variable containing the times of the measurements of the endpoint. Argument `repeated=timyrcls` specifies that variable `timyrcls` is to be used as a factor defining the order of the measurements of the surrogate endpoint within each patient.

The structure of the longitudinal data model (8.1) is defined by arguments `W1` and `Xlong`. In particular, `W1=int timeyr timysqrt` specifies the random-effects structure (8.10) of model (8.9), i.e., the random intercept and the random slopes of the measurement time and its square root. The fixed-effects part of the model is specified by the string given in the `Xlong` argument. In particular, group-by-treatment-specific slopes for the measurement time and the square root of the time are assumed, as specified in (8.9).

The structure of the survival data model (8.2) is defined by arguments `ysurv`, `censvar`, `xsurv`, and `classurv`. In particular, `ysurv=survyr` and `censvar=survcens` indicate the variables containing, respectively, the failure-time true endpoint and the corresponding event indicator. Argument `xsurv=countryn treat*countryn` defines the fixed-effects part of (8.2), while `classurv=countryn` indicates that `countryn` is to be treated as a factor (class-variable). Hence, `xsurv=countryn treat*countryn` implies the use of group-specific intercepts and treatment effects. Finally, the random-effect structure W_2 of (8.2) is fixed to be equal to (8.11).

Arguments `r2t_lg0`, `r2t_lg1`, and `r2t_lg2` specify the terms in the `Xlong` argument that define the group-specific treatment effects on the surrogate endpoint. In our case, we have group-specific overall effects (`r2t_lg0=treat*countryn`), linear-time-dependent treatment effects (`r2t_lg1=timeyr*treat*countryn`), and square root-time-dependent treatment effects (`r2t_lg2=timysqrt*treat*countryn`). Similarly, `r2t_sv=treat*countryn` specifies the terms in the `xsurv` argument that define the group-specific treatment effects on the true endpoint. In our case, these are group-specific overall effects (`r2t_sv=treat*countryn`).

Finally, argument `noint=1` implies that no intercept is to be used in the construction of the design matrices for the LMM and the PH model, while the maximum number of iterations of the EM algorithm is fixed at `niter=500`. Argument `label` provides the prefix for the names of the output datasets that are produced by the macro. It is also possible to specify a suffix by using the `suff` argument.

The macro produces several output datasets. Treatment effects are stored in a dataset named *label_trt_effect_suff*. Estimates of the fixed-effects coefficients and variance components of the longitudinal model (8.1) are stored in a file named *label_long_est_suff*, while the estimates of the fixed- and random-effects coefficients of the PH model (8.2) are stored in a file named *label_surv_est_suff*. The file named *label_expect_suff* contains the predicted values of the random effects $U_{k,ij}$ of $W_{1,ij}$. Finally, the file named *label_r2indiv_suff* contains the estimates of $R^2_{\text{indiv}}(\tau, \tau)$ for a grid of values of τ between `tbeg=0` and `tend=9` in steps of `step=0.05`. In particular, two estimates of $R^2_{\text{indiv}}(\tau,\tau)$ are provided. One (stored in variable "R2IND") is computed by using the estimated values of coefficients γ and the variance-covariance matrix G. The other (stored in variable "R2INDH") is obtained from the sample variance-covariance matrix of the predicted values of the random-effects vector $(W_{1,ij}, W_{2,ij})'$. Note that all the output files are supposed to be stored in the (permanent) SAS library named `longsurv`. Thus, before running the SAS macro `longsurvtst2_2stage.sas`, library `longsurv` should be created by using an appropriate `libname` statement.

The estimated values of γ_1, γ_2, γ_3, and γ_4 for model (8.11) are equal to 0.191, 0.288, 0.321, 0.198, respectively. The estimated value of matrix G is

$$\begin{pmatrix} 1.66 & 0.01 & -0.41 \\ 0.01 & 10.45 & -9.08 \\ -0.41 & -9.08 & 12.02 \end{pmatrix},$$

and the residual variance $\sigma^2_e = 0.128$. Using these values and equations similar to (8.6)–(8.8), it is possible to compute the values of $R^2_{\text{indiv}}(\tau_1,\tau_2)$, capturing the strength of the individual-level association between the longitudinal surrogate and clinical event processes. The solid curve in Figure 8.2 presents the estimated values of the section $R^2_{\text{indiv}}(\tau,\tau) \equiv R^2_{\text{indiv}}(\tau)$. The dashed curve presents the estimates obtained from the sample variance-covariance matrix of the predicted values of the random-effects vector $(W_{1,ij}, W_{2,ij})'$. The two estimates are close to each other. They both suggest that, initially, the strength of the association is low, but it increases in time, reaching a plateau at a value of about 0.9 at one year. Thus, one could conclude that PSA levels measured close to the initiation of a therapy provide relatively little information about patient survival (Renard et al., 2003). With passing time, especially during the first year of treatment, the levels become more informative; afterward, there is no further gain in information.

As mentioned in Section 8.2, the $R^2_{\text{indiv}}(\tau)$ curve should be interpreted with caution as it is strongly dependent on the assumed form of the model.

The estimated treatment effects for the LMM and the PH models are given in Table 8.1.

Figure 8.3 presents the scatter plot matrix of the estimates (the sizes of the circles are proportional to the sample sizes of the corresponding trial-by-country groups). The bottom row contains the plots illustrating the association between $\widehat{\alpha}_{0,i}$, $\widehat{\alpha}_{1,i}$ and $\widehat{\alpha}_{2,i}$ (on the horizontal axis) and $\widehat{\beta}_i$ (on the vertical axis). The plots suggest that there is not much association between the treatment-effect estimates. The value of $R^2_{\text{trial(f)}}$, obtained from regressing $\widehat{\beta}_i$ on $(\widehat{\alpha}_{0,i}, \widehat{\alpha}_{1,i}, \widehat{\alpha}_{2,i})'$, is equal to 0.52 (delta-method-based 95% CI: [0.18,0.86]). The estimated linear regression equation (8.5) is

$$\beta_i = 0.467 + 0.543 \times \alpha_{0,i} + 0.407 \times \alpha_{1,i} + 0.683 \times \alpha_{2,i},$$

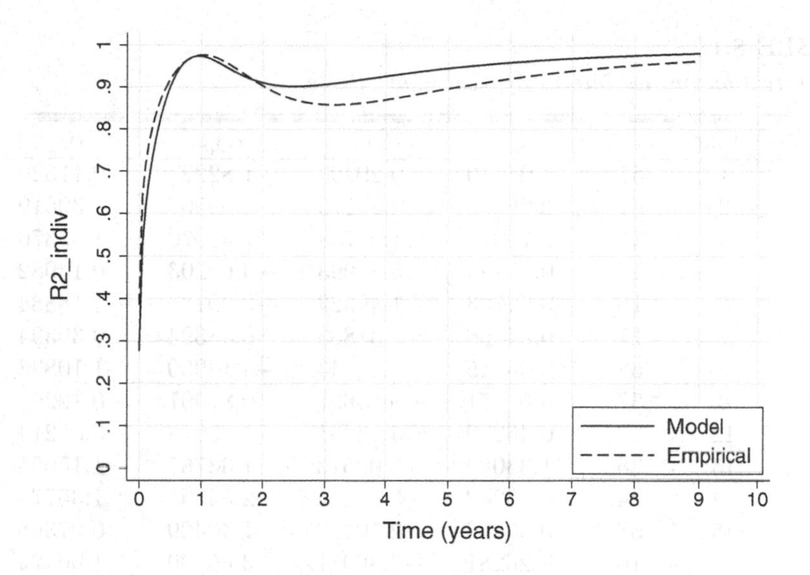

FIGURE 8.2
Prostate Cancer. Individual-level association, as measured by $R^2_{indiv}(\tau)$.

with standard errors of the estimated coefficients λ_0–λ_3 equal to 0.236, 0.336, 0.137, and 0.189, respectively.

The value of $R^2_{\text{trial(f)}}$, obtained from a linear regression model weighted by the group-specific sample size, is equal to 0.61 (delta-method-based 95% CI: [0.31,0.91]). The estimated linear regression equation (8.5) is

$$\beta_i = 0.342 + 0.656 \times \alpha_{0,i} + 0.422 \times \alpha_{1,i} + 0.663 \times \alpha_{2,i},$$

with standard errors of the estimated coefficients λ_0–λ_3 equal to 0.186, 0.263, 0.128, and 0.158, respectively.

Neither of the $R^2_{\text{trial(f)}}$ values is large enough to allow concluding that PSA measurements can be considered a valid surrogate for OS.

8.3.1.2 Marginal Models

The analysis presented in Section 8.3.1.1 allows evaluating both the individual- and trial-level surrogacy. However, fitting the joint model (8.1)–(8.2) is not trivial and requires specialized software.

A simpler analysis would result from using marginal models for the longitudinal surrogate and failure-time endpoint. In particular, using the `psadat` dataset described in Section 8.3.1.1, the LMM (8.9)–(8.10) can be fitted by using a call to `PROC MIXED` similar to the following one:

```
PROC MIXED data=psadat method=ml;
```

TABLE 8.1
Prostate Cancer. Estimates of treatment effects.

Group	N	$\widehat{\alpha}_{0,i}$	$\widehat{\alpha}_{1,i}$	$\widehat{\alpha}_{2,i}$	$\widehat{\beta}_i$
1	51	1.07150	0.29793	−1.82227	−0.11320
2	64	−0.06582	4.27175	−4.02507	−0.39519
3	19	−0.11073	1.04748	1.45070	1.43370
4	12	0.97395	5.84993	−3.62203	−0.13982
6	16	−0.02703	1.49523	−3.39183	−1.18884
7	17	−0.04868	−2.31853	0.48394	0.39394
8	68	0.05255	3.41043	−4.13950	−1.10833
9	57	0.01571	−0.85608	0.87997	−0.12267
12	15	−0.46289	4.13031	−1.80918	3.05214
13	35	−1.33082	−3.02613	1.33767	−1.15655
14	24	0.49202	5.14484	−2.54004	1.35772
15	37	0.30646	−2.10418	1.40429	0.27368
17	16	−0.26281	−6.36071	3.66200	1.06424
18	30	−0.08881	2.08421	−2.24416	−0.45748
20	19	−1.23598	4.66113	−3.34404	−1.25542
21	37	−1.13152	−2.69907	3.09017	0.46413
24	50	0.71554	0.72275	−0.90372	1.00531

```
    CLASS patid countryn timyrcls;
    MODEL logpsa = countryn timeyr*countryn timysqrt*countryn
                   treat*countryn treat*timeyr*countryn
                   treat*timysqrt*countryn / noint;
    RANDOM int timeyr timysqrt / subject = patid type = un;
    REPEATED timyrcls / subject = patid;
RUN;
```

Note that we use the ML estimation (`method = ml`) for compatibility with the joint-model analysis presented in Section 8.3.1.1, which was based on using the EM algorithm.

Treatment effects on OS can be estimated by the following SAS syntax:

```
PROC SORT data=psadat;
    BY patid timeyr;
RUN;

DATA survdat;
    SET psadat;
    BY patid timeyr;
```

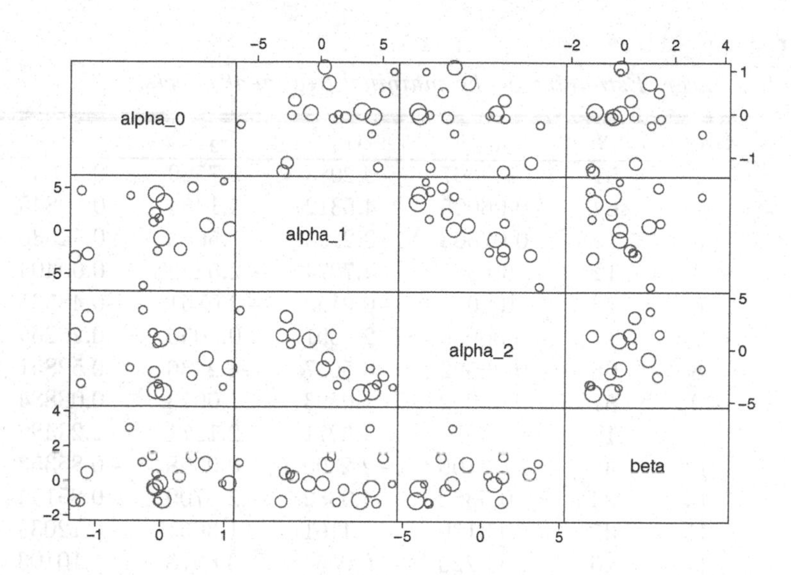

FIGURE 8.3
Prostate Cancer. Scatter plot matrix of the estimated treatment effects for the longitudinal log-PSA measurements ($\alpha_{0,i}$, $\alpha_{1,i}$, $\alpha_{2,i}$) and overall survival time (β_i). The circles' areas are proportional to the trial size.

```
    IF first.patid=1;
RUN;

PROC PHREG data=survdat;
    CLASS countryn;
    MODEL survyr*survcens(0) = treat(countryn);
    STRATA countryn;
RUN;
```

Note that, in the syntax, we specify trial-by-country-specific hazards (`STRATA countryn`) rather than assuming that the hazards are proportional, as in (8.2).

The estimated treatment effects for the LMM and the PH model are given in Table 8.2.

The value of $R^2_{\text{trial(f)}}$, obtained from regressing $\widehat{\beta}_i$ on $(\widehat{\alpha}_{0,i}, \widehat{\alpha}_{1,i}, \widehat{\alpha}_{2,i})'$, is equal to 0.33 (delta-method-based 95% CI: $[-0.05, 0.70]$). When the group-specific sample sizes are used as weights, the resulting value of $R^2_{\text{trial(f)}}$ is equal to 0.40 (delta-method-based 95% CI: [0.03,0.77]). The estimates are consistent with, though somewhat smaller than, the corresponding estimates obtained in the joint-model analysis presented in Section 8.3.1.1.

TABLE 8.2
Prostate Cancer. Estimates of the marginal treatment effects.

Group	N	$\widehat{\alpha}_{0,i}$	$\widehat{\alpha}_{1,i}$	$\widehat{\alpha}_{2,i}$	$\widehat{\beta}_i$
1	51	1.0667	0.2083	−1.7529	−0.37639
2	64	−0.06095	4.5312	−4.1454	−0.29845
3	19	0.07563	0.2193	1.5656	0.54536
4	12	0.8381	4.7874	−2.5423	0.00404
6	16	−0.2011	−0.2152	−2.0851	−0.48535
7	17	−0.06936	−2.2591	0.5050	0.26265
8	68	0.09522	3.5037	−4.2436	−0.52851
9	57	0.02962	−1.0893	1.0013	−0.08884
12	15	−0.4634	4.6271	−2.1271	2.23486
13	35	−1.3106	−2.2500	0.9558	−0.85353
14	24	0.5362	4.9382	−2.6709	0.85144
15	37	0.3170	−2.1101	1.3651	−0.12038
17	16	−0.3220	−6.0554	3.6978	1.10103
18	30	−0.09799	2.2145	−2.3323	−0.02217
20	19	−1.2290	5.8949	−3.9451	−1.42056
21	37	−1.1031	−4.1257	3.7887	0.35782
24	50	0.7034	0.6324	−0.9446	0.49801

8.3.2 Using R

Currently, there are no specific tools available in R for evaluation of a longitudinal surrogate for a failure-true endpoint. One could consider using the *JM* package (Rizopoulos, 2010), which does allow fitting a range of joint models for longitudinal and failure-time data. However, by default, in the joint models available in the package, the fixed-effects part of the LMM (8.1) is included in the PH model (8.2). As a result, the effect of treatment on the failure-time endpoint is estimated while already taking into account the treatment effect on the longitudinal process. Additionally, with, e.g., $W_1(\tau) = U_1 + U_2\tau + U_3\sqrt{\tau}$, the PH model (8.2) can include random effects of the form $W_2(\tau) = \gamma_2 U_2 + \gamma_3 U_3 + \gamma_4 W_1(\tau)$, but not $W_2(\tau) = \gamma_1 U_1 + \gamma_2 U_2 + \gamma_3 U_3 + \gamma_4 W_1(\tau)$. Thus, the flexibility of modeling of the association between the longitudinal and failure-time processes is somewhat restricted.

On the other hand, conducting an analysis based on the marginal models for the longitudinal and failure-time endpoints can be conducted in R without much problem with existing tools. Toward this aim, the *nlme* and *survival* packages can be used, for instance. In particular, function `lme` can be used to fit the LMM (8.1). On the other hand, the marginal PH model can be fitted by using function `coxph`.

More specifically, assume availability of a data frame **psadat**, say, that corresponds to the dataset **psadat** used in the SAS analysis presented in Section 8.3.1.1. Then the following R command fits the LMM (8.9)–(8.10) by using the ML estimation:

```
lme(logpsa ~ -1 + factor(countryn) + timeyr:factor(countryn)
             + timysqrt:factor(countryn)
             + treat:factor(countryn)
             + treat:timeyr:factor(countryn)
             + treat:timysqrt:factor(countryn),
random = ~ 1 + timeyr + timysqrt | patid,
                                   method = "ML", data=psadat)
```

On the other hand, assume availability of a data frame **survdat**, say, that corresponds to the dataset **survdat** used in the SAS analysis presented in Section 8.3.1.1. Then the following R command fits the marginal PH model:

```
coxph(Surv(survyr,survcens) ~ treat:factor(countryn)
                              + strata(countryn),
ties="breslow", data=survdat)
```

The option **ties="breslow"** implies using the Breslow method for the construction of the partial likelihood function, which is the default method in SAS' PROC PHREG.

The so-obtained treatment-effect estimates for the LMM and PH models correspond to those reported in Table 8.2.

8.4 Concluding Remarks

Longitudinal measurements contain the full information about the dynamics of a continuous biomarker, including the magnitude and timing of changes. Hence, it could be argued that such a biomarker could offer the greatest potential for becoming a surrogate for a clinical endpoint that may be distant in time.

Longitudinal measurements of PSA were evaluated as a candidate surrogate for OS by several authors. In particular, Buyse et al. (2003), Renard et al. (2003), and Collette et al. (2005) applied the meta-analytic approach, presented in the current chapter, to various sets of data from prostate cancer clinical trials. In none of the analyses was PSA found to be an acceptable surrogate for OS. Given this result, it is not surprising that none of the other PSA-based endpoints (such as, e.g., PSA response, time to PSA progression, etc.) was found to be a valid surrogate either (Buyse et al., 2003; Collette et al., 2005).

As illustrated in this chapter, evaluation of a continuous, normally distributed, longitudinal surrogate for a failure-time true endpoint is not trivial due to the need to use a joint model for the two longitudinal and failure-time processes. The model is needed if one wants to assess the strength of both the individual- and trial-level associations. However, if the former is not of interest, then the marginal linear mixed-effects and proportional-hazards models can be used to evaluate the strength of the trial-level association. The marginal analysis can be easily implemented with existing software tools.

9

Evaluation of Surrogate Endpoints from an Information-Theoretic Perspective

Ariel Alonso Abad

KU Leuven, Belgium

CONTENTS

9.1 Introduction

Buyse et al. (2000) developed an elegant formalism to assess the validity of surrogate endpoints in a meta-analytic context. However, these authors only considered the simplest setting where both endpoints are Gaussian random variables measured cross-sectionally. Over the years, work was done to extend the meta-analytic methodology to other outcome types and in the preceding chapters, some of these methods were described in detail.

Assessing surrogacy in more complex scenarios raises a number of difficult challenges. First, one needs to deal with highly complicated hierarchical models that frequently suffer from severe numerical issues. Second, based on the outputs of these models, one needs to define meaningful metrics to quantify surrogacy at both trial and individual levels. If one is willing to consider only a linear relationship between the expected causal treatment effect on the surrogate and the true endpoint, then the methodology described in Chapter 4 can be applied in a straightforward fashion to quantify trial-level surrogacy. At the individual level, however, abandoning the realm of normality has much deeper implications. Indeed, within the meta-analytic paradigm, several individual-level metrics of surrogacy have been proposed. For instance, in the binary-binary setting, Renard et al. (2002) assumed that the observed dichotomous outcomes emerge from two latent and normally distributed variables $(\tilde{S},\tilde{T})$. Essentially, it is assumed that the surrogate (true endpoint) takes value 1 when the corresponding latent variable is positive and 0 otherwise. In this framework, using a bivariate probit model, these authors defined individual-level surrogacy as $R^2_{\text{indiv}} = \text{corr}(\tilde{S},\tilde{T})^2$, i.e., the squared correlation at the latent level. Alternatively, they also defined $R^2_{\text{indiv}} = \psi$, the global odds ratio between both binary endpoints estimated from a bivariate Plackett-Dale model.

When the true endpoint is a survival time and the surrogate is a longitudinal sequence, Renard et al. (2003), using Henderson's model, proposed to study the individual-level surrogacy based on a time function defined as $R^2_{\text{indiv}}(t) = \text{corr}[W_1(t), W_2(t)]^2$, where $(W_1(t), W_2(t))$ is a latent bivariate Gaussian process. Burzykowski et al. (2001) approached the case of two failure-time endpoints based on copula models and quantified the individual-level surrogacy using Kendall's τ. Spearman's rho has also been used in this scenario.

In addition, using multivariate ideas, the so-called R^2_{Λ} was proposed to evaluate surrogacy when both responses are measured longitudinally (Alonso et al., 2006). The R^2_{Λ} coefficient quantifies the association between both longitudinal sequences, after adjustment by treatment and trial, and is defined using the covariance matrices emanating from a longitudinal model that characterizes the joint distribution of both endpoints. Furthermore, R^2_{Λ} can be incorporated into a more general framework allowing for interpretation in terms of canonical correlations of the error vectors, based on which, a family of individual-level parameters can be defined (Alonso et al., 2006).

These examples underscore a limitation of the meta-analytic methodology so far: different settings require different definitions. Even though it seems logical that different settings require different approaches, some of these metrics are defined at a latent level, which hampers their clinical interpretation. Actually, as previously illustrated, the meta-analytic methodology may lead to different metrics even within one single setting and these metrics do not necessarily have the same interpretation or lead to the same conclusion. Clearly, this could bring problems when different surrogates need to be compared. In addition, the need for complex hierarchical models hinders the use of the methodology and causes important numerical issues. In the next section, a unified approach to the validation of surrogate endpoints will be introduced based on information theory. Furthermore, it will be argued that this approach may help to overcome some of the aforementioned problems.

9.2 An Information-Theoretic Unification

In spirit and concepts, information theory has its mathematical roots connected with the idea of disorder or entropy used in thermodynamics and statistical mechanics. An early attempt to formalize the theory was made by Nyquist in 1924 who recognized the logarithmic nature of information (Nyquist, 1924). Claude Shannon (?), together with Warren Weaver in 1949 wrote the definitive, classic work in information theory: *The Mathematical Theory of Communication*. Divided into separated treatments for continuous-time and discrete-time signals, systems, and channels, this book laid out all the key concepts and relationships that define the field today.

R.A. Fisher's well-known measure of the amount of information supplied by data about an unknown parameter is the first use of information in statistics. Kullback and Leibler (1951) studied another statistical information measure involving two probability distributions, the so-called Kullback-Leibler information.

The concept of entropy lies at the center of information theory and can be interpreted as a measure of the uncertainty associated with a random variable. If Y is a discrete random variable taking values $\{k_1, k_2, \ldots, k_m\}$ with probability function $P(Y = k_i) = p_i$, then the entropy of Y is defined as

$$H(Y) = -E_Y[\log P(Y)] = -\sum_i p_i \log p_i.$$

The joint and conditional entropies are defined in an analogous fashion as $H(X,Y) = -E_{X,Y}\left[P(X,Y)\right]$ and $H(Y|X) = -E_X\left[E_Y(P(Y|X))\right]$, with $P(x,y)$ and $P(y|x)$ denoting the joint and conditional probability functions, respectively. Entropy is always non-negative and satisfies $H(Y|X) \leq H(Y)$ for any pair of random variables (X,Y), with equality holding under independence. Basically, the previous inequality states that, as an average, uncertainty about Y can only decrease if additional information (X) becomes available. Furthermore, entropy is invariant under a bijective transformation.

Similarly, the so-called differential entropy $h_d(Y)$ of a continuous random variable Y with density $f(y)$ and support S_Y is defined as

$$h_d(Y) = -E_Y[\log f(Y)] = -\int_{S_Y} f(y) \log f(y)\, dy.$$

Differential entropy enjoys some but not all properties of entropy, it can be infinitely large, negative, or positive, and is coordinate dependent. For a bijective transformation $W = v(Y)$, it follows that $h_d(W) = h_d(Y) - \mathrm{E}_W\left(\log\left|\frac{dv^{-1}}{dw}(W)\right|\right)$.

The amount of uncertainty in Y, expected to be removed if the value of X were known, is quantified by the so-called *mutual information* $I(X,Y) =$

$h(Y) - h(Y|X)$, where $h = H$ in the discrete case and $h = h_d$ for continuous random variables. It is always non-negative, zero if and only if X and Y are independent, symmetric, invariant under bijective transformations of X and Y, and $I(X, X) = h(X)$. Moreover, mutual information approaches infinity as the distribution of (X, Y) approaches a singular distribution; that is, $I(X, Y)$ is large if there is an approximate functional relationship among X and Y (Joe, 1989; Cover and Tomas, 1991).

Alonso and Molenberghs (2007) proposed to assess the validity of a surrogate endpoint in terms of uncertainty reduction. In fact, these authors stated that S is a valid surrogate for T at the individual (trial) level, if uncertainty about T (the expected causal treatment effect on T) is reduced by a "large" amount when S (the expected causal treatment effect on S) is known. This definition conceptualizes, in a simple yet formal way, what is intuitively expected from a valid surrogate endpoint. Indeed, often in practice, at the individual level, surrogate endpoints are used to gain information about the outcome on the true endpoint. For instance, a treating physician may measure cholesterol level to gain information about the risk of heart attack for a given patient. Similarly, at the trial level, it is expected that studying the treatment effect on the surrogate may provide information on the effect of the treatment on the true endpoint. For instance, a trialist may study the impact of a treatment on progression-free survival hoping to gain information on its impact on overall survival. In the following sections, the use of the previous definition at the trial level will be illustrated.

9.3 Information-Theoretic Approach: Trial Level

As in Chapter 4, let us assume that data from $i = 1, \ldots, N$ clinical trials are available, in the ith of which $j = 1, \ldots, n_i$ subjects are enrolled, and let β_i and α_i denote the trial-specific expected causal treatment effects on the true and surrogate endpoints, respectively. Furthermore, let us assume that (α_i, β_i) follows a distribution characterized by the density function $f(\alpha, \beta)$.

The mutual information between both expected causal treatment effects $I(\alpha, \beta)$ quantifies the amount of uncertainty in β, expected to be removed if the value of α becomes known and hence, it seems sensible to use this measure to quantitatively assess the previous definition of surrogacy. However, the absence of an upper bound for $I(\alpha, \beta)$ hinders its interpretation. To solve this problem, Alonso and Molenberghs (2007) proposed to use instead a normalized version of the mutual information, the so-called squared informational coefficient of correlation (SICC) introduced by Linfoot (1957) and Joe (1989):

$$R^2_{ht} = 1 - e^{-2I(\alpha,\beta)}, \quad \text{where} \quad I(\alpha, \beta) = \int\int f(\alpha, \beta) \log\left(\frac{f(\alpha, \beta)}{f(\alpha)f(\beta)}\right) d\alpha d\beta.$$

If $f(\alpha, \beta)$ is a bivariate normal distribution, then $I(\alpha, \beta) = -\frac{1}{2}\log(1-\rho^2_{\alpha\beta})$ where $\rho_{\alpha\beta} = \text{corr}(\alpha, \beta)$ and, therefore, $R^2_{ht} = R^2_{\text{trial}}$ in this scenario. The SICC is always in the interval $[0, 1]$, is invariant under bijective transformations, and takes value zero if and only if α and β are independent. As previously mentioned, mutual information approaches infinity when the distribution of (α, β) approaches a singular distribution, i.e., $R^2_{ht} \approx 1$ if and only if there exists an approximate functional relationship among α and β (Joe, 1989). In addition, the randomness of β can be defined using the so-called entropy-power:

$$\text{EP}(\beta) = \frac{1}{2\pi e} e^{2h(\beta)}. \tag{9.1}$$

The previous definition is motivated by the functional form of the normal distribution. Indeed, the differential entropy of a continuous normal random variable X is $h(X) = \log\sqrt{(2\pi e\sigma^2)}$ and, thus, for the normal distribution the differential entropy is just a function of the variance. Measuring information in nats (using the natural logarithm) leads to $\text{EP}(X) = \sigma^2$, i.e., the larger the variability, the larger the uncertainty or "randomness." Although valid for the normal distribution, the previous equivalence between variability and uncertainty does not hold in other scenarios.

The residual randomness of β given α can be quantified using $\text{EP}(\beta|\alpha)$, obtained by substituting $h(\beta)$ by $h(\beta|\alpha)$ in (9.1) and R^2_{ht} can then be interpreted as the proportion of the randomness in β, which is explained by α (Kent, 1983):

$$R^2_{ht} = \frac{\text{EP}(\beta) - \text{EP}(\beta|\alpha)}{\text{EP}(\beta)}.$$

9.3.1 Plausibility of Finding a Valid Surrogate: Trial Level

Fano's inequality relates prediction accuracy with different information-theoretic concepts and, when applied to the evaluation of surrogate endpoints at the trial level, this inequality sets a limit for our capacity to successfully predict the expected causal treatment effect on the true endpoint using the expected causal treatment effect on the surrogate (Cover and Tomas, 1991; Alonso and Molenberghs, 2007). In fact, applying Fano's inequality to the validation problem at the trial level leads to

$$\text{E}\left[(\beta - g(\alpha))^2\right] \geq \text{EP}(\beta)(1 - R^2_{ht}). \tag{9.2}$$

This inequality raises some interesting issues. First, note that nothing has been assumed about the distribution of (α, β) and no specific form has been considered for the prediction function g. Second, (9.2) clearly shows that the quality of the prediction strongly depends on the characteristics of the true endpoint and the treatments under study, more specifically, on the power-entropy $\text{EP}(\beta)$. Essentially, Fano's inequality defines a lower bound for the prediction error and this lower bound can be decomposed in two different elements. The second element on the right side of (9.2) depends on the surrogate through the value of R^2_{ht}; the first element, however, is an intrinsic characteristic of the true-endpoint-treatment pair and it is independent of the surrogate. It is clear from (9.2) that the prediction error increases with $\text{EP}(\beta)$. Consequently, if the true endpoint has a large power-entropy at the trial level, then a surrogate should produce an R^2_{ht} close to one to have some predictive value. In other words, the expected causal treatment effect on the surrogate would need to be almost deterministically related to the expected causal treatment effect on the true endpoint to have some predictive power. Essentially, this inequality hints at the fact that, for some true endpoints and treatments, the search for a valid surrogate at the trial level may not be viable.

When $f(\alpha, \beta)$ is a bivariate normal distribution Fano's lower bound is reached, i.e., (9.2) becomes an equality and the right-hand side takes the simpler form $\sigma^2_{\beta\beta}\left(1 - R^2_{\text{trial}}\right)$. Based on this equality, Burzykowski and Buyse (2006) introduced a new measure of surrogacy at the trial level for normally distributed (α, β), the so-called surrogate threshold effect (STE). For details, see Section 4.5.

9.3.2 Estimating R^2_{ht}

Finding an estimator for R^2_{ht} can be essentially reduced to finding one for $I(\alpha, \beta)$. The estimation of the mutual information between two random variables is a complex problem that has received a lot of attention in the literature see, for example, Brillinger (2004), Kent (1983), and the references there in. However, there are some general results allowing the estimation of the mutual information using the likelihood function. To that end, let us consider the random variables $\boldsymbol{X}$ and $\boldsymbol{Y}$ with density function of $f(\boldsymbol{x}, \boldsymbol{y}|\boldsymbol{\theta})$ and suppose that the realizations $(\boldsymbol{x}_i, \boldsymbol{y}_i)$, $i = 1, 2, \ldots n$ are available. Suppose further that the parameter $\boldsymbol{\theta}$ has the form $\boldsymbol{\theta} = (\boldsymbol{\theta}_0, \boldsymbol{\theta}_1)$ and let $\hat{\boldsymbol{\theta}}_0$ denote the maximum likelihood estimator (mle) of $\boldsymbol{\theta}_0$ under the null hypothesis of independence $(\boldsymbol{\theta}_1 = \boldsymbol{0})$. Consider the estimate

$$\frac{1}{n}G^2 = \frac{1}{n}\sum_i \left(\log[f(\boldsymbol{y}_i|\boldsymbol{x}_i, \hat{\boldsymbol{\theta}})] - \log[f(\boldsymbol{y}_i|\hat{\boldsymbol{\theta}}_0)]\right), \tag{9.3}$$

with $\hat{\boldsymbol{\theta}}$ the full model maximum likelihood estimator. Notice that (9.3) is just the classical log-likelihood ratio test statistic for the hypothesis of independence divided by n, i.e., $G^2 = \log(\text{likelihood ratio test})$ comparing the models $f(\boldsymbol{y}_i|\boldsymbol{x}_i, \boldsymbol{\theta})$ and $f(\boldsymbol{y}_i|\boldsymbol{\theta}_0)$ or, equivalently, testing $H_0 : \boldsymbol{\theta}_1 = 0$. If $\hat{\boldsymbol{\theta}}_0 \to \boldsymbol{\theta}_0$ in probability, then, under general regularity conditions, the statistic (9.3) will tend to $I(\boldsymbol{X}, \boldsymbol{Y})$, i.e., (9.3) provides a consistent estimator for the mutual information (Kent, 1983; Brillinger, 2004). The use of (9.3) has two important advantages. First, no integrals need to be evaluated, and second, no joint models need to be considered for $\boldsymbol{X}$ and $\boldsymbol{Y}$.

The aforementioned properties can help to consider more complex dependencies at the trial level with no additional cost. Indeed, although elegant, the hierarchical models considered by Buyse et al. (2000) often pose a considerable computational challenge (Burzykowski, Molenberghs, and Buyse, 2005). To address this problem, Tibaldi et al. (2003) suggested several simplifications, like treating the trial-specific parameters (α_i, β_i) as fixed effects in a two-stage approach. In the first stage the vectors (α_i, β_i) are estimated within each trial using a bivariate linear model for the surrogate and true endpoints, and at the second stage, the estimated treatment effect on the true endpoint is regressed on the estimated treatment effect on the surrogate using a linear regression model. Essentially, the trial-level surrogacy R^2_{trial} is assessed by regressing $\widehat{\beta}_i$ on $\widehat{\alpha}_i$.

The information-theoretic approach allows considering more general regression models at the trial-level without substantially increasing the computational burden, for instance, one could now use two general regression models $f(\beta_i|\alpha_i, \boldsymbol{\theta})$ and $f(\beta_i|\boldsymbol{\theta}_0)$, not necessarily linear. The parameters $\boldsymbol{\theta}$ and $\boldsymbol{\theta}_0$ can then be estimated using maximum likelihood and based on the estimates $(\widehat{\alpha}_i, \widehat{\beta}_i)$ obtained at the first stage of the previously described two-stage procedure. Finally, (9.3) can be used to obtain an estimate of $I(\alpha, \beta)$ and R^2_{ht}.

9.3.3 Asymptotic Confidence Interval for R^2_{ht}

In this section we will follow the ideas of Kent (1983) to construct an asymptotic confidence interval for $2I(\alpha, \beta)$. An asymptotic confidence interval for R^2_{ht} can then be constructed using a proper transformation. If the model describing the association between β and α is correctly specified, then Kent (1983) showed that

$$2\hat{I}(\alpha, \beta) = \frac{2}{n}G^2 \sim n^{-1}\chi^2_p(a),$$

where a can be estimated by $\hat{a} = 2n\hat{I}(\alpha, \beta)$, with n the total number of trials, $p = 1$, and $\hat{I}(\alpha, \beta) = G^2/n$ calculated as in (9.3). Therefore,

$$2\hat{I}(\alpha, \beta) = \frac{2}{n}G^2 \sim n^{-1}\chi^2_1(\hat{a}).$$

The previous expressions and the tables for the non-central χ^2 distribution can now be used to construct confidence intervals. Let us define $\kappa_{1:\alpha}(a)$ and $\delta_{1:\alpha}(a)$ by

$$P\left(\chi^2_1(\kappa_{1:\alpha/2}(a)) \geq a\right) = \frac{\alpha}{2},$$
$$P\left(\chi^2_1(\delta_{1:\alpha/2}(a)) \leq a\right) = \frac{\alpha}{2}.$$

If $P\left(\chi^2_1(0) \geq a\right) = \alpha/2$, then we set $\kappa_{1:\alpha/2}(a) = 0$. A two-sided $1 - \alpha$ asymptotic confidence interval for $2I(T, S)$ is then given by the closed interval

$$I_{1-\alpha} = \left[n^{-1}\kappa_{1:\alpha/2}(\hat{a}), n^{-1}\delta_{1:\alpha/2}(\hat{a})\right].$$

Notice further than under the null hypothesis of no association $H_0 : I(\alpha, \beta) = 0$ classical maximum likelihood theory indicates that, asymptotically,

$$2\hat{I}(\alpha, \beta) = \frac{2}{n}G^2 \sim n^{-1}\chi_1^2.$$

Using the previous distribution, a test can be constructed for evaluating the validity of the surrogate at the trial level, i.e., the hypothesis $H_0 : R_{ht}^2 = 0$.

10

Information-Theoretic Approach: Individual-Level Surrogacy

Ariel Alonso Abad

KU Leuven, Belgium

CONTENTS

Similar to the trial level, at the individual level the mutual information between both endpoints, $I(T, S)$, quantifies the amount of uncertainty in T, expected to be removed if the value of S becomes known, and hence, it seems sensible to use this measure again to quantitatively assess the definition of surrogacy given in Chapter 9. However, unlike at the trial level where both α and β are always continuous random variables, at the individual level, S and T may be both binary, time-to-event, continuous, or have different levels of measurement. This additional complexity brings some problems that need to be addressed in the information-theoretic approach but, at the same time, make this methodology more appealing at this level.

10.1 General Setting

Finding suitable estimators for $I(\boldsymbol{T}, \mathbf{S})$, where $\boldsymbol{T}$ and $\mathbf{S}$ are vector-valued true and surrogate endpoints, is a fundamental step when using the information-theoretic approach at the individual level. Importantly, the same line of reasoning employed in Chapter 9 to estimate mutual information at the trial level can be followed at the individual level as well. To illustrate this, let us consider the random vectors $\boldsymbol{T}$ and $\mathbf{S}$ with density function $f(\boldsymbol{t}, \boldsymbol{s}|\boldsymbol{\psi})$ and suppose that the realizations $(\boldsymbol{t}_i, \boldsymbol{s}_i)$, $i = 1, 2, \ldots n$, are available. In addition, it will be assumed that $\boldsymbol{\psi} = (\boldsymbol{\psi}_0, \boldsymbol{\psi}_1)$ and let $\widehat{\boldsymbol{\psi}}_0$ denote the maximum likelihood estimator of $\boldsymbol{\psi}_0$ under the null hypothesis of independence ($\boldsymbol{\psi}_1 = \mathbf{0}$). We define the estimator

$$\frac{1}{n}G^2 = \frac{1}{n}\sum_i \left(\log[f(\boldsymbol{t}_i|\boldsymbol{s}_i, \widehat{\boldsymbol{\psi}})] - \log[f(\boldsymbol{t}_i|\widehat{\boldsymbol{\psi}}_0)]\right) \tag{10.1}$$

with $\widehat{\boldsymbol{\psi}}$ the full model maximum likelihood estimator. Here again (10.1) is the classical likelihood ratio test statistic for the hypothesis of independence ($H_0 : \boldsymbol{\psi}_1 = 0$) divided by n. Actually, in (10.1), $G^2 = \log(\text{likelihood ratio test})$ comparing $f(\boldsymbol{t}_i|\boldsymbol{s}_i, \boldsymbol{\psi})$ and $f(\boldsymbol{t}_i|\boldsymbol{\psi}_0)$. Moreover, if $\widehat{\boldsymbol{\psi}}_0 \to \boldsymbol{\psi}_0$, in probability then, under general regularity conditions, the statistic (10.1) will tend to $I(\boldsymbol{T}, \mathbf{S})$, i.e., (10.1) provides a consistent estimator for the mutual information (Kent, 1983; Brillinger, 2004). A confidence interval for $I(\boldsymbol{T}, \mathbf{S})$ can be obtained along the lines presented in Section 9.3.3.

Based on (10.1), Alonso et al. (2004b) proposed to quantify the individual-level surrogacy using the so-called *likelihood reduction factor* (*LRF*). Later, Alonso and Molenberghs (2007) introduced a unified framework for the evaluation of surrogate endpoints based on the squared informational coefficient of correlation (SICC) proposed by Linfoot (1957) and Joe (1989) and, along the lines previously discussed, showed that the *LRF* is a consistent estimator of the SICC.

One of the major problems associated with the assessment of the individual-level surrogacy in the meta-analytic approach, is the need for complex joint models to characterize $f(\boldsymbol{t}, \boldsymbol{s}|\boldsymbol{\psi})$ and to describe the association between both endpoints. The use of (10.1) completely avoids this issue by only considering the conditional and marginal models $f(\boldsymbol{t}_i|\boldsymbol{s}_i, \boldsymbol{\psi})$ and $f(\boldsymbol{t}_i|\boldsymbol{\psi}_0)$, respectively. Note further that, although the expression $I(\boldsymbol{T}, \mathbf{S})$ involves a possibly high-dimensional integral, in (10.1) no integrals need to be evaluated.

In the next section the information-theoretic approach will be explained in detail for some relevant and frequently encountered outcome types.

10.2 S and T Both Continuous

Let us recall the setting in which both endpoints are continuous and normally distributed random variables. In this setting, T_{ij} and S_{ij} denote the true and surrogate endpoints for patient j in trial i, respectively, and Z_{ij} is the treatment indicator variable taking values 0/1 for the control/treated groups. The random treatment allocation in a clinical trial context naturally leads to the following bivariate model (Buyse et al., 2000)

$$\begin{cases} T_{ij} = \mu_{Ti} + \beta_i Z_{ij} + \varepsilon_{Tij}, \\ S_{ij} = \mu_{Si} + \alpha_i Z_{ij} + \varepsilon_{Sij}, \end{cases} \tag{10.2}$$

where μ_{Ti} and μ_{Si} are trial-specific intercepts quantifying the average response in the control group, β_i and α_i are trial-specific expected causal treatment effects and ε_{Tij} and ε_{Sij} are correlated error terms, assumed to be zero-mean normally distributed with covariance matrix

$$\Sigma = \begin{pmatrix} \sigma_{TT} & \sigma_{TS} \\ \sigma_{TS} & \sigma_{SS} \end{pmatrix}, \tag{10.3}$$

i.e., (10.3) denotes the within-trial covariance matrix of T and S after adjusting by treatment and considering the patient as the level of analysis. In this setting, Buyse et al. (2000) proposed to assess the individual-level surrogacy using the coefficient of determination

$$R^2_{\text{indiv}} = \rho^2_{TS} = \frac{\sigma^2_{ST}}{\sigma_{SS}\sigma_{TT}}.$$

Given the bivariate normality of $(\varepsilon_S, \varepsilon_T)$ it seems sensible to quantify the association at the individual level using the SICC, i.e.,

$$R^2_{h\text{indiv}} = 1 - e^{-2I(\varepsilon_S,\varepsilon_T)},$$

with $I(\varepsilon_S, \varepsilon_T)$ denoting the mutual information between both residuals. Furthermore, for the normal distribution, $I(\varepsilon_S, \varepsilon_T) = -\frac{1}{2}\log(1 - \rho^2_{TS})$ and, therefore, $R^2_{h\text{indiv}} = \rho^2_{TS} = R^2_{\text{indiv}}$. This result, together with the ones presented in Section 9.3 for the trial level, show that the methodology introduced by Buyse et al. (2000) can basically be seen as a special case of the information-theoretic approach at the trial and individual level.

10.2.1 Case Study Analysis: The Age-Related Macular Degeneration Trial

In the ARMD study, the efficacy of interferon-α to treat age-related macular degeneration (ARMD) was evaluated in a multi-trial setting (for details, see

Section 2.2.1). The true endpoint is the change in visual acuity 52 weeks after the start of the treatment and the candidate surrogate endpoint is the change in visual acuity after 24 weeks. Center is used as the trial-level unit of analysis. The results of the case study are discussed without reference to the software tools that can be used to conduct the analyses. In Section 13.2.2 it is detailed how the analyses can be conducted in R.

The analysis showed that $\widehat{R}^2_{h\text{ind}} = 0.5339$, with 95% confidence interval [0.4315; 0.6292]. It can thus be concluded that the amount of uncertainty in T = visual acuity after 52 weeks that is removed when the value of S = visual acuity after 24 weeks becomes known is moderate. This conclusion is in line with the results of the meta-analytic analysis (see Section 4.6).

10.3 S and T Longitudinal

Alonso et al. (2003, 2004a) studied the scenario where both endpoints are longitudinal random variables. In the rest of this section, the following model will be considered to describe the joint time evolution of S and T

$$\begin{cases} \boldsymbol{T}_{ij} = \boldsymbol{f}_i\left(\boldsymbol{X}_{Tij}^T, \boldsymbol{\beta}_i\right) + \boldsymbol{\varepsilon}_{Tij}, \\ \mathbf{S}_{ij} = \boldsymbol{g}_i\left(\boldsymbol{X}_{Sij}^T, \boldsymbol{\alpha}_i\right) + \boldsymbol{\varepsilon}_{Sij}, \end{cases} \tag{10.4}$$

where $\boldsymbol{T}_{ij}^T = (T_{ijt_1}, T_{ijt_2}, \ldots, T_{ijt_{p_i}})$, $\mathbf{S}_{ij}^T = (S_{ijt_1}, S_{ijt_2}, \ldots, S_{ijt_{q_i}})$, denote the true and surrogate endpoint vectors, describing the time evolution of both variables for patient j in trial i; t_k is the kth time point; p_i, q_i are the number of time points in the ith trial for the true and surrogate endpoint respectively; $\boldsymbol{X}_{Tij}$, $\boldsymbol{X}_{Sij}$, $\boldsymbol{\beta}_i$ and $\boldsymbol{\alpha}_i$ are the associated design matrices and effects; $\boldsymbol{f}_i$, $\boldsymbol{g}_i$ are two general and sufficiently smooth vector functions describing the average time evolution of patient j in trial i, and $\boldsymbol{\varepsilon}_{Tij}$, $\boldsymbol{\varepsilon}_{Sij}$ are the associated error vectors. For the sake of simplicity, in the following it will be assumed that in all trials patients were evaluated at the same time points and had the same number of evaluations, thus, $p_i = p$ and $q_i = q$ for all i. Further, it will be assumed that

$$\begin{pmatrix} \boldsymbol{\varepsilon}_{Tij} \\ \boldsymbol{\varepsilon}_{Sij} \end{pmatrix} \sim N(\mathbf{0}, \Sigma),$$

and

$$\Sigma = \begin{pmatrix} \Sigma_{TT} & \Sigma_{TS} \\ \Sigma_{TS}^T & \Sigma_{SS} \end{pmatrix}. \tag{10.5}$$

In this context, Alonso et al. (2003, 2004a), proposed the following measure of surrogacy at the individual level:

$$R_\Lambda^2 = 1 - \Lambda, \quad \text{where} \quad \Lambda = \frac{|\Sigma|}{|\Sigma_{TT}|\,|\Sigma_{SS}|}. \tag{10.6}$$

The residual vector $(\boldsymbol{\varepsilon}_T^T, \boldsymbol{\varepsilon}_S^T)$ follows a multivariate normal distribution and, therefore, it seems sensible to quantify the association at the individual-level using the SICC

$$R^2_{h\text{indiv}} = 1 - e^{-2I(\boldsymbol{\varepsilon}_T,\boldsymbol{\varepsilon}_S)}, \tag{10.7}$$

with $I(\boldsymbol{\varepsilon}_T, \boldsymbol{\varepsilon}_S)$ denoting the mutual information between both vectors of residuals. Furthermore, for the multivariate normal distribution,

$$I(\boldsymbol{\varepsilon}_T, \boldsymbol{\varepsilon}_S) = -\frac{1}{2}\log\frac{|\Sigma|}{|\Sigma_{TT}|\,|\Sigma_{SS}|} \quad \text{and, hence,} \quad R^2_{h\text{indiv}} = R^2_\Lambda.$$

If ρ_i, with $i = 1, \ldots \min(p,q)$, denote the canonical correlations between $\boldsymbol{\varepsilon}_T$ and $\boldsymbol{\varepsilon}_S$, then it can be shown that $I(\boldsymbol{\varepsilon}_T, \boldsymbol{\varepsilon}_S) = \frac{1}{2}\sum_i \log(1-\rho_i^2)$ and, consequently, (Alonso et al., 2003, 2004a)

$$R^2_{h\text{indiv}} = R^2_\Lambda = 1 - \prod_i \left(1 - \rho_i^2\right).$$

10.3.1 Asymptotic Confidence Interval for R^2_Λ

In what follows, let $\widehat{\Sigma}$, $\widehat{\Sigma}_{TT}$ and $\widehat{\Sigma}_{SS}$ denote the maximum likelihood estimator of the corresponding matrices the maximum likelihood estimator of the mutual information is then given by

$$\widehat{I}(\boldsymbol{\varepsilon}_T, \boldsymbol{\varepsilon}_S) = -\frac{1}{2}\log\frac{\left|\widehat{\Sigma}\right|}{\left|\widehat{\Sigma}_{TT}\right|\left|\widehat{\Sigma}_{SS}\right|}. \tag{10.8}$$

Notice that in this Gaussian scenario, the maximum likelihood ratio test to assess the independence of $\boldsymbol{\varepsilon}_T$ and $\boldsymbol{\varepsilon}_S$ equals (Kendall and Stuart, 1966)

$$\frac{n}{2}\log\frac{\left|\widehat{\Sigma}\right|}{\left|\widehat{\Sigma}_{TT}\right|\left|\widehat{\Sigma}_{SS}\right|}, \tag{10.9}$$

where n denotes the number of patients. The statistic (10.9) is proportional to the plug-in estimate (10.8) and, hence, from classical likelihood ratio test theory, it follows that the large-sample null distribution of (10.8) is χ^2_{pq}. Using the previous distribution, a test can be constructed to evaluate the quality of the surrogate at the individual level, i.e., the hypothesis $H_0 : R^2_\Lambda = 0$.

To obtain the asymptotic distribution of (10.8) in the non-null scenario, notice first that

$$\widehat{I}(\boldsymbol{\varepsilon}_T, \boldsymbol{\varepsilon}_S) = \frac{1}{2}\sum_i \log(1-\widehat{\rho}_i^2),$$

where the $\widehat{\rho}_i$ denote the sample canonical correlations. If ρ_i are all distinct and non-zero, then $\widehat{\rho}_i$ are asymptotically independent and normally distributed with means ρ_i and variances $\frac{1}{n}(1-\rho_i^2)^2$ (Hsu, 1941; Brillinger, 2004). It then follows that, asymptotically, $\widehat{I}(\varepsilon_T, \varepsilon_S) \sim N\left(I(\varepsilon_T, \varepsilon_S), \sum_i \rho_i^2/n\right)$ and a confidence interval for R_Λ^2 can be obtained using (10.7). If some of the ρ_i are equal or some of them are zero, then the asymptotic distribution becomes much more complex and a bootstrap confidence interval may be a more viable option (Hsu, 1941).

10.3.2 Remarks

At the beginning of this section it was assumed, for the sake of simplicity, that in all trials patients were evaluated at the same time points and had the same number of evaluations, i.e., $p_i = p$ and $q_i = q$ for all i. Additionally, it was assumed that matrix (10.5), characterizing the association at the individual level, was constant across trials. We will now relax these assumptions by considering the setting in which trials are nested within M clusters. Trials belonging to the same cluster have the same evaluation moments and number of evaluations and it will be further assumed that the matrix (10.5) varies across clusters but is constant within a cluster, i.e., the association structure is characterized by Σ_j , with $j = 1, \ldots, M$. Similarly, $R_{\Lambda j}^2$ will be constant within clusters as well. A global individual-level measure of surrogacy can then be defined as

$$R_\Lambda^2 = \sum_j^M \gamma_j R_{\Lambda j}^2 = 1 - \sum_j^M \gamma_j \Lambda_j,$$

where $\gamma_j > 0$ for all j and $\sum_j \gamma_j = 1$. The weights γ_j can be chosen based on scientific arguments, for instance, in some settings, clusters with large sample sizes may receive more weight. Furthermore, like before, we can construct an asymptotic confidence interval for $R_{\Lambda j}^2$ for all j and using Bonferroni correction one gets

$$P\left(R_{\Lambda 1}^2 \in I_{1-\alpha^*}^1, R_{\Lambda 2}^2 \in I_{1-\alpha^*}^2, \ldots, R_{\Lambda M}^2 \in I_{1-\alpha^*}^M\right) \geq 1-\alpha,$$

where $1-\alpha^*$ is the Bonferroni confidence level for the cluster-specific intervals ($\alpha^* = \alpha/M$). Moreover, if $\left\{R_{\Lambda 1}^2 \in I_{1-\alpha^*}^1, R_{\Lambda 2}^2 \in I_{1-\alpha^*}^2, \ldots, R_{\Lambda M}^2 \in I_{1-\alpha^*}^M\right\}$, then $R_\Lambda^2 = \sum_j \gamma_j R_{\Lambda j}^2 \in I = \sum_j \gamma_j I_{1-\alpha}^j$ and, therefore, $P\left(R_\Lambda^2 \in I\right) \geq 1-\alpha$. So, I can be used as a conservative confidence interval for R_Λ^2.

Alonso et al. (2003) proposed another metric of surrogacy in this setting, the so-called variance reduction fraction (VRF), defined as

$$VRF_{\text{indiv}} = \frac{\text{tr}\left(\Sigma_{TT}\right) - \text{tr}\left(\Sigma_{T|S}\right)}{\text{tr}\left(\Sigma_{TT}\right)}, \tag{10.10}$$

where $\Sigma_{T|S} = \Sigma_{TT} - \Sigma_{TS}\Sigma_{SS}^{-1}\Sigma_{TS}^T$ denotes the variance-covariance matrix of $\varepsilon_T|\varepsilon_S$. Intuitively, expression (10.10) tries to quantify how much of the total variability around the repeated measurements on the true endpoint is explained by adjusting for the treatment effects and the repeated measurements on the surrogate endpoint. The VRF_{indiv} satisfies a set of properties that make it a plausible extension of the R^2_{indiv}. Indeed, it is always in the unit interval, $VRF_{\text{indiv}} = 0$ if and only if $\boldsymbol{\varepsilon}_T$ and $\boldsymbol{\varepsilon}_S$ are independent, and $VRF_{\text{indiv}} = 1$ if and only if there exists a non-singular matrix A so that $P(\boldsymbol{\varepsilon}_T = A\boldsymbol{\varepsilon}_S) = 1$. Moreover, in the cross-sectional case, $VRF_{\text{indiv}} = R^2_{\text{indiv}}$.

The VRF_{indiv} can also be expressed as a function of the canonical correlations. In fact, Alonso et al. (2004a) showed that $VRF_{\text{indiv}} = \sum \omega_i \rho_i^2$ with $\omega_i > 0$ for all i and $\sum_i \omega_i = 1$. Notice that, if $VRF_{\text{indiv}} = 1$, then $R^2_{\Lambda} = 1$, but the reciprocal is not true in general. Actually, $R^2_{\Lambda} = 1$ if and only if there exist vectors $\boldsymbol{a}$ and $\boldsymbol{b}$ so that $P(\boldsymbol{a}\boldsymbol{\varepsilon}_T = \boldsymbol{b}\boldsymbol{\varepsilon}_S) = 1$ and, therefore, R^2_{Λ} can detect more general and weaker patterns of dependence than the VRF_{indiv}.

Finally, it is important to point out that, although originally proposed in a longitudinal scenario, the previous methods can be applied in more general multivariate settings. For instance, Alonso et al. (2003) considered the case in which two surrogate endpoints are available in a cross-sectional framework. Using a theoretical example and the VRF, these authors showed that even though the treatment effect on each surrogate may not be able to predict the treatment effect on the true endpoint (β) with a high level of accuracy, both treatment effects combined could precisely predict β. This example illustrates how much can be gained when multivariate surrogates are used, however, this promising area of research has been so far little explored.

10.4 S and T Time-to-Event Variables

Prior to describing the assessment of the individual-level surrogacy in this scenario, let us introduce some general notation for time-to-event outcomes. The random variables of interest in this setting are represented by the vector $(Y, C, \boldsymbol{X}^T)$, where Y is a time-to-event variable, C the censoring time, and $\boldsymbol{X}$ is a p-dimensional column vector of possibly time-dependent explanatory variables. Time dependency is sometimes indicated through $\boldsymbol{X} = \boldsymbol{X}(t)$.

The response variable for individual j is given by the vector (T_j, δ_j), where $T_j = \min(Y_j, C_j)$ and $\delta_j = I(Y_j \leq C_j)$, with $I(\cdot)$ an indicator function. Furthermore, let $K_j(t)$ denote a function indicating whether subject j is at risk ($K_j(t) = 1$) or not ($K_j(t) = 0$) at time t. The regression model for T, given the observed values of the covariates $\boldsymbol{X} = \boldsymbol{x}$, tries to describe the conditional density $f(t|\boldsymbol{x})$, although it is more frequently expressed equivalently in terms of the hazard function, also referred to as the intensity function. The proportional hazard (PH) model specifies the intensity function as (Cox, 1972)

$$\lambda[t|\boldsymbol{x}(t)] = K(t)\lambda_0(t)\exp\{\boldsymbol{\beta}\boldsymbol{x}(t)\}, \tag{10.11}$$

where $\lambda_0(t)$ is a fixed but unknown baseline hazard function, and $\boldsymbol{\beta}$ is a p-dimensional vector of unknown coefficients. For a binary covariate x_q, β_q can be interpreted as the log-relative risk, conditional on the values of all other covariates. The baseline hazard function $\lambda_0(t)$ can be specified using a power form or a constant, in which cases the Weibull and exponential models are recovered (Cox and Oakes, 1984; Kalbfleisch and Prentice, 1980). In the following it will be assumed that censoring is non-informative, i.e., the censoring and failure times are statistically independent. The parameters of interest in (10.11) are estimated based on the so-called *partial likelihood* introduced by Cox (1972).

Given the continuous nature of time-to-event variables, Alonso and Molenberghs (2008) proposed to quantify the individual-level surrogacy in this scenario using the SICC, i.e., $R^2_{h\text{indiv}} = 1 - e^{-2I(T,S)}$, where $I(T,S)$ is the mutual information between both endpoints after adjusting by trial and treatment. The estimation of the mutual information $I(T,S)$ is particularly challenging in this setting for two main reasons: i) both endpoints S and T are potentially censored and ii) the estimation of the parameters in (10.11) is carried out using a non-likelihood procedure, i.e., it is based on the partial likelihood function. In the next section two estimation strategies will be discussed.

10.4.1 Estimating $R^2_{h,\text{ind}}$

Alonso and Molenberghs (2008) proposed to redefine the surrogate endpoint S as a time-dependent covariate $S(t)$, taking value 0 until the surrogate endpoint occurs and 1 thereafter. Furthermore, these authors considered the models

$$\lambda[t|\boldsymbol{x}_{ij}, \boldsymbol{\beta}] = K_{ij}(t)\lambda_{0i}(t)\exp\{\boldsymbol{\beta}\boldsymbol{x}_{ij}\}, \tag{10.12}$$

$$\lambda[t|\boldsymbol{x}_{ij}, S_{ij}, \boldsymbol{\beta}, \psi] = K_{ij}(t)\lambda_{0i}(t)\exp\{\boldsymbol{\beta}\boldsymbol{x}_{ij} + \psi S_{ij}\}, \tag{10.13}$$

where $K_{ij}(t)$ is the risk function of patient j in trial i, $\boldsymbol{x}_{ij}$ is a p-dimensional vector of possibly time-dependent covariates, $\boldsymbol{\beta}$ is a p-dimensional vectors of unknown coefficients, $\lambda_{0i}(t)$ is a trial-specific baseline hazard function, and S_{ij} is a time-dependent covariate version of the surrogate endpoint and ψ its associated effect. The vector $\boldsymbol{x}_{ij}$ may contain covariates like treatment, trial, country, etc.

Along the lines presented in Section 10.1, Alonso and Molenberghs (2008) proposed to estimate the mutual information between both endpoints using $\widehat{I}(T,S) = \frac{1}{n}G^2$, where n is the number of patients and $G^2 =$ log(partial likelihood ratio test) comparing (10.12) and (10.13). The SICC can then be estimated as

$$\widehat{R}^2_{h\text{indiv}} = LRF = 1 - e^{-\frac{1}{n}G^2}.$$

O'Quigley and Flandre (2006) pointed out that the previous estimator depends upon the censoring mechanism, even when the censoring mechanism is non-informative. For low levels of censoring, this may not be an issue of much concern, but for high levels it could lead to biased results. To properly cope with the censoring mechanism in time-to-event outcomes, O'Quigley and Flandre (2006) proposed to estimate the mutual information as $\widehat{I}(T, S) = \frac{1}{k}G^2$, where k is the total number of events experienced in the studies. The SICC is then estimated as

$$\widehat{R}^2_{h\text{indiv}} = LRF_a = 1 - e^{-\frac{1}{k}G^2}.$$

Approximate asymptotic confidence intervals can be calculated using the method introduced by Kent (1983) or via bootstrap. It is important to point out that the information-theoretic approach can be applied when there are more than two arms in the clinical trials, as well as to assess the joint effect of multiple surrogate endpoints on a true endpoint. Furthermore, the information-theoretic approach is able to elegantly deal with time-ordered endpoints. For instance, when progression-free survival S is used as a surrogate for overall survival T, then naturally $S \leq T$, with equality either when survival censors progression, or when censoring occurs on both endpoints simultaneously. In the classical meta-analytic approach, a bivariate model for (S, T) is required, on which it may be difficult to impose this restriction. However, in the information-theoretic approach, rather the conditional model for T given S is required. When this is replaced by $T - S|S$, for instance, the constraint is immediate, yet neither the computations nor the derived measures are affected (Assam et al., 2011).

10.5 Case Study Analysis: Four Ovarian Cancer Trials

The ovarian dataset combines the data that were collected in four double-blind randomized clinical trials in advanced ovarian cancer (for details, see Section 2.2.3). Two treatments were considered, i.e., cyclophosphamide plus cisplatin (control treatment) and cyclophosphamide plus adriamycin plus cisplatin (experimental treatment). The candidate surrogate endpoint S is progression-free survival time, defined as the time (in years) from randomization to clinical progression of the disease or death. The true endpoint T is survival time, defined as the time (in years) from randomization to death of any cause. The results of the case study are discussed without reference to the software tools that can be used to conduct the analyses. Section 13.3 provides full details on how the analyses can be conducted in R.

The estimated LRF was 0.7446, with 95% confidence interval [0.7152; 0.7720]. When the censoring mechanism is taken into account, the estimated LRF_a was 0.8193, with 95% confidence interval [0.7928; 0.8433]. Overall, these results indicate that the amount of uncertainty in T that is expected to be removed when the value of S becomes known is quite high, suggesting that progression-free survival time is a relatively good surrogate for survival time.

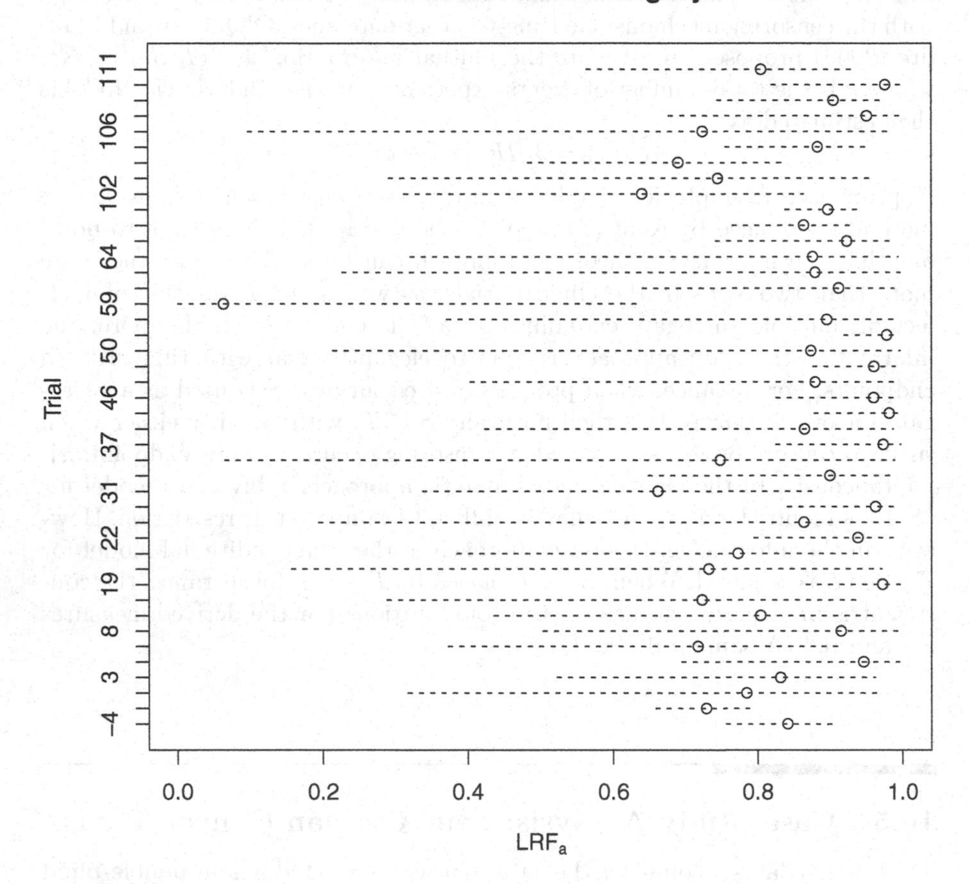

FIGURE 10.1

Ovarian Cancer Data. Plot of the estimated LRF_a (and their 95% confidence intervals) per cluster.

Figure 10.1 provides the estimated LRF_a and their 95% confidence intervals in each of the clusters. As can be seen, the point estimates for LRF_a were similar in most clusters (units) and they were typically above 0.65. In cluster 59, the point estimate of the LRF_a was only 0.0639, though its 95% confidence interval overlapped with those of many other clusters. This indicates that the individual-level association between progression-free survival and overall survival is of the same magnitude across the different clusters.

10.6 S and T: Binary-Binary or Continuous-Binary

Like in all previous scenarios, the evaluation of the individual-level surrogacy in this setting will be based on $I(T,S)$, i.e., the mutual information between both endpoints after adjusting by trial and treatment. To this end, in the following, three generalized linear models will be considered

$$g_T[E(T_{ij}|\boldsymbol{x}_{ij})] = \boldsymbol{\beta x}_{ij}, \quad (10.14)$$

$$g_T[E(T_{ij}|\boldsymbol{x}_{ij}, S_{ij})] = \boldsymbol{\beta x}_{ij} + \theta S_{ij}, \quad (10.15)$$

$$g_S[E(S_{ij}|\boldsymbol{x}_{ij})] = \boldsymbol{\alpha z}_{ij}, \quad (10.16)$$

where T_{ij} and S_{ij} denote the true and surrogate endpoints for patient j in trial i; g_T and g_S are known link functions, $\boldsymbol{x}_{ij}$ is a p-dimensional vector of covariates that may include variables like trial, treatment, etc., and $\boldsymbol{\beta}$, $\boldsymbol{\alpha}$ and θ are the corresponding effects. Based on the results presented in Section 10.1, Alonso et al. (2006) and Alonso and Molenberghs (2007) proposed to estimate the mutual information between both endpoints using $\widehat{I}(T,S) = \frac{1}{n}G^2$, where n is the number of patients and G^2 = log(likelihood ratio test) comparing (10.14) and (10.15).

As stated in Section 9.3, the absence of an upper bound for $I(T,S)$ hinders its interpretation and, to solve this problem, in all previous scenarios a scaled version of the mutual information was used, namely, the squared informational coefficient of correlation introduced by Linfoot (1957) and Joe (1989). However, if T has a fixed discrete distribution and if T given S is modeled by a family of discrete distributions, then the SICC is bounded above by a number strictly less than 1, even in the case where T and S are deterministically related. To illustrate this issue notice that, given the non-negative nature of entropy,

$$I(T,S) = H(T) - H(T|S) \leq H(T).$$

Furthermore, $H(T) \leq \log|\Im|$, where $\Im$ denotes the domain of T and $|\Im|$ is its cardinality, i.e., the number of elements in the range of T. The equality is obtained if and only T has a uniform distribution over $\Im$ (Cover and Tomas, 1991). The previous inequality implies $I(T,S) \leq \log|\Im|$ and, thus,

$$R^2_{h\text{indiv}} \leq 1 - \frac{1}{|\Im|^2}.$$

The upper bound reaches its minimum value when $|\Im| = 2$, i.e., when T is binary and, in this case, $R^2_{h\text{indiv}} \leq 0.75$. Kent (1983) claims that 0.75 is a reasonably high upper bound and, hence, except for very high values, the SICC can usually be interpreted without paying special attention to the discreteness of T.

Alternately, to address this upper bound problem, we will also follow Joe

(1989) and propose another scaled version of the mutual information to quantify the individual-level surrogacy, when both the surrogate and true endpoint are binary outcomes,

$$R^2_{b\text{indiv}} = \frac{I(T,S)}{\min\left[H(T), H(S)\right]}. \tag{10.17}$$

Along the lines discussed in Joe (1989), it can be shown that $R^2_{b\text{indiv}}$ is invariant under one-to-one transformations and that it always lies in the unit interval, taking value zero when T and S are independent and value one when there is a non-trivial transformation ψ so that $P\left[T = \psi(S)\right] = 1$. The entropy of T and S in the denominator of (10.17) can be estimated using the log likelihood function of the models (10.14) and (10.15), respectively. The confidence interval can be computed via bootstrap.

10.7 Case Study Analysis: Five Trials in Schizophrenia

The schizophrenia dataset combines the data that were collected in five double-blind randomized clinical trials (for details, see Section 2.2.2). In each of these trials, the efficacy of the experimental treatment risperidone was compared to an active control. Schizophrenic symptomatology was assessed using the Brief Psychiatric Rating Scale (BPRS), the Positive and Negative Syndrome Scale (PANSS), and the Clinical Global Impression (CGI). The main endpoints of interest were the change in the BPRS (= BPRS posttreatment score − BPRS baseline score), PANSS, and CGI scores. These endpoints can be analyzed as (semi)continuous normally distributed variables, but they are also often dichotomized to reflect clinically relevant change. In the latter case, the BPRS/PANSS scores are dichotomized as 1 = 20% reduction in posttreatment scores relative to baseline scores and 0 = otherwise, and CGI is dichotomized as 1 = a change of more than 3 points on the original CGI scale and 0 = otherwise. The results of the case study are discussed without reference to the software tools that can be used to conduct the analyses. Sections 13.4 and 13.5 provide details on how the analyses in the binary-binary and continuous-binary settings can be conducted in R, respectively.

The binary-binary setting

Here, it is examined whether the dichotomized BPRS is an appropriate surrogate for the dichotomized PANSS. The $\widehat{R}^2_{h\text{ind}}$ equaled 0.5392, with 95% confidence interval [0.5089; 0.5688]. The results thus indicate that the uncertainty about T = clinically relevant change on the PANSS that is reduced when S = clinically relevant change on the BPRS becomes known (individual-level surrogacy) is moderate.

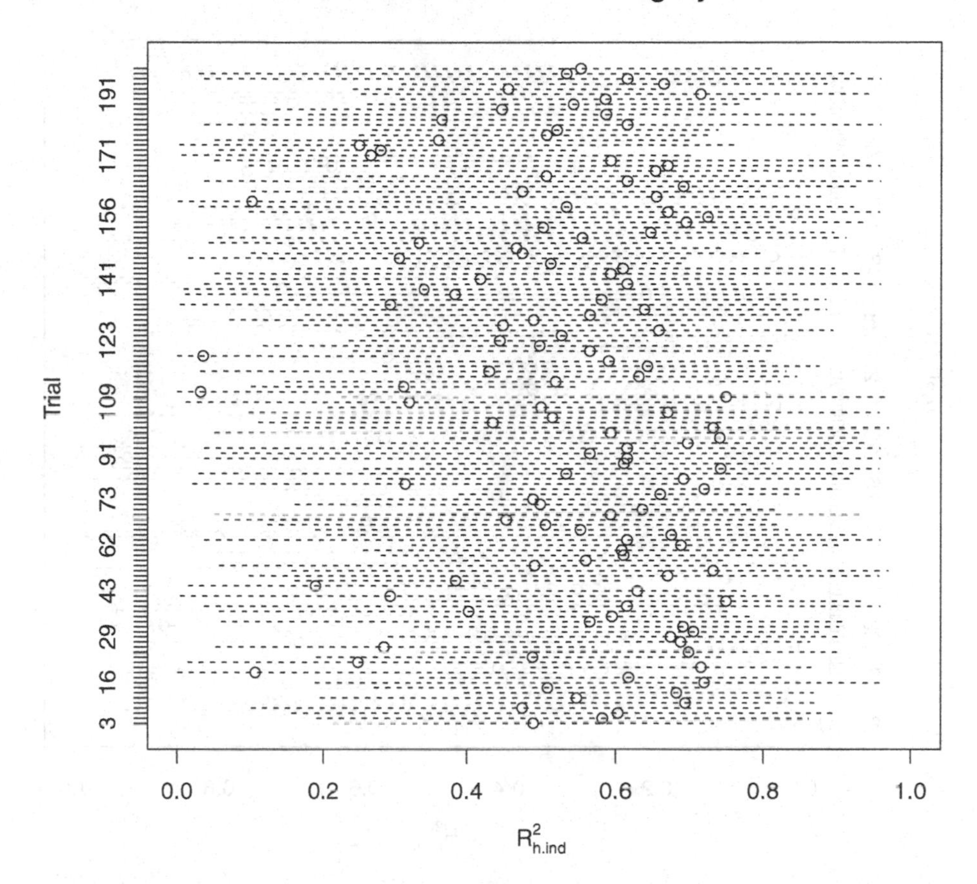

FIGURE 10.2

Schizophrenia Data. Binary-binary setting. Plot of the estimated $R^2_{h_{ind}}$ *(and their 95% confidence intervals) per cluster (treating physician) for S = clinically relevant change on the BPRS and T = clinically relevant change on the PANSS.*

Figure 10.2 shows the estimated $R^2_{h_{\text{ind}}}$ and their 95% confidence intervals for each of the clusters (treating psychiatrists) separately. As can be seen, there was substantial variability in the point estimates for $R^2_{h_{\text{ind}}}$ across clusters. Nonetheless, the 95% confidence intervals for most clusters overlapped, indicating that the individual-level surrogacy estimates were of similar magnitude for the different clusters.

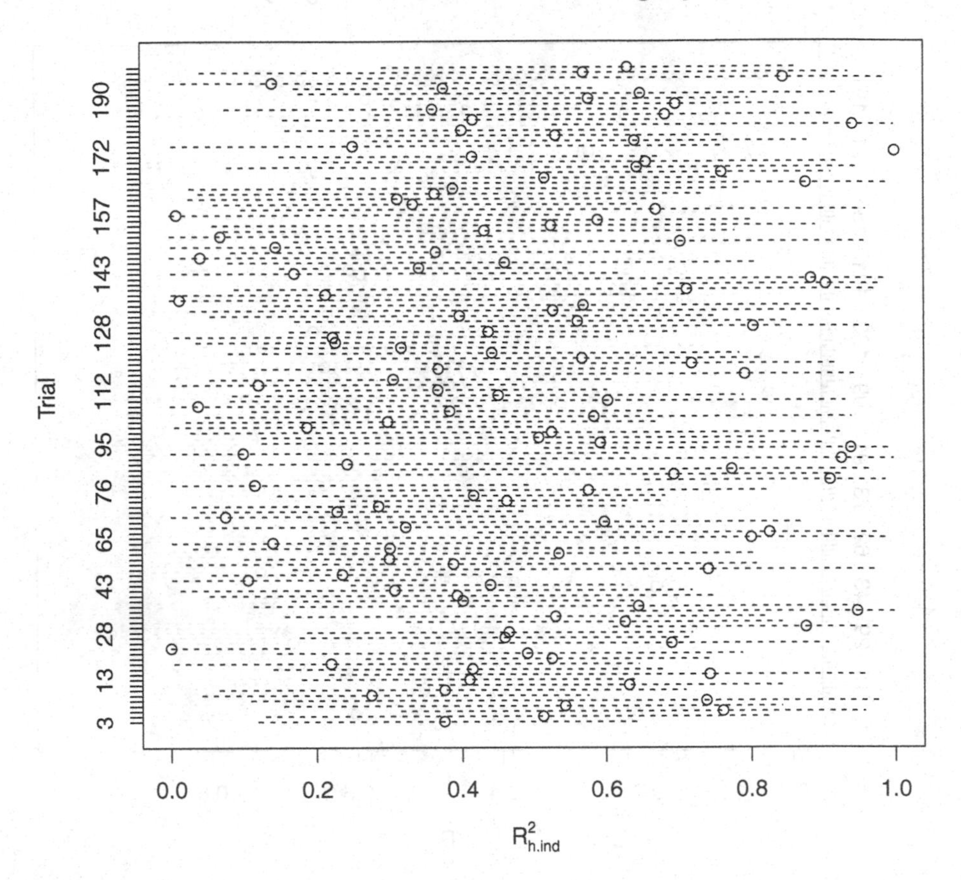

FIGURE 10.3

Schizophrenia Data. Continuous-binary setting. Plot of the estimated R^2_{hind} (and their 95% confidence intervals) per cluster (treating physician) for S = clinically relevant change on the CGI and T = PANSS.

The continuous-binary setting

Here, it is examined whether the dichotomized CGI is an appropriate surrogate for the change in PANSS scores (measurement on the original scale). The $\widehat{R}^2_{h\text{ind}}$ equaled 0.4545, with 95% confidence interval [0.4229; 0.4859]. It can thus be concluded that the uncertainty about T = change on the PANSS that is reduced when S = clinically relevant change on the CGI becomes known (individual-level surrogacy) is low to moderate.

Figure 10.3 shows the estimated $R^2_{h\text{ind}}$ (and 95% confidence intervals) in each of the clusters (treating psychiatrists). As can be seen, there was quite some variability in the point estimates for $R^2_{h\text{ind}}$ across clusters, though their

95% confidence intervals largely overlapped. This indicates that the individual-level surrogacy estimates across clusters were of the same magnitude.

11

Two Categorical Endpoints

Hannah Ensor

Biomathematics and Statistics Scotland, United Kingdom

Christopher J. Weir

University of Edinburgh, United Kingdom

CONTENTS

11.1 Introduction

In this chapter, we extend the information-theoretic approaches introduced in Chapters 9 and 10 to the general categorical outcome context, where one or both of the surrogate and true outcomes is ordinal. With categorical outcomes, computational issues come to the fore when implementing the information-theoretic approach to surrogate evaluation. We address these at the individual and trial levels in turn.

Section 11.2 covers the scenario of binary surrogate S and ordinal true endpoint T, considers relevant computational aspects, and illustrates it using a case study. Section 11.3 addresses, in a similar format, the situation where S is ordinal and T is either binary or ordinal. Concluding remarks are offered in Section 11.4.

11.2 S and T: Binary-Ordinal

11.2.1 Information-Theoretic Approach

11.2.1.1 Individual-Level Surrogacy: Binary-Ordinal

At the individual level we apply the *likelihood reduction factor* (LRF) in the same manner as in the continuous case in Chapter 9, but now G_i is based on the difference in $-2\times$log-likelihood of two proportional odds models for trial i, modeling the effect of treatment on T, with and without adjustment for S:

$$\text{logit}(P[T_{ij} \leq w]) = \mu_{T_{w_i}} + \beta_i Z_{ij}, \quad (11.1)$$
$$\text{logit}(P[T_{ij} \leq w|S_{ij}]) = \theta_{0_{w_i}} + \theta_{1i} Z_{ij} + \theta_{2i} S_{ij}. \quad (11.2)$$

Here, $w = 1, \ldots, W-1$ and W is the number of categories in the ordinal true outcome T_{ij} measured on patient j in trial i. $\mu_{T_{w_i}}$ and $\theta_{0_{w_i}}$ are intercept parameters in each trial for each cut point of the ordinal true outcome; β_i and θ_{1i} are treatment effect parameters (where Z_{ij} is the treatment group indicator) and θ_{2i} the surrogate parameter. The LRF represents the amount of information gained on the true outcome in each trial with knowledge of the surrogate.

Since (11.1) and (11.2) are based on discrete outcomes and conditional on Z, the information theory measure of individual-level surrogacy is bounded above by: $R_h^2 \leq 1 - e^{-2H(T)}$, where $H(T)$ represents the entropy of T and $H(T)$ is calculated as $E_T[-\log P(T)] = -\sum p_i \log p_i$. Hence, R_h^2 is usually rescaled (Alonso and Molenberghs, 2007):

$$\widehat{R_h^2} = \frac{R_h^2}{1 - e^{-2H(T)}}. \tag{11.3}$$

11.2.1.2 Trial-Level Surrogacy: Binary-Ordinal Setting

A two-stage approach to determining trial-level surrogacy enables the computational issues, such as those illustrated in Section 11.2.2, to be overcome. In stage one, a generalized linear model is fitted to the binary S regressed on treatment Z separately for each trial i, as in (11.4). Similarly, a proportional odds model is fitted, for each trial i, to the ordinal T regressed on treatment Z in (11.5). This estimates the trial-specific treatment effects β_i and α_i:

$$\text{logit}[P(S_{ij}] = \mu_{Si} + \alpha_i Z_{ij}, \tag{11.4}$$

$$\text{logit}[P(T_{ij} \leq w)] = \mu_{T_{w_i}} + \beta_i Z_{ij}, \tag{11.5}$$

where $w = 1, \ldots, W-1$; W is the number of categories in T, $\mu_{T_{w_i}}$ is the set of intercept parameters for each of the $W-1$ cut points of T; and all other parameters are the same as in the continuous case (Section 10.2).

In stage two, the estimates of the trial-specific treatment effects β_i and α_i are regressed on each other to estimate R_{ht}^2:

$$\widehat{\beta_i} = \gamma_0 + \gamma_1 \widehat{\mu_{Si}} + \gamma_2 \widehat{\alpha_i}, \tag{11.6}$$

$$LRF = \widehat{R_{ht}^2} = 1 - \exp\left(-\frac{G^2}{N_T}\right). \tag{11.7}$$

In (11.7), N_T is the total sample size across all trials. G^2, the difference in $-2\times$log-likelihood between (11.6) and a null (intercept only) model, can be calculated and the LRF applied as in (11.7) to estimate R_{ht}^2.

11.2.1.3 Confidence Intervals

The standard approach to confidence interval estimation introduced in Chapter 4 also applies in this context, although the rescaling that takes place for individual-level surrogacy (11.3) also needs to be applied to the individual-level confidence intervals.

11.2.2 Computational Aspects

11.2.2.1 Separation: Categorical Variables

Where separation or quasi-complete separation of categorical variables occur, no unique maximum likelihood estimates exist.

TABLE 11.1
No separation.

		Treatment	Placebo
Surrogate	Y	$A \neq 0$	$B \neq 0$
	N	$C \neq 0$	$D \neq 0$

TABLE 11.2
Complete separation.

		Treatment	Placebo
Surrogate	Y	$A \neq 0$	0
	N	0	$D \neq 0$

11.2.2.2 Separation: Binary Variables

Let us consider the case of two binary variables, for example, where a binary surrogate S is regressed on a binary treatment variable Z, as in (11.4). Complete and quasi-complete separation relate to the existence of empty cells in the cross-tabulation of S and Z. Table 11.1 shows no separation, as there are no empty cells. Table 11.2 gives an example of complete separation, when the binary variable Z perfectly predicts S. Table 11.3 illustrates quasi-complete separation, as one table cell is empty.

For complete or quasi-complete separation, the likelihood has no maximum, although it is bounded above by a number less than zero (Allison, 2008). For two binary variables we estimate the log-odds ratio φ as

$$\widehat{\varphi} = \log\left(\frac{A \cdot D}{B \cdot C}\right). \tag{11.8}$$

Here, we can see that if a zero occurs in the denominator but not in the numerator, then $\widehat{\varphi} = +\infty$; if a zero occurs in the numerator but not in the denominator, then $\widehat{\varphi} = -\infty$. Both are limiting cases. If a zero value occurs in both, then φ is undefined.

11.2.2.3 Separation: Ordinal Variables

At the first stage of calculating R^2_{ht}, we model ordinal T on binary Z for each trial, as in (11.5). Separation can also occur in this circumstance, with the same consequences as in the binary case. Imagine that we collapse the categories of an ordinal variable into a binary variable at each possible threshold. For each collapse in which one or more of the cells in the binary cross-tabulation is zero, quasi-complete separation exists (Agresti, 2014).

In Table 11.4, dichotomizing the seven-point scale into binary groups at

TABLE 11.3
Quasi-complete separation.

		Treatment	Placebo
Surrogate	Y	$A \neq 0$	$B \neq 0$
	N	$C \neq 0$	0

TABLE 11.4
Quasi-complete separation for an ordinal variable. A_1, A_2, B_1, C_1, D_1, E_1, F_1, and G_1 are all greater than zero.

1	2	3	4	5	6	7
A_1	B_1	C_1	D_1	E_1	F_1	G_1
A_2	$B_2 = 0$	0	0	0	0	0

any threshold would result in a cross-tabulation containing an empty cell, similar to the quasi-complete separation seen in Table 11.3. However, if $B_2 \neq 0$ in Table 11.4, dichotomizing at 1 would give a similar pattern to Table 11.1. In this case, since dichotomization at one or more thresholds gives no separation, there is no quasi-complete separation.

An ordinal variable may also have quasi-complete separation if there "exists a pair of rows for which all observations on one row never fall above any observation in the other row" (Agresti, 2014); see Table 11.5.

11.2.2.4 Impact of Separation on Surrogate Evaluation

When complete or quasi-complete separation occurs, this typically causes problems with maximum likelihood estimation for generalized linear models. The typical scenario (Allison, 2008) is that the model-fitting algorithm goes through several iterations, while attempting to converge. Upon each iteration the affected parameter estimate increases and this continues until a fixed iteration limit is exceeded. At this point the parameter estimate will typically be large and its standard error very large. Statistical software generally does not highlight this issue via error messages.

At the first stage of trial-level surrogacy estimation, two binary (S, Z) or an ordinal and a binary variable (T, Z) are regressed on one another for each trial in (11.4) and (11.5). This returns treatment effect estimates on the binary surrogate and ordinal true outcome. However, separation causes outlying data points at stage 2, where the effects of treatment on T are regressed on those on S as in (11.6). The LRF (11.7) is then based on a model with potentially highly influential outliers. This leads to unreliable estimation of R^2_{ht}, with a tendency to underestimate the true value.

TABLE 11.5

Quasi-complete separation example for an ordinal variable. A_1, B_1, C_1, D_1, D_2, E_2, F_2, and G_2 are all greater than zero.

1	2	3	4	5	6	7
A_1	B_1	C_1	D_1	0	0	0
0	0	0	D_2	E_2	F_2	G_2

11.2.2.5 Solution to Separation Issues

Without correction for separation, the trials where separation occurs would need to be removed from analysis to avoid the bias in estimating R^2_{ht} previously mentioned. This would lead to large loss of information where many trials are small and therefore prone to separation.

An alternative, more promising solution to the issue of separation is the use of penalized maximum likelihood (Firth, 1993). Although originally introduced to reduce small sample bias in maximum likelihood estimates, it has been found to be useful in dealing with separation (Heinze and Schemper, 2002). Firth (1993) found that bias occurred in estimates when trying to derive the score function (first derivative of the log-likelihood), which has no maximum in the case of separation, and suggested adding a bias term to the score function to resolve this.

Heinze and Schemper (2002) applied the technique of Firth (1993) to deal with separation. The bias term they applied to the score function was based on the information matrix of the parameter affected by separation, and produces finite parameter estimates that are superior to uncorrected estimates.

11.2.2.6 Separation: Final Considerations

Firth's approach works best for small samples: to calculate the Firth-corrected estimate of R^2_{ht}, models for each trial will need to be fitted rather than full models incorporating all trials. In the case of complete or quasi-separation, parameter estimates but not values of the log-likelihood function are affected, hence individual-level surrogacy, which does not rely on parameter estimation, can be determined without using penalized likelihood.

Penalized likelihood may be implemented for generalized linear models using the `logistf` command in the `logistf` R package. There is also a command available to provide this bias reduction for cumulative logit models called `pordlogist` in package `OrdinalLogisticBiplot` (Sanchez and Vicente-Villardon, 2013). This uses a similar penalized likelihood technique to Firth (1993) based on le Cessie and Van Houwelingen (1992). `pordlogist` does however fail where empty cells are present in both treatment arms for any outcome category.

11.2.3 Surrogate Package: Binary-Ordinal Setting

In the `Surrogate` package, the function `FixedDiscrDiscrIT()` investigates surrogacy where both the surrogate and true outcome are ordinal or one is ordinal and the other binary. This function estimates both trial- and individual-level surrogacy using the fixed-effects information theory approach summarized in this chapter.

11.2.3.1 Case Study Analysis: Five Trials in Schizophrenia

In this analysis of the Schizophrenia dataset (introduced in Section 2.2.2), we investigate the dichotomized Positive and Negative Syndrome Scale (PANSS) change score as a possible surrogate for Clinical Global Impression (CGI, an ordinal measure of the change in schizophrenia symptoms on a seven-point scale). Hence, we evaluate binary S for an ordinal T. PANSS change was dichotomized according to convention as 1: an improvement of 20% or more in the PANSS score from beginning to end of treatment, and 0: otherwise. Lower CGI scores represent an improved psychiatric outcome. We would therefore anticipate a negative association between the binary PANSS surrogate and the ordinal CGI.

The Schizophrenia dataset includes five trials - too few to use as the clustering unit in surrogacy evaluation – and so the 198 treating physicians were instead considered as "trials" in the analysis (see Section 2.2.2). As in other settings, observations are deleted if any outcome has a missing value; and if only one treatment group exists for a particular trial, then that trial cannot be included in the calculation of R_h^2 or R_{ht}^2. Occasionally models may fail at either level due to very small trial size, again leading to exclusion of a trial. In the current analysis, 47 clusters have only one treatment group and there is further model failure in nine very small trials for R_h^2 and in one trial for R_{ht}^2. Therefore, 141 trials are included in calculating R_h^2 and 150 in R_{ht}^2. Among trials included in the analysis, there are 88 instances of separation in the trials for binary PANSS and 63 instances for ordinal CGI. These trials are retained in the analysis thanks to the use of penalized likelihood in model estimation.

At the trial level, $R_{ht}^2 = 0.45$ with 95% confidence interval [0.32; 0.59], indicating that little uncertainty in the treatment effect on CGI is removed through knowledge of binary PANSS. Figure 11.1 illustrates this moderate strength of relationship between treatment effects on the binary PANSS and ordinal CGI. At the individual level, $R_h^2 = 0.46$ with 95% confidence interval [0.10; 0.82]. The reduction in uncertainty about CGI through knowledge of binary PANSS is again limited. The wide confidence intervals for R_h^2 demonstrate diminished certainty in the findings due to the loss of information in the binary PANSS versus its continuous counterpart. Overall, a binary interpretation of PANSS does not have strong legitimacy as a surrogate for the ordinal CGI measure. Full details of how to run the above analysis in the `Surrogate` package in R, including the relevant commands, function arguments, and software output, may be found in Chapter 13.

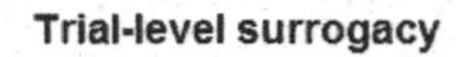

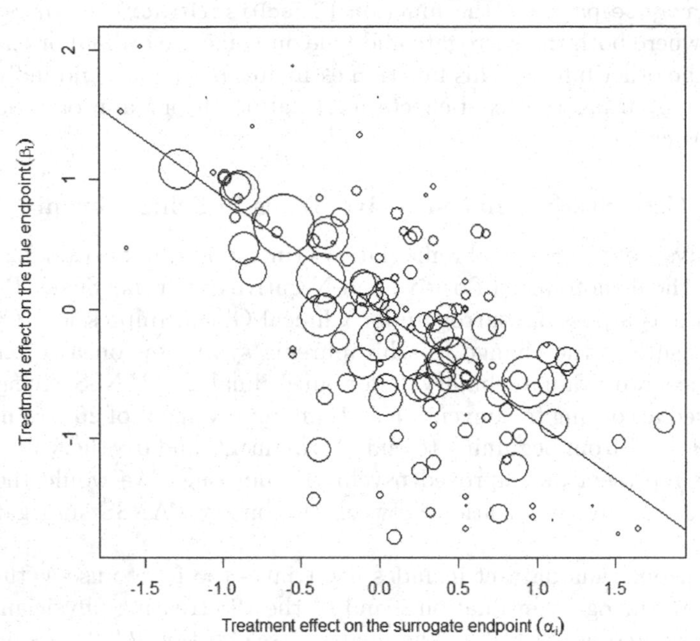

FIGURE 11.1
Assessing trial-level surrogacy of binary PANSS change for the ordinal CGI true outcome. Treatment effects are log-odds ratios.

11.2.4 Summary: Binary-Ordinal Setting

The preceding sections demonstrate that despite the additional computational problems associated with binary and ordinal outcomes in relatively small trials, the information-theoretic approach may be readily applied to binary S and ordinal T with the aid of the penalized likelihood technique. This in turn may be easily implemented in the `Surrogate` R package.

11.3 S and T: Ordinal-Binary or Ordinal-Ordinal

11.3.1 Information-Theoretic Approach

11.3.1.1 Individual-Level Surrogacy: Ordinal-Binary or Ordinal-Ordinal Settings

For the extension to the case of an ordinal S and binary T, we replace (11.1) and (11.2) with two logistic regression models, for each trial i, as the response variable is binary:

$$\begin{aligned}\text{logit}[P(T_{ij})] &= \mu_i + \beta_i Z_{ij}, &(11.9)\\ \text{logit}[P(T_{ij}|S_{ij})] &= \theta_{0i} + \theta_{1i} Z_{ij} + \theta_{2i} S_{ij}. &(11.10)\end{aligned}$$

For the situation of ordinal S and ordinal T, the proportional odds models of (11.1) and (11.2) would again be used. In each of these, the ordinal surrogate may be modeled in one of two ways. The first, as represented in (11.10), is to treat S as if it were continuous. The alternative would be to model S as a factor using dummy variables, but this ignores the ordering of the categories of the surrogate and is not parsimonious. Hence, modeling the ordinal surrogate as an interval scale variable is preferable.

At the individual level we apply the *likelihood reduction factor* (LRF) as before, basing G_i on the difference in $-2\times$log-likelihood of (11.9) and (11.10) for ordinal S, binary T, and (11.1) and (11.2) for ordinal S and ordinal T. As T is discrete, the individual-level R_h^2 is bounded above by $1 - e^{-2H(T)}$ and should again be rescaled (Alonso and Molenberghs, 2007) using (11.3).

11.3.1.2 Trial-Level Surrogacy: Ordinal-Binary or Ordinal-Ordinal Settings

The only substantial difference in modeling the ordinal-binary and ordinal-ordinal settings, compared to the binary-ordinal setting, is in the way intercepts are handled. With an ordinal surrogate, the first-stage models (11.11)–(11.12) return one intercept for each cut-point on the ordinal surrogate. These intercepts are then averaged for use in the penalized likelihood approach of the second stage, as described in detail in Section 11.3.2.

11.3.2 Computational Aspects

11.3.2.1 Separation: Ordinal-Binary/Ordinal Setting

Separation causes the same problems for ordinal S as for binary S and ordinal T, but the penalized likelihood technique again offers a solution. As the currently available penalized likelihood software for ordinal outcomes cannot handle the large datasets and hierarchical data structures we need to use, for each trial i, separate models of S and T are regressed on treatment Z in stage one of trial-level estimation:

$$\begin{aligned}\text{logit}[P(S_{ij} \leq v)] &= \mu_{S_{v_i}} + \alpha_i Z_{ij}, &(11.11)\\ \text{logit}[P(T_{ij})] &= \mu_{T_i} + \beta_i Z_{ij}, &(11.12)\end{aligned}$$

where $v = 1, \ldots, V-1$; V is the number of categories in the ordinal true outcome; $\mu_{S_{v_i}}$ is the set of intercept parameters for each of the $V-1$ cut-points on the ordinal surrogate outcome in trial i; and all other parameters are the same as in the continuous case.

For the information-theoretic approach, the second-stage model (11.6) can be replaced with the following model, using all the surrogate intercept variables of (11.11):

$$\widehat{\beta}_i = \rho_0 + \rho_1 \overline{\mu_{S_{1i}}} + \rho_2 \overline{\mu_{S_{2i}}} + \cdots + \rho_{V-1} \overline{\mu_{S_{(V-1)i}}} + \rho_S \widehat{\alpha}_i. \tag{11.13}$$

Here, $\overline{\mu_{S_{1i}}}, \ldots, \overline{\mu_{S_{(V-1)i}}}$ are the intercept variables for each cut-point modeled alongside a treatment effect estimate, $\widehat{\alpha}_i$. However, we can see that in the case of few trials, this model would lead to over-fitting. One way to resolve this would be to calculate the mean intercept value for each trial over all cut-points to give a single estimate of the intercept for each trial, $\overline{\mu_{S_{v_i}}}$. Then the stage 2 model of trial-level surrogacy would become:

$$\widehat{\beta}_i = \gamma_0 + \gamma_1 \overline{\mu_{S_{v_i}}} + \gamma_2 \widehat{\alpha}_i. \tag{11.14}$$

The difference in $-2\times$log-likelihood between (11.14) and a null (intercept only) model can be used to determine the LRF (11.7) and estimate R^2_{ht}.

11.3.3 Summary: Ordinal-Binary or Ordinal-Ordinal Setting

Only two additional considerations are required where S is ordinal. First, for individual-level surrogacy, one must define how the surrogate is handled as a covariate in a generalized linear model. We recommend that treating it as a continuous measure is preferable to comparing a series of dummy variables to a reference category. The second change, which is required for evaluating trial-level surrogacy, is to derive a single intercept estimate $\overline{\mu_{S_{v_i}}}$ which summarizes the multiple intercepts generated in the proportional odds modeling for the various cut points in the ordinal outcome. As in Section 11.2, penalized likelihood may be used to correct for any bias due to occurrences of separation.

11.4 Concluding Remarks

We have outlined the extension of the information-theoretic approach to categorical surrogate and true outcomes. This was done without using joint modeling of the surrogate and true outcomes, thus avoiding additional computational complexities. The penalized likelihood approach provides an effective solution to prevent problems of bias due to separation or quasi-separation of categorical outcomes. As penalized likelihood does not readily handle large or hierarchically structured datasets, it may be implemented instead by separate modeling of the data for each trial.

hierarchically structured data—[illegible] by separate
modelling of the data [illegible]

Part III

Software Tools

12

SAS Software

Theophile Bigirumurame

Hasselt University, Belgium

Ziv Shkedy

Hasselt University, Belgium

Tomasz Burzykowski

Hasselt University, Belgium, and IDDI, Belgium

CONTENTS

12.1 Introduction

A set of SAS macros was developed for the analysis presented in previous chapters. Tables 12.1 and 12.2 present the different surrogacy settings and models implemented in the SAS macros. Most of the surrogacy settings presented in Tables 12.1 and 12.2 were discussed previously in the book but some of the settings will be presented in this chapter for the first time. The use of each SAS macro is illustrated using a case study for a specific setting and a reference to a section in the book in which the surrogacy setting is presented is given whenever relevant.

The SAS macros presented in this chapter do not require the user to formulate a model in SAS, but rather to specify a surrogacy setting, and the macro then automatically formulates the model in SAS. However, for readers who wish to get deeper insight about the models and SAS procedures behind the macros, an equivalent analysis in which the explicit SAS procedure for a surrogacy setting of interest is given as well.

12.2 General Structure of the SAS Macros Available for the Analysis of Surrogate Endpoints

The SAS macros, developed for the analysis presented in the book, have the same general form. Depending on the surrogacy setting, the macros require the user to prepare a dataset with a specific structure. Note that different macros require different dataset structures. A generic call of a surrogacy SAS macro has the following form:

```
% macroname (data=,true=,surrog=,trial=,treatment=,patid=,
            optional-arguments)
```

The following arguments are used in all macros:

- `data`: a dataset containing one record per patient with measurements for both the true and the surrogate endpoints.
- `true`: a measurement of the true endpoint.
- `surrog`: a measurement of the surrogate endpoint.
- `treatment`: treatment indicator variable (1= active, -1=control).
- `trial`: the unit of the study for which trial-level surrogacy will be estimated.
- `patid`: the patient's identification number.
- `optional-arguments`: optional arguments that should be provided to conduct a specific analysis (for example, the leave-one-out trial analysis or the exploratory plots); all of this will be discussed further in Section 12.3.1.

Graphical and numerical outputs are customized in such a way that users only see relevant information, depending on the surrogacy setting. Note that the standard SAS output tables are not produced and that it is recommended to check the SAS log window for possible problems.

For the remainder of the chapter we present different surrogacy settings and their corresponding macros, case studies, and output. Note that, for some surrogacy settings, the models are only briefly presented and we refer to the relevant section elsewhere in the book, where the necessary technical details and model formulations are presented and explained.

12.3 Validation of Surrogacy Using a Joint Modeling Approach for Two Normally Distributed Endpoints

In this section, we present SAS macros for the setting in which both endpoints are continuous. For all models discussed in this section the age-related macular degeneration (ARMD) data is used for illustration. Visual acuity at week 52 (`Diff52`) and visual acuity at week 24 (`Diff24`) are the true and the surrogate endpoints, respectively. Each line in the data contains information about one patient. A partial print of the data is shown in Figure 12.1.

TABLE 12.1
SAS macros available for the evaluation of surrogate endpoints in randomized clinical trials. Part I.

Surrogacy Setting	Macro name	Model	Surrogacy measures	Chapter 12	Rest of the book	Case study
1. Normal/Normal	CONTCONTFULL	Full fixed	R^2_{trial}, R^2_{indiv}	12.3.1	4.3.1	ARMD data
	CONTCONTRED	Reduced fixed	R^2_{trial}, R^2_{indiv}	12.3.2	4.3.2	True endpoint= Diff52
	CONTRANFULL	Full random	R^2_{trial}, R^2_{indiv}	12.3.3	4.2	Surrogate endpoint=Diff24
	CONTRANRED	Reduced random	R^2_{trial}, R^2_{indiv}	12.3.4	4.3.2	
2. Survival/Survival	TWOSTAGEKM	Two-stage	R^2_{indiv}	12.4.1		Ovarian data
	TWOSTAGECOX	Two-stage	R^2_{trial}	12.4.2	13.3	True endpoint= OS
	COPULA	joint model	R^2_{trial}, R^2_{indiv}	12.4.3	5.2	Surrogate endpoint=PFS
3. Survival/Binary	SURVBIN	Joint model	R^2_{trial}, Gl. odds	12.5	6.2	Colorectal data True endpoint=OS Surrogate endpoint=Remission
4. Survival/Normal	NORMSURV	Two-stage model	Kendall's τ R^2_{trial}	12.7	Ch. 7	Prostate cancer True endpoint=OS Surrogate endpoint=ln(PSA)
5. Normal/Binary	NORMALBIN	Joint model Normal-binary	R^2_{trial}, R^2_{indiv}	12.7		Schizo data True endpoint=PANSS Surrogate endpoint=CGI

TABLE 12.2
SAS macros available for the evaluation of surrogate endpoints in randomized clinical trials. Part II.

Surrogacy Setting	Macro name	Model	Surrogacy measures	Chapter 12	Rest of the book	Case study
6. Binary/Binary	`BINBIN`	Bivariate probit	R^2_{trial}, R^2_{indiv}	12.8		Schizo data True endpoint=CGI Surrogate endpoint=PANSS
7. Survival/Binary	`SURVBINIT` `SURVBININFO`	Information theory	R^2_{ht}, R^2_h	12.9		Colorectal data True endpoint=OS Surrogate endpoint=Remission
8. Normal/Binary	`NORMBINIT`	Information theory	R^2_{ht}, R^2_h	12.9	10.6	Schizo data True endpoint=PANSS Surrogate endpoint=CGI
9. Binary/Binary	`BINBINIT`	Information theory	R^2_{ht}, R^2_h	12.9	10.6	Schizo data True endpoint=CGI Surrogate endpoint=PANSS
10. Normal/Normal	`NORMNORMIT`	Information theory	R^2_{ht}, R^2_h	12.9	13.2.2.1 10.2	ARMD data True endpoint=Diff52 Surrogate endpoint=Diff24

Obs	Id	Center	Treat	Diff24	Diff52
1	1	13395	1	0	-10
2	2	13395	-1	-3	1
3	3	13396	1	-6	-17
4	4	13396	-1	8	1
5	5	13396	-1	-2	-2
6	6	13396	1	-5	-1
7	7	13745	1	-19	-22
8	8	13745	1	2	17
9	9	13745	-1	3	0
10	10	13746	1	2	3

FIGURE 12.1
Data snapshot for some patients, when the true and the surrogate endpoints are normally distributed.

12.3.1 The Full Fixed-Effects Model

12.3.1.1 Model Formulation

The two-stage approach for two normally distributed endpoints was discussed in Chapter 4. Briefly, the first stage consists of a joint model for the surrogate and true endpoints given by

$$\begin{cases} S_{ij} = \mu_{Si} + \alpha_i Z_{ij} + \varepsilon_{Sij}, \\ T_{ij} = \mu_{Ti} + \beta_i Z_{ij} + \varepsilon_{Tij}, \end{cases} \tag{12.1}$$

where μ_{Si} and μ_{Ti} are trial-specific intercepts for S and T, α_i and β_i are trial-specific treatment effects on the surrogate and the true endpoint, respectively. The error terms, ε_{Sij} and ε_{Tij}, are bivariate normally distributed with zero mean and covariance matrix given by

$$\Sigma = \begin{pmatrix} \sigma_{SS} & \sigma_{ST} \\ & \sigma_{TT} \end{pmatrix}. \tag{12.2}$$

As pointed out in Chapter 4, individual-level surrogacy is assessed by the squared correlation between S and T after adjusting for trial-specific treat-

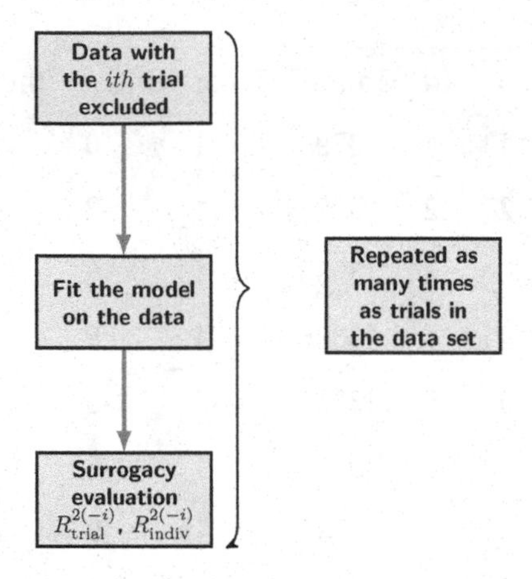

FIGURE 12.2
A leave-one-out evaluation procedure.

ment effects, that is,

$$R^2_{\text{indiv}} = \frac{\sigma^2_{ST}}{\sigma_{SS}\sigma_{TT}}. \tag{12.3}$$

For the full fixed-effects model, the trial-level surrogacy is estimated using the coefficient of determination obtained by fitting the following model:

$$\widehat{\beta}_i = \lambda_0 + \lambda_1 \widehat{\mu}_{Si} + \lambda_2 \widehat{\alpha}_i + \varepsilon_i, \tag{12.4}$$

where $\widehat{\beta}_i$, $\widehat{\mu}_{Si}$, and $\widehat{\alpha}_i$ are the parameter estimates obtained from the joint model specified in (12.1). A weighted analysis, which takes into account the sample size in each trial (see also Section 4.3.4), can be used as well. The standard error for R^2_{indiv} and R^2_{trial} can be calculated using the delta method.

12.3.1.2 Sensitivity Analysis: Leave-One-Out Evaluation

The surrogacy measures estimated in the previous section are derived using all units in the study (i.e., all trials, centers, etc.). To check the stability of the estimated measures, we propose to use a "leave-one-out" evaluation procedure as a sensitivity analysis approach. It is an iterative procedure in which at each iteration, one trial is left out and the surrogacy measures are estimated using the remaining trials in the data. The procedure is shown in Figure 12.2. At the end of the run, parameter estimates for both R^2_{trial} and R^2_{indiv} are obtained for each trial and influential trials can be identified.

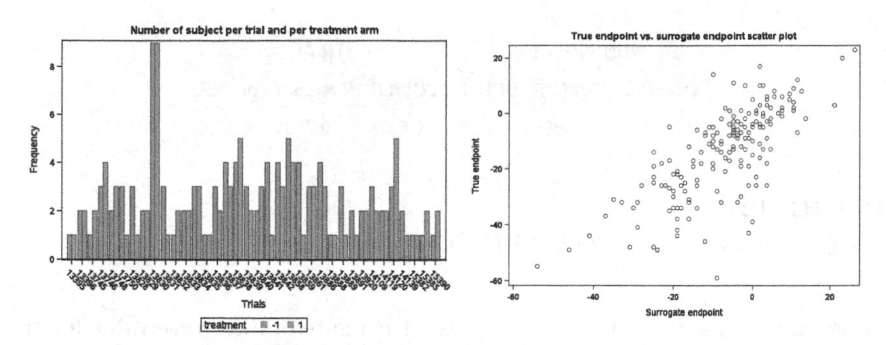

FIGURE 12.3
Age-Related Macular Degeneration Trial. Descriptive plots. Left panel: Patient distribution in the trials by treatment arm. Right panel: Scatter plot between the true and the surrogate endpoints.

12.3.1.3 The SAS Macro %CONTCONTFULL

The SAS macro %CONTCONTFULL can be used to conduct the analysis for a setting with two normally distributed endpoints using the full fixed-effects model. The following macro call is used:

```
%CONTCONTFULL(data=armd,true=diff52,surrog=diff24,trt=treat,
              trial=center,patid=patientId,weighted=1,
              looa=1)
```

The optional arguments that we use are:

- `weighted`: an option which allows the use of weighted regression (weighted=1) in the computation of the trial-level surrogacy. The number of patients in the trial is used as the weight.
- `looa`: an option to perform a leave-one-trial-out analysis (looa=1). Both surrogacy measures are computed by leaving each one of the trials out, so as to check the influence of the trial on the surrogacy measures.

12.3.1.4 Data Analysis and Output

The macro %CONTCONTFULL produces default numerical and graphical output. The first part of the output, shown in Figure 12.3, consists of two descriptive plots, which show the distribution of the patients in the trials by treatment arm (Figure 12.3, left panel) and a scatter plot between the true and the surrogate endpoints (Figure 12.3, right panel).

As shown in Figure 12.4, for the ARMD study, individual and trial-level surrogacy are equal, respectively, to R^2_{indiv} = 0.4866 (0.3814, 0.5919) and R^2_{trial} = 0.7031 (0.5333, 0.8730). Both surrogacy measures indicate that the

INDIVIDUAL			TRIAL		
LOWER	Individual	UPPER	LOWER	R square	UPPER
0.3814	0.4866	0.5919	0.5333	0.7031	0.8730

FIGURE 12.4
Surrogacy measures with their 95% confidence intervals (C.I.).

change in visual acuity after 24 weeks is a surrogate of moderate value for the visual acuity at 52 weeks after starting the interferon treatment.

The results for the leave-one-out sensitivity analysis are presented in Figure 12.5. Note how the value of R^2_{trial} is dropping when center 13830 is left out ($R^{2(-13830)}_{\text{trial}} = 0.6295$). We can see in Figure 12.3 (left panel) that this center is the one with highest number of patients in both treatment arms. Leaving out this center has an impact on the estimated trial-level surrogacy, since it has the highest weight.

A table containing the surrogacy measures estimated using the leave-one-out sensitivity analysis is presented in Figure 12.6.

12.3.1.5 SAS Code for the First Step

Although not visible to the users, the analysis implemented in the `%CONTCONTFULL` macro is based on procedure MIXED. In this section we discuss in more detail the implementation of the joint model specified in (12.1) in SAS. Using procedure MIXED, the following code can be used to fit the joint model in (12.1).

```
proc mixed data=dataset covtest;
class endp patid trial;
model outcome = endp*trial endp*treat*trial / solution noint;
repeated endp / type=un subject=patid(trial);
ods output solutionF=eb CovParms=covar;
run;
```

The above code presumes that there are two records per subject in the input dataset, one corresponding to the surrogate endpoint and the other to the true endpoint. The variable `endp` (endpoint) is an indicator variable for the endpoint (coded -1 for surrogate and 1 for true endpoint), the variable `outcome` contains measurements obtained from each endpoint and the variable `treat` is assumed to be $-1/1$ coded (Burzykowski, Molenberghs, and Buyse, 2005).

The `REPEATED` statement is used for the estimation of the residual covariance matrix Σ in (12.2). For the mean structure, the interaction term `endp*trial` in the model statement allows us to fit trial-specific intercepts on both endpoints while the three-way interaction `endp*treat*trial` produces the trial-specific treatment effects on both endpoints.

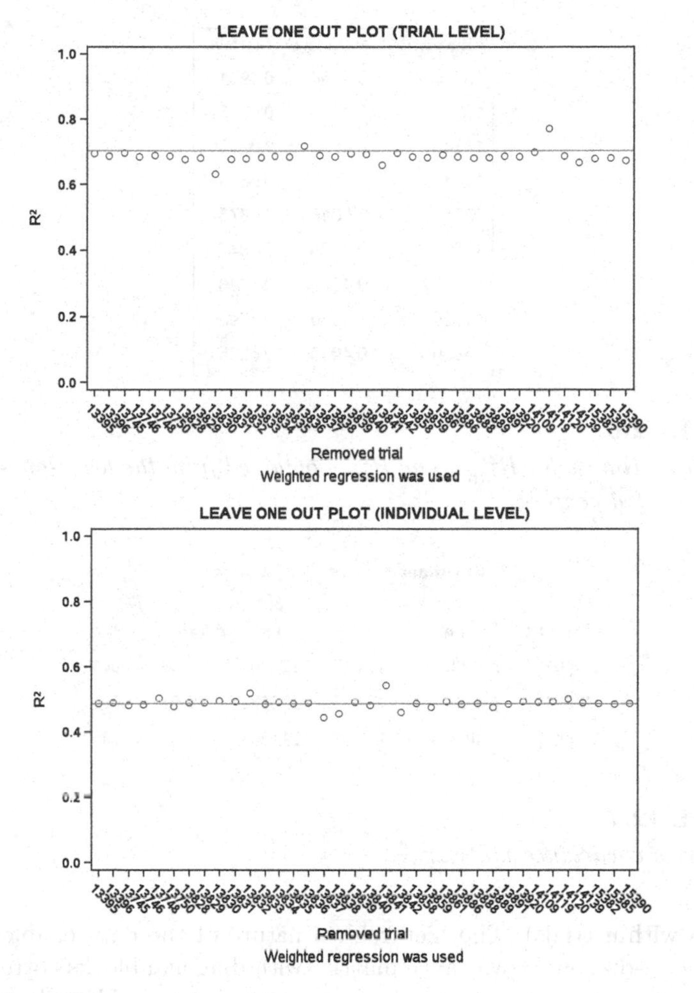

FIGURE 12.5
Age-Related Macular Degeneration Trial. Sensitivity analysis. Top panel: trial-level surrogacy. Bottom panel: individual-level surrogacy.

The options `solutionF` and `CovParms` in the `ODS OUTPUT` statement allow to output datasets containing the fixed-effects estimates and the errors covariance matrix, respectively, for further analysis. The estimated covariance matrix is shown in Figure 12.7. Individual-level surrogacy measure is estimated by

$$\widehat{R}^2_{\text{indiv}} = \frac{133.26^2}{166.77 \times 218.80} = 0.4866. \tag{12.5}$$

Note that the nesting notation in the `subject=patid(trial)` option is necessary for SAS to recognize the nested structure of the data (subjects are

Removed trial	Indiv. level	Trial level
13395	0.4866	0.6931
13396	0.4892	0.6845
13745	0.4806	0.6946
13746	0.4825	0.6838
13748	0.5015	0.6875
13750	0.4765	0.6845
13828	0.4879	0.6748
13829	0.4880	0.6798
13830	0.4940	0.6295

FIGURE 12.6
Parameter estimate for R^2_{indiv} and R^2_{trial} obtained from the leave-one-out analysis for selected centers.

Covariance Parameter Estimates					
Cov Parm	Subject	Estimate	Standard Error	Z Value	Pr Z
UN(1,1)	patid(trial)	166.77	22.5903	7.38	<.0001
UN(2,1)	patid(trial)	133.26	22.3088	5.97	<.0001
UN(2,2)	patid(trial)	218.80	29.6383	7.38	<.0001

FIGURE 12.7
Error terms covariance matrix.

clustered within trials). The hierarchical nature of the data enables SAS to build a block-diagonal covariance matrix, with diagonal blocks corresponding to the different trials, which speeds up computations considerably.

12.3.1.6 SAS Code for the Second Step

The second-stage model, from which trial-level surrogacy is estimated, is based on procedure `REG`.

```
proc reg data=secondstage;
model true=surrinterc surrogate;
weight n;
ods output FitStatistics=rsq;
run;
```

Here, `true` is the parameter estimate for the treatment effect on the true endpoint ($\widehat{\beta}_i$), `surrinterc`, and `surrogate` are the parameter estimates for trial-specific intercept ($\widehat{\mu}_{S_i}$) and treatment effects ($\widehat{\alpha}_i$) on the surrogate endpoint,

Root MSE	10.17175	R-Square	0.7031
Dependent Mean	-2.23029	Adj R-Sq	0.6851
Coeff Var	-456.07202		

Parameter Estimates					
Variable	DF	Parameter Estimate	Standard Error	t Value	Pr > |t|
Intercept	1	-0.21941	1.17985	-0.19	0.8536
Surrinterc	1	0.06588	0.13236	0.50	0.6220
Surr	1	1.17595	0.13671	8.60	<.0001

FIGURE 12.8
SAS output for the second-stage model.

respectively. The statement `WEIGHT n;` is used to account for the variability in trial sizes as discussed in Section 12.3.1.

SAS output from the second-stage model is shown in Figure 12.8. The estimated regression line is $\widehat{\beta}_i = -0.22 + 0.07\widehat{\mu_{S_i}} + 1.18\widehat{\alpha}_i$ with the trial-level surrogacy $\widehat{R}^2_{\text{trial(f)}} = 0.7031$.

12.3.2 The Reduced Fixed-Effects Model

12.3.2.1 Model Formulation

The reduced fixed-effects model approach assumes common intercepts for S and T in (12.1). Hence, trial-specific μ_{Si} and μ_{Ti} are replaced by μ_S and μ_T, respectively. The full fixed-effects model in (12.1) can be rewritten as

$$\begin{cases} S_{ij} = \mu_S + \alpha_i Z_{ij} + \varepsilon_{Sij}, \\ T_{ij} = \mu_T + \beta_i Z_{ij} + \varepsilon_{Tij}. \end{cases} \tag{12.6}$$

The term $\widehat{\mu}_{S_i}$ is dropped from the second-stage model, which implies that trial-level surrogacy is assessed using the coefficient of determination obtained for the model

$$\widehat{\beta}_i = \lambda_0 + \lambda_1 \widehat{\alpha}_i + \varepsilon_i. \tag{12.7}$$

Individual-level surrogacy can be assessed using the adjusted association in (12.3).

12.3.2.2 The SAS Macro %CONTCONTRED

The SAS macro `%CONTCONTRED` can be used to fit the reduced joint model specified in (12.6). For the ARMD data we use

INDIVIDUAL			TRIAL		
LOWER	Individual	UPPER	LOWER	R square	UPPER
0.4315	0.5318	0.6321	0.4695	0.6585	0.8476

FIGURE 12.9
Surrogacy measures with 95% C.I; reduced fixed effects model.

```
%CONTCONTRED(data=armd,true=diff52,surrog=diff24,trt=treat,
             trial=center,patid=patientId,weighted=1,
             looa=1)
```

The specification of the macro's arguments is the same as the specification presented in Section 12.2.

12.3.2.3 Data Analysis and Output

Surrogacy measures obtained from the reduced fixed-effect model are shown below. Similar to the results presented in Section 12.3.1, the surrogacy measures $R^2_{\text{indiv}} = 0.5318$ (0.4315,0.6321) and $R^2_{\text{trial(r)}} = 0.6585$ (0.4695,0.8476) indicated that visual acuity after 24 weeks after starting the interferon-α treatment is a surrogate of moderate value for the visual acuity at 52 weeks after starting the interferon-α treatment. Trial-specific parameter estimates for treatment effects are shown in Figure 12.10. The regression line fitted at the second stage is added. The circle sizes in the plot are proportional to the number of patients from a given trial. Similar to the analysis presented in the previous section, if the argument `looa=1` is used, a "leave-one-out" analysis is performed.

12.3.2.4 SAS Code for the First Step

The joint model formulated in (12.6) can be fitted using the SAS procedure `MIXED` in the following way:

```
proc mixed data=dataset covtest;
class endp patid trial;
model outcome = endp endp*treat*trial / S noint;
repeated endp / type=un subject=patid(trial);
ods output solutionF=eb CovParms=covar;
run;
```

Note that the two-way interaction term `endp*treat` is dropped from the `MODEL` statement and instead we use the variable `endp`; as a result, a common intercept is fitted to the two endpoints. The panel in Figure 12.12 shows the parameter estimates for the first-stage model. The individual-level surro-

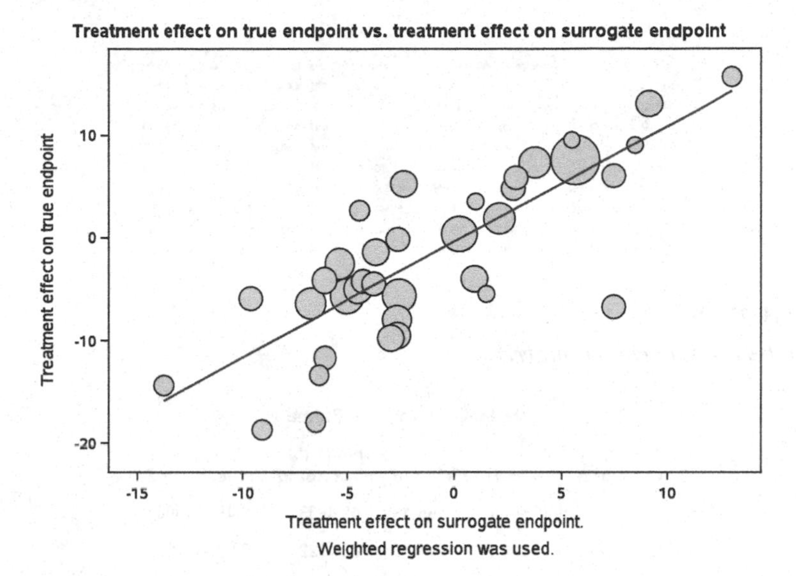

FIGURE 12.10
Age-Related Macular Degeneration Trial. Estimation of trial-level surrogacy using a two-stage model. Trial-specific treatment effects obtained from the reduced fixed-effects model. Circle areas are proportional to trial size.

gacy measure can be estimated using the residual covariance matrix shown in Figure 12.12,

$$\widehat{R}^2_{\text{indiv}} = \frac{144.75^2}{165.15 \times 238.56} = 0.5318. \tag{12.8}$$

The second-stage model, from which trial-level surrogacy is estimated, can be fitted in the same way as in Section (12.3.1).

12.3.3 The Full Mixed-Effects Model

The full mixed-effects model, discussed in Chapter 4, is a joint model for the surrogate and true endpoint given by

$$\begin{cases} S_{ij} = \mu_S + m_{Si} + (\alpha + a_i)Z_{ij} + \varepsilon_{Sij}, \\ T_{ij} = \mu_T + m_{Ti} + (\beta + b_i)Z_{ij} + \varepsilon_{Tij}. \end{cases} \tag{12.9}$$

Here, μ_S and μ_T are fixed intercepts, α and β are the fixed treatment effects on the two endpoints, m_{Si} and m_{Ti} are random intercepts, and a_i and b_i are trial-specific random treatment effects. As pointed out in Chapter 4, the vector of random effects $(m_{Si}, m_{Ti}, a_i, b_i)$ is assumed to follow a normal distribution with zero mean and covariance matrix (4.2). The error terms, ε_{Sij} and ε_{Tij}, are assumed to follow a bivariate normal distribution with covariance matrix

Solution for Fixed Effects										
Effect	endpoint	Center	Estimate	Standard Error	DF	t Value	Pr > |t|	Alpha	Lower	Upper
endpoint	-1		-6.7471	0.9882	181	-6.83	<.0001	0.05	-8.6970	-4.7971
endpoint	1		-12.8799	1.1877	181	-10.84	<.0001	0.05	-15.2235	-10.5363
trt1*endpoint*Center	-1	13395	1.5000	9.0871	181	0.17	0.8691	0.05	-16.4303	19.4303
trt1*endpoint*Center	-1	13396	-4.2500	6.4256	181	-0.66	0.5092	0.05	-16.9287	8.4287
trt1*endpoint*Center	-1	13745	-4.4176	7.4269	181	-0.59	0.5527	0.05	-19.0721	10.2368
trt1*endpoint*Center	-1	13746	2.1067	4.8593	181	0.43	0.6651	0.05	-7.4815	11.6949
trt1*endpoint*Center	-1	13748	0.9494	5.7506	181	0.17	0.8691	0.05	-10.3974	12.2962
trt1*endpoint*Center	-1	13750	-9.6235	6.4445	181	-1.49	0.1371	0.05	-22.3396	3.0926
trt1*endpoint*Center	-1	13828	-6.1235	6.4445	181	-0.95	0.3433	0.05	-18.8396	6.5926

FIGURE 12.11
Error terms covariance matrix.

Covariance Parameter Estimates					
Cov Parm	Subject	Estimate	Standard Error	Z Value	Pr Z
UN(1,1)	Id(Center)	165.15	19.4633	8.49	<.0001
UN(2,1)	Id(Center)	144.75	20.4722	7.07	<.0001
UN(2,2)	Id(Center)	238.56	28.1146	8.49	<.0001

FIGURE 12.12
Error terms covariance matrix.

given in (4.3). Trial- and individual-level surrogacy can be estimated using the variance-covariance elements in the covariance matrices (4.2) and (4.3), respectively. For more detail, see Chapter 4.

12.3.3.1 The SAS Macro %CONTRANFULL

The `%CONTRANFULL` macro can be used to perform the analysis and it can be invoked using the following call:

```
%CONTRANFULL(data=simdata,true=true,surrog=surr,trt=treat,
trial=trial,patid=patientId,looa=1).
```

The macro's arguments are the same as those presented in Section 12.2.

12.3.3.2 Data Analysis and Output

Due to convergence problems with the full random effects, a simulated set of data was used to generate numerical and graphical outputs. The following parameters were used to simulate the data: 1000 observations from 50 trials were generated from a multivariate normal distribution with the mean vector

INDIVIDUAL			TRIAL		
LOWER	Individual	UPPER	LOWER	R square	UPPER
0.5893	0.6260	0.6628	0.6483	0.7655	0.8828

FIGURE 12.13
Surrogacy measures with their 95% C.I., full mixed-effects model.

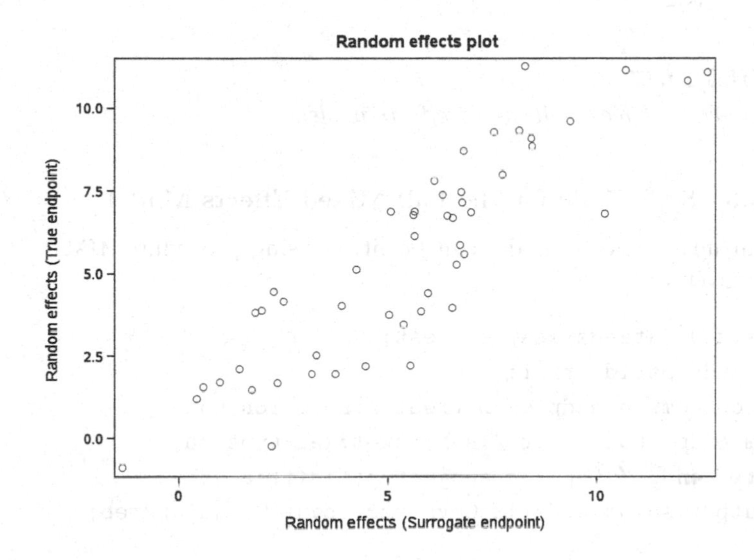

FIGURE 12.14
Trial-specific random-effects plot.

$(\mu_S, \mu_T, \alpha, \beta) = (5, 5, 5, 5)$, and covariance matrices given by

$$D = \begin{pmatrix} 10 & 8 & 0 & 0 \\ & 10 & 0 & 0 \\ & & 10 & 9 \\ & & & 10 \end{pmatrix}, \quad \Sigma = \begin{pmatrix} 10 & 8 \\ & 10 \end{pmatrix}.$$

As shown in Figure 12.13, the surrogacy measures are equal to $\widehat{R}^2_{\text{indiv}} = 0.6260$ (0.5893, 06628) and $\widehat{R}^2_{\text{trial}} = 0.7655$ (0.6483, 0.8828). Figure 12.14 shows the empirical Bayes estimates for the trial-specific random treatment effects.

	ERROR SURROGATE	ERROR TRUE
ERROR_SURROG	9.3313	7.4406
ERROR_TRUE	.	9.4772

	INTERCEPT SURROGATE	INTERCEPT TRUE	SLOPE SURROGATE	SLOPE_TRUE
INTER_SURROG	12.4363	9.0861	-0.4732	-0.3845
INTER_TRUE	.	9.6945	-0.4146	-0.2926
SLOPE_SURROG	.	.	9.6047	8.7171
SLOPE_TRUE	.	.	.	10.3347

FIGURE 12.15
Covariance matrices, full mixed-effects model.

12.3.3.3 SAS Code for the Full Mixed-Effects Model

The full mixed-effects model can be fitted using procedure MIXED. Possible code is given by

```
proc mixed data=dataset covtest;
class endp patid trial;
model outcome = endp endp*treat / solution noint;
random endp endp*treat / subject=trial type=un;
repeated endp / type=un subject=patid(trial);
ods output solutionF=fix CovParms=covar SolutionR=eb;
run;
```

The data structure and variables are identical to those outlined in Section 12.3.1. The MODEL statement defines the 4 fixed effects in the mean structure, $(\mu_T, \mu_S, \alpha, \beta)$, while the RANDOM statement defines the structure of the covariance matrix D for the random effects, and the REPEATED statement builds up the error covariance matrix Σ in (12.2). The estimated covariance matrices are shown in Figure 12.15. The lower panel presents the parameter estimates of the covariance matrix D (given in 4.2).

$$\widehat{D} = \begin{pmatrix} 12.4363 & 9.0861 & -0.4732 & -0.3845 \\ & 9.6945 & -0.4146 & -0.2926 \\ & & 9.6047 & 8.7171 \\ & & & 10.3347 \end{pmatrix}. \tag{12.10}$$

The trial-level surrogacy measure is estimated by (4.4):

$$\widehat{R}^2_{\text{trial(f)}} = \frac{\begin{pmatrix} -0.3845 \\ 8.7171 \end{pmatrix}^T \begin{pmatrix} 12.4363 & -0.4732 \\ -0.4732 & 9.6047 \end{pmatrix}^{-1} \begin{pmatrix} -0.3845 \\ 8.7171 \end{pmatrix}}{10.3347} = 0.7655. \tag{12.11}$$

The estimated covariance matrix for the residuals (defined in (12.2)) is given by

$$\widehat{\Sigma} = \begin{pmatrix} 9.3313 & 7.4406 \\ & 9.4772 \end{pmatrix}, \tag{12.12}$$

and individual-level surrogacy is derived according to (4.9):

$$\widehat{R}^2_{\text{indiv}} = \frac{7.4406^2}{9.3313 \times 9.4772} = 0.6260. \tag{12.13}$$

12.3.4 Reduced Mixed-Effects Model

An elaborate discussion about the reduced mixed-effects model is given in Chapter 4. Briefly, a joint model if formulated for the true and the surrogate endpoints in which trial-specific treatment effects are assumed to be random:

$$\begin{cases} S_{ij} = \mu_S + (\alpha + a_i)Z_{ij} + \varepsilon_{Sij}, \\ T_{ij} = \mu_T + (\beta + b_i)Z_{ij} + \varepsilon_{Tij}, \end{cases} \tag{12.14}$$

is used to estimate the surrogacy measures. Trial- and individual-level surrogacy measures are given, respectively, by (see 4.14 and 4.9 for more details):

$$R^2_{\text{trial(r)}} = \frac{d^2_{ab}}{d_{aa}d_{bb}}, \text{ and } R^2_{\text{indiv}} = \frac{d^2_{ST}}{d_{SS}d_{TT}}. \tag{12.15}$$

12.3.4.1 The SAS Macro %CONTRANRED

The macro `%CONTRANRED` is used to conduct the analysis.

```
%CONTRANRED(data=simreduced,true=true,surrog=surr,trt=treat,
trial=trial,patid=patientId,looa=0).
```

The macro's arguments are presented in Section 12.2.

INDIVIDUAL			TRIAL		
LOWER	Individual	UPPER	LOWER	R square	UPPER
0.5872	0.6241	0.6609	0.7186	0.8144	0.9102

FIGURE 12.16
Surrogacy measures with their 95% C.I, reduced mixed-effects model.

12.3.4.2 Data Analysis and Output

Similar to full random effects models, convergence problems arise. Simulated data were used to generate numerical and graphical output. The following parameters were used to simulate the data: 1000 observations from 50 trials were generated from a multivariate normal distribution with the mean vector $(\mu_S, \alpha, \beta) = (5, 3, 5, 4)$, and covariance matrices given by

$$D = \begin{pmatrix} 10 & 9 \\ & 10 \end{pmatrix}, \quad \Sigma = \begin{pmatrix} 3 & 2.4 \\ & 3 \end{pmatrix}.$$

Parameter estimates for trial- and individual-level surrogacy measures obtained for the reduced mixed-effects model are equal to $\widehat{R}^2_{\text{trial(r)}} = 0.8144$ (0.7186, 0.9102) and $\widehat{R}^2_{\text{indiv}} = 0.6241$ (0.5872, 0.6609), respectively (Figure 12.16). Figure 12.17 shows the empirical Bayes estimates for the random effects.

12.3.4.3 SAS Code for the Reduced Mixed-Effects Model

The SAS code to fit the reduced mixed-effects model is:

```
proc mixed data=dataset covtest;
class endp patid trial;
model outcome = endp endp*treat / solution noint;
random endp*treat / subject=trial type=un;
repeated endp / type=un subject=patid(trial);
ods output solutionF=fix CovParms=covar SolutionR=eb;
run;
```

Note that, compared with the full mixed-effects model, the `RANDOM` statement was changed from `RANDOM endp endp*treat / subject=trial type=un` to `RANDOM endp*treat / subject=trial type=un`, while the `MODEL` and `REPEATED` statements remain the same. This implies that the covariance matrix for the trial-specific treatment effects is a 2×2 covariance matrix, while the `repeated` statement defines the error covariance matrix Σ in (12.2). The estimated matrices are shown in Figure 12.18. Trial-level surrogacy is esti-

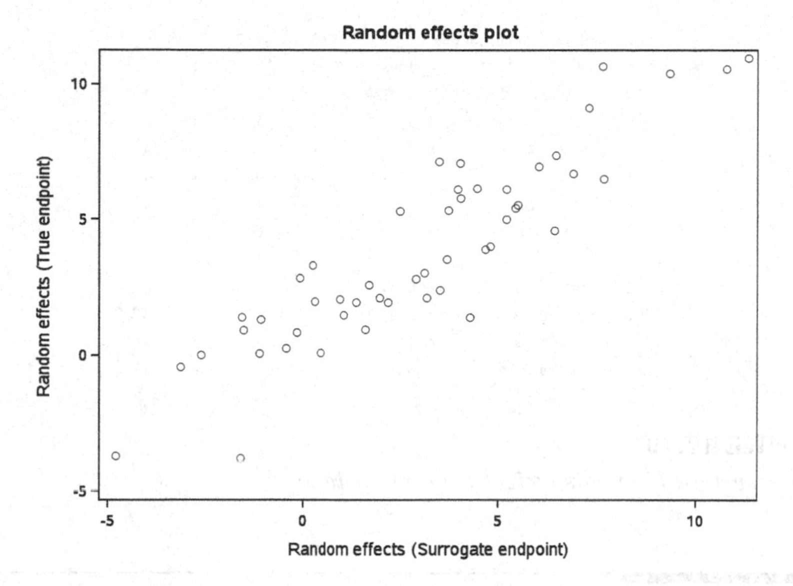

FIGURE 12.17
Empirical Bayes estimates for the trial-specific random effects.

	SLOPE SURR	SLOPE TRUE
TRTSUR	12.6148	10.9702
TRTTRU	.	11.7144

	ERROR SURROGATE	ERROR TRUE
ERRSUR	2.7696	2.1859
ERRTRU	.	2.7644

FIGURE 12.18
Covariance matrices, reduced mixed-effects model.

mated using equation (12.15).

$$\widehat{R}^2_{\text{trial(r)}} = \frac{10.9702^2}{12.6148 \times 11.7144} = 0.8144, \tag{12.16}$$

and individual-level surrogacy is derived as follows (see equation 12.15):

$$\widehat{R}^2_{\text{indiv}} = \frac{2.1859^2}{2.7696 \times 2.7644} = 0.6241. \tag{12.17}$$

Obs	PATIENT	SURV	SURVIND	PFS	PFSIND	TREAT	CENTER	TRIAL
1	1074	0.18571	1	0.10516	1	0	-4	-4
2	1075	1.40873	1	0.89524	1	0	-4	-4
3	1076	0.12619	1	0.07897	1	0	-4	-4
4	1077	1.73929	0	1.73929	0	1	-4	-4
5	1078	0.12738	1	0.09127	1	0	-4	-4
6	1079	0.22540	1	0.16984	1	1	-4	-4
7	1080	0.73810	1	0.36944	1	0	-4	-4
8	1081	0.74802	1	0.26071	1	0	-4	-4
9	1082	0.38929	1	0.14405	1	1	-4	-4
10	1083	0.17381	1	0.13373	1	1	-4	-4
11	1084	1.39484	0	1.39484	0	0	-4	-4
12	1085	0.31190	1	0.11825	1	1	-4	-4

FIGURE 12.19
Data structure for two survival time endpoints.

12.4 Analysis for a Surrogacy Setting with Two Survival Endpoints

Analysis strategies for a surrogacy setting in which the two endpoints are time-to-event variables were discussed in Chapter 5. In this section, we focus on three applications. In the first two, the analysis is based on a two-stage approach (see Section 5.3) while the third application is based on the joint modeling of two time-to-event endpoints (see Section 5.2).

For illustration, we used the ovarian study with overall survival and progression-free survival as the true and surrogate endpoints, respectively. Overall, 1153 patients from 39 trials are included in the analysis (569 in the treatment arm and 584 in the control arm). Throughout this section, we briefly discuss the technical details and we refer to Chapter 5 for an elaborate discussion about the modeling approaches and surrogacy measures. A partial print of the data is given in Figure 12.19. The data for each patient appear as a single line.

12.4.1 A Two-Stage Approach (I)

As pointed out in Chapter 5, the first-stage model consists of trial-specific Cox proportional hazard models for the two endpoints given by

$$\begin{cases} S_{ij}(t) = S_{i0}(t)\exp(\alpha_i Z_{ij}), \\ T_{ij}(t) = T_{i0}(t)\exp(\beta_i Z_{ij}), \end{cases} \tag{12.18}$$

where $S_{i0}(t)$ and $T_{i0}(t)$ are the trial-specific baseline hazard functions, and Z_{ij} is a treatment indicator for the jth individual in the ith trial. The parameters β_i and α_i are the trial-specific treatment effects.

One way to account for variation in trial size is to use the number of patients in each trial in a weighted linear regression of the form

$$\widehat{\beta}_i = \lambda_0 + \lambda_1 \widehat{\alpha}_i + \varepsilon_i. \tag{12.19}$$

A second approach to account for the variability between trials is to use a robust sandwich estimator of Lin and Wei (1989) for the covariance matrix of the parameter estimates for treatment effects in (12.18) and follow the approach proposed by van Houwelingen et al. (2002). The two approaches are implemented in the macro `%TWOSTAGECOX` discussed below. As before, the coefficient of determination from (12.19) is used as a trial-level surrogacy measure. A leave-one-out analysis can be performed in order to assess model accuracy.

12.4.1.1 The SAS Macro %TWOSTAGECOX

The model discussed in the previous section can be fitted using the SAS macro `%TWOSTAGECOX`, which has the following generic form:

```
%TWOSTAGECOX(data=ovarian,true=surv,trueind=survind,
             surrog=pfs,surrogind=pfsind,trt=treat,
             trial=center,patid=patient,common=1,
             robust=1,looa=1);
```

The macro's specific arguments are;

- `trueind`: censoring indicator for the true endpoint (1=event, 0=censoring).
- `surrogind`: censoring indicator for the surrogate (1=event, 0=censoring).
- `common`: an option that allows the user to choose between the trial-specific baseline hazard function (common=0), or the common baseline hazard function (common=1) in the first stage.
- `robust`: an option that allows the user to obtain the robust (or adjusted) R^2_{trial} in the output (1 for robust; 0 for non-robust).

12.4.1.2 Data Analysis and Output

The macro `%TWOSTAGECOX` produces two exploratory plots: the patients' distribution in the trials by treatment arm (shown in Figure 12.20, top panel) and the Kaplan-Meier curves for the true and surrogate endpoints (shown in Figure 12.20, bottom panel).

As shown in Figure 12.21, the estimated trial-level surrogacy is equal to $R^2_{\text{trial}} = 0.9184$ (0.8674, 0.9695), which implies that progression-free survival time is a good surrogate for overall survival, which can be clearly seen in Figure 12.22. The result of the leave-one-out analysis is shown in Figure 12.23.

12.4.1.3 SAS Code for the First-Stage Model

The Cox proportional hazard model formulated in (12.18) can be fitted using SAS procedure PHREG.

```
proc phreg data=firststage covs(aggregate) covout outest=mat;
class  center endpoint/param=glm;
model outcome*status(0)=  endpoint*treat*center;
strata center endpoint;
id patid;
run;
```

It is assumed that there are two records per subject in the input dataset, the first one corresponding to the surrogate endpoint and the second one to the true endpoint. The option covs(aggregate) applies the robust sandwich estimator of Lin and Wei (1989) for the covariance matrix that will be used in the second stage to correct for the uncertainty in the estimated parameters. The outest option creates an output SAS dataset containing estimates of the regression coefficients and the option covout adds the estimated covariance matrix of the parameter estimates to the outest dataset. In the MODEL statement, status is the censoring indicator variable (0=censoring, 1=event). In the strata statement we specify the variables that determine the stratification.

The parameter estimates obtained from model (12.18) are shown in Figure 12.24.

12.4.2 A Two-Stage Approach (II)

In this section, we discuss the evaluation approach, proposed by Buyse et al. (2011), to compute the individual-level surrogacy. The underlying idea behind this evaluation approach is that S_{ij} can be considered as a valid surrogate for T_{ij} with respect to a new treatment if the pair of endpoints scores sufficiently high on the validation measures. Buyse et al. (2011) proposed the use of the Kaplan-Meier (KM) estimates (for both endpoints) at a fixed time point and to estimate the correlation between the KM estimates of the two endpoints. Kaplan-Meier estimates per trial and per endpoint are estimated using the following formula:

$$S(t_i) = \prod_{t_i \leq t} \left(1 - \frac{d_i}{n_i}\right). \quad (12.20)$$

Here, $S(t_i)$ is the estimated survival probability, d_i is the number of patients who had an event at time t_i, and n_i is the number of patients who are at risk at that time. The estimated values are denoted by $\widehat{\beta}_i$, $\widehat{\alpha}_i$ for the true and surrogate endpoints, respectively.

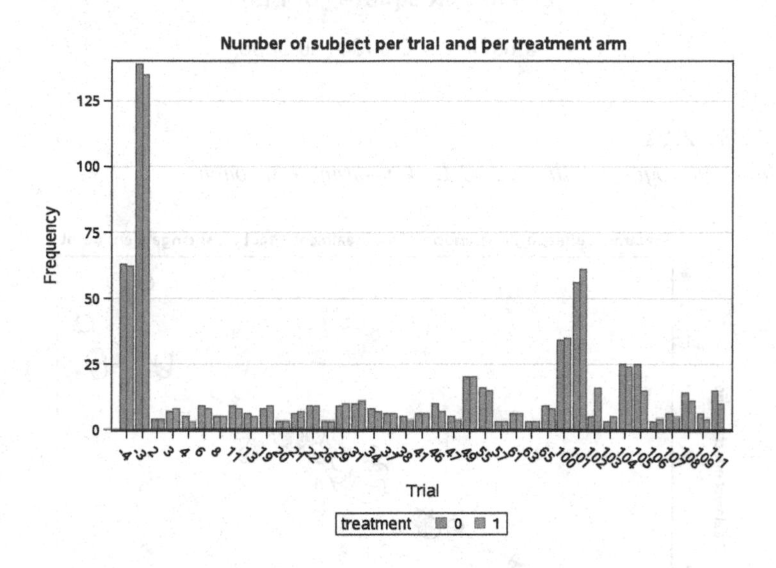

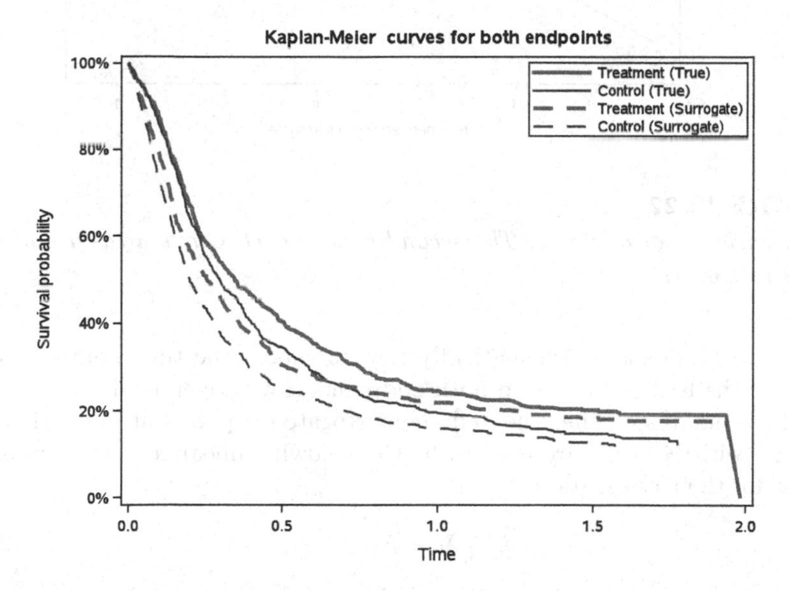

FIGURE 12.20

The Ovarian Cancer Study. Top panel: Patient distribution by treatment arms within centers. Bottom panel: Kaplan-Meier curves for the survival time (true endpoint) and progression-free survival (surrogate endpoint) for the two treatment groups CP and CAP.

LOWER	R square	UPPER
0.8674	0.9184	0.9695

FIGURE 12.21
Trial-level surrogacy with 95% C.I., two-stage approach.

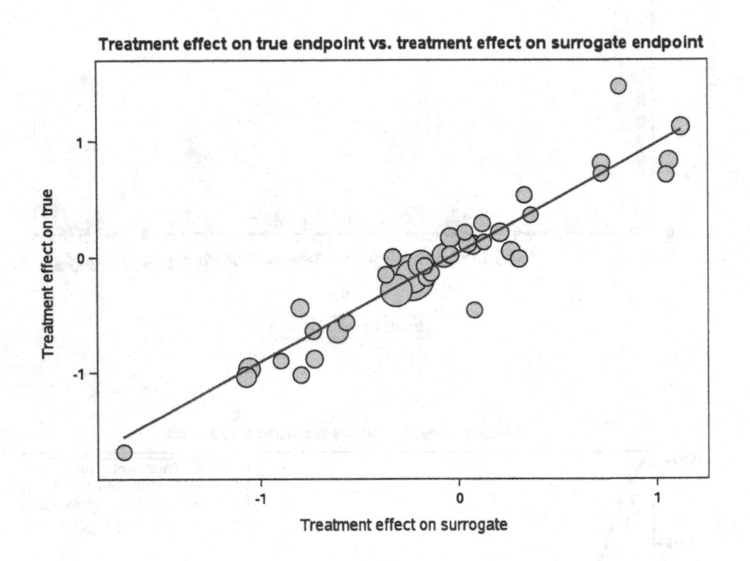

FIGURE 12.22
The Ovarian Cancer Study. The second-stage model. Circle areas are proportional to trial size.

Figure 12.25 shows schematically how to choose the time points used to compute the KM estimates on both endpoints (for a given trial).

KM estimates on the true and the surrogate endpoints at given time t_T, and t_S , with $t_T > t_S$, are used to fit the following linear regression in order to test for their association.

$$\widehat{\beta}_i = \lambda_0 + \lambda_1 \widehat{\alpha}_i + \varepsilon_i. \tag{12.21}$$

The effective sample size at the time point considered for KM estimates (the number of deaths prior to the time point plus the number of patients at risk at the time point) can be used for each trial as a weight. The coefficient of determination, R^2, obtained for the linear regression model in (12.21) can be used to quantify the surrogacy measure at individual level.

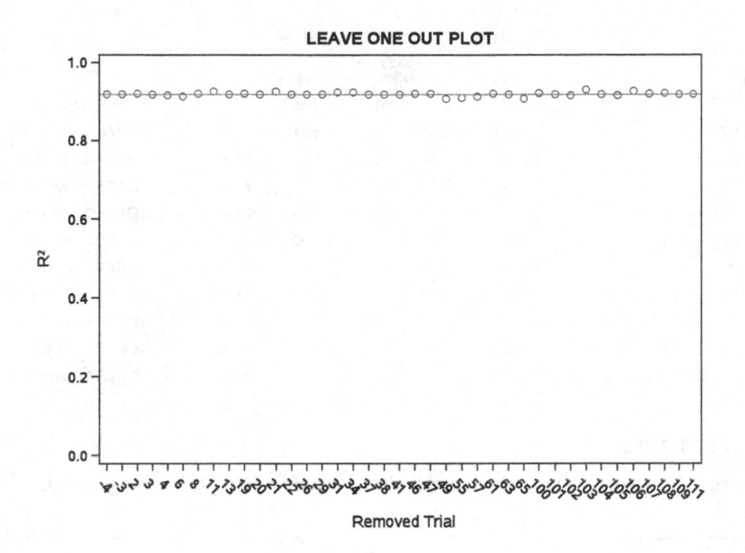

FIGURE 12.23
The Ovarian Cancer Study. Leave-one-out analysis plot.

12.4.2.1 The SAS Macro %TWOSTAGEKM

The model discussed in this section can be fitted using the SAS macro %TWOSTAGEKM. The macro has the general form of

```
%TWOSTAGEKM(data=ovarian,true=surv,trueind=survind,surrog=pfs,
            surrogind=pfsind,trt=treat,trial=center,
            upsurr=1,uptrue=2)
```

The macro's arguments are:

- `upsurr`: the time point at which the KM estimates are computed on the surrogate endpoint.
- `uptrue`: the time point at which the KM estimates are computed on the true endpoint.

The rest of the arguments were defined in Section 12.2.

12.4.2.2 Data Analysis and Output

The %TWOSTAGEKM macro produces the Kaplan-Meier curves for both endpoints (Figure 12.26). For the example in this section, we use the KM estimates at 1 year for progression-free survival and the KM estimates at 2 years for overall survival. Our aim is to compute the correlation between the KM estimates of the two endpoints. The estimated individual-level surrogacy measure for

Analysis of Maximum Likelihood Estimates										
Parameter			DF	Parameter Estimate	Standard Error	StdErr Ratio	Chi-Square	Pr > ChiSq	Hazard Ratio	Label
TREAT*CENTER*endpoin	-4	-1	1	-0.23281	0.19966	0.990	1.3595	0.2436	.	CENTER -4 * endpoint -1 * TREAT
TREAT*CENTER*endpoin	-4	1	1	-0.16965	0.20392	0.991	0.6921	0.4055	.	CENTER -4 * endpoint 1 * TREAT
TREAT*CENTER*endpoin	-3	-1	1	-0.23613	0.12780	1.003	3.4140	0.0646	.	CENTER -3 * endpoint -1 * TREAT
TREAT*CENTER*endpoin	-3	1	1	-0.17740	0.12852	1.001	1.9054	0.1675	.	CENTER -3 * endpoint 1 * TREAT
TREAT*CENTER*endpoin	2	-1	1	0.03336	0.74965	0.959	0.0020	0.9645	.	CENTER 2 * endpoint -1 * TREAT
TREAT*CENTER*endpoin	2	1	1	0.21356	0.69948	0.906	0.0932	0.7601	.	CENTER 2 * endpoint 1 * TREAT
TREAT*CENTER*endpoin	3	-1	1	-0.04031	0.52329	0.885	0.0059	0.9386	.	CENTER 3 * endpoint -1 * TREAT
TREAT*CENTER*endpoin	3	1	1	0.01961	0.51873	0.877	0.0014	0.9699	.	CENTER 3 * endpoint 1 * TREAT
TREAT*CENTER*endpoin	4	-1	1	0.71928	0.67213	0.818	1.1452	0.2846	.	CENTER 4 * endpoint -1 * TREAT
TREAT*CENTER*endpoin	4	1	1	0.71928	0.67213	0.818	1.1452	0.2846	.	CENTER 4 * endpoint 1 * TREAT
TREAT*CENTER*endpoin	6	-1	1	0.72007	0.49831	0.883	2.0881	0.1485	.	CENTER 6 * endpoint -1 * TREAT

FIGURE 12.24
Parameter estimates from the first-stage model (for selected trials).

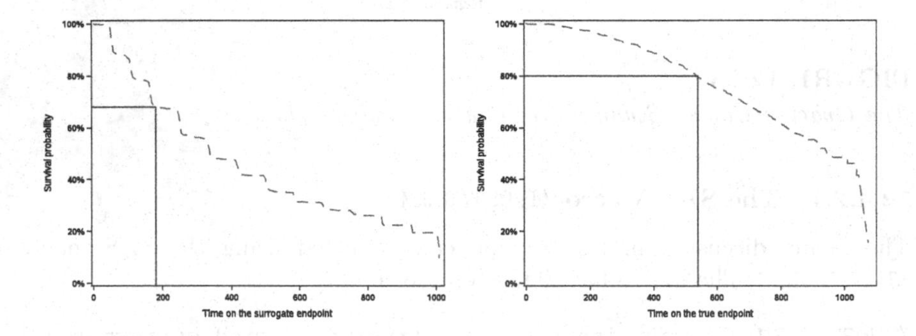

FIGURE 12.25
Kaplan-Meier curves for the true and the surrogate endpoints for a given time point.

the ovarian data is shown in Figure 12.27 and is equal to $\widehat{R}^2_{\text{indiv}} = 0.6431$ (0.6101, 0.6762). This indicates that that progression-free survival at 1 year is a moderate surrogate for overall survival at two years. This can be seen in Figure 12.28, which presents the KM estimates of progression-free survival at 1 year versus the KM estimates for overall survival at two years.

12.4.2.3 SAS Code for Trial-Specific KM Estimates (at a Given Time Point)

The survival probability based on the KM curves can be estimated using SAS procedure LIFETEST in the following way:

```
proc lifetest data=ovar;
time surv * survind(0);
```

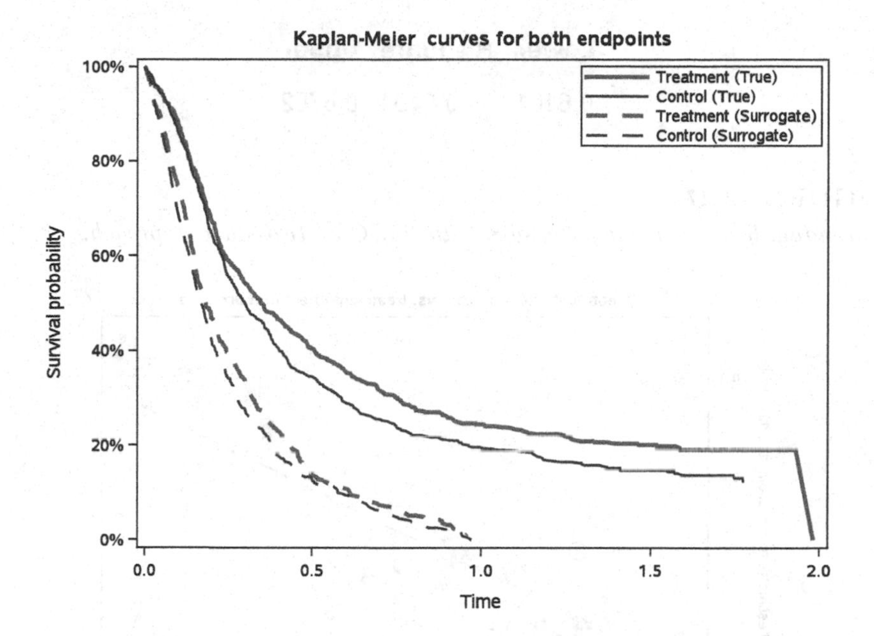

FIGURE 12.26
Kaplan-Meier curve for the true endpoint at 2 years and for the surrogate endpoint at 1 year.

```
strata treat;
where surv<=2;
by trial;
run;
```

The variables `surv` and `survind` are the survival time and the censoring indicator, respectively. The `STRATA` statement produces the results for the active treatment and control groups separately. The `WHERE` statement allows us to select observations for which the survival time is less or equal to 2 years (for the true endpoint). Figure 12.29 presents Kaplan-Meier estimates for one trial.

12.4.3 A Joint Model for Survival Endpoints

As explained in Chapter 5, a joint survival function of (S_{ij}, T_{ij}) can be written as

$$F(s,t) = P(S_{ij} \geq s, T_{ij} \geq t) = C_\theta\{F_{Sij}(s), F_{Tij}(t)\}, \quad s,t \geq 0, \qquad (12.22)$$

where F_{Sij} and F_{Tij} denote marginal survival functions for both endpoints (overall survival and progression free survival) and C_θ is a copula, i.e., a

Lower	R square	Upper
0.6101	0.6431	0.6762

FIGURE 12.27
Individual-level surrogacy measure with 95%C.I., two-stage approach.

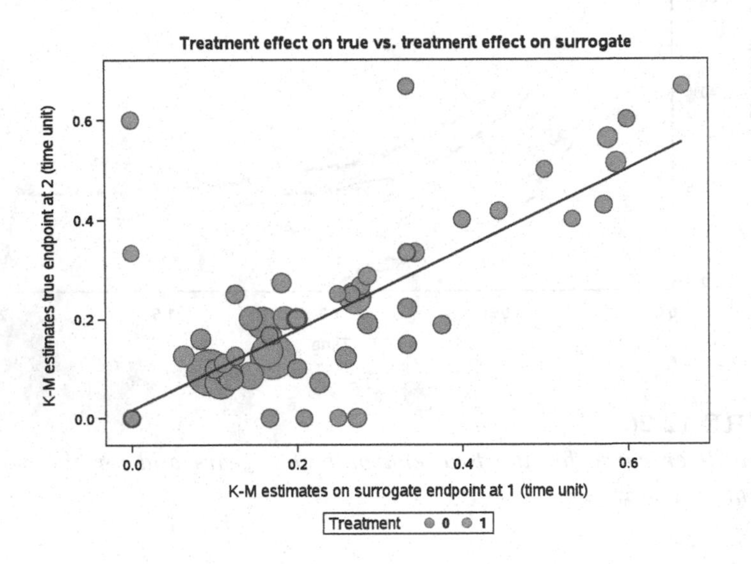

FIGURE 12.28
Kaplan-Meier estimates at 2 years on the true endpoint versus at 1 year on the surrogate endpoint.

bivariate distribution function on $[0,1]^2$ which allows correlated probabilities to be modeled. In Chapter 5, we use marginal survival functions given by

$$\begin{cases} F_{S_{ij}}(s) = \exp\{-\int_0^s \lambda_{Si}(x)\exp(\alpha_i Z_{ij})\,dx\}, \\ F_{T_{ij}}(t) = \exp\{-\int_0^t \lambda_{Ti}(x)\exp(\beta_i Z_{ij})\,dx\}, \end{cases} \tag{12.23}$$

where λ_{Si} and λ_{Ti} are trial-specific marginal baseline hazard functions and α_i and β_i are trial-specific treatment effects. At the second stage, a joint model is formulated to the treatment effects

$$\begin{pmatrix} \alpha_i \\ \beta_i \end{pmatrix} = \begin{pmatrix} \alpha \\ \beta \end{pmatrix} + \begin{pmatrix} a_i \\ b_i \end{pmatrix}, \tag{12.24}$$

Product-Limit Survival Estimates						
surv2		Survival	Failure	Survival Standard Error	Number Failed	Number Left
0.00000		1.0000	0	0	0	10
0.03056		0.9000	0.1000	0.0949	1	9
0.05198		0.8000	0.2000	0.1265	2	8
0.05794		0.7000	0.3000	0.1449	3	7
0.13690		0.6000	0.4000	0.1549	4	6
0.15873		0.5000	0.5000	0.1581	5	5
0.21508		0.4000	0.6000	0.1549	6	4
0.22619		0.3000	0.7000	0.1449	7	3
0.24563		0.2000	0.8000	0.1265	8	2
1.50635	*	.	.	.	8	1
1.76944	*	.	.	.	8	0

FIGURE 12.29
Kaplan-Meier estimates for the treated group for a selected trial.

where the second term on the right-hand side of (12.24) is assumed to follow a zero mean normal distribution with a covariance matrix given by

$$D = \begin{pmatrix} d_{aa} & d_{ab} \\ & d_{bb} \end{pmatrix}. \tag{12.25}$$

The quality of the surrogate S at the trial level is assessed based on the coefficient of determination given by:

$$R^2_{\text{trial}} = \frac{d^2_{ab}}{d_{aa}d_{bb}}. \tag{12.26}$$

To assess the quality of the surrogate at the individual level, a measure of association between S_{ij} and T_{ij}, calculated while adjusting the marginal distributions of the two endpoints for both the trial and treatment effects, is needed. Burzykowski et al. (2001) proposed to used Kendall's τ as it depends only on the copula function C_θ and is independent of the marginal distribution of S_{ij} and T_{ij}:

$$\tau = 4\int_0^1\int_0^1 C_\theta(F_{S_{ij}}, F_{T_{ij}})C_\theta(dF_S, dF_T) - 1. \tag{12.27}$$

It describes the strength of the association between the two endpoints remaining after adjustment, through the marginal models (12.23), for the trial and the treatment effects.

INDIVIDUAL			TRIAL		
LOWER	TAU	UPPER	LOWER	R square	UPPER
0.8596	0.8711	0.8826	0.7989	0.8733	0.9476

FIGURE 12.30
Surrogacy measures at trial and individual levels with the 95%C.I.

12.4.3.1 The SAS Macro %COPULA

The SAS macro `%COPULA` can be used to conduct the analysis discussed above in the following way:

```
%COPULA(data=covar,true=Surv,trueind=survind,surrog=pfs,
        surrogind=pfsind,trt=treat,center=center,trial=center,
        vars=,patid=patientid,copula=clayton,
        adjustment=weighted)
```

The macro's arguments are:

- `center`: unique id (continuous) for units, for which specific treatment effects are estimated.
- `trial`: unique id (continuous) for groups of the units, for which common baselines are used.
- `vars`: macro variable containing possible covariates for adjustment of the Weibull and proportional odds models. The names of these covariates have to be passed to the program through the macro variable `vars`.
- `copula`: variable allowing the user to choose one of the three different copulas (`clayton`, `hougaard`, `plackett`).
- `eda`: option choice (1=yes, 0=no) to display the exploratory data analysis plots.
- `adjustment`: adjustment method used to compute the R^2_{trial} (weighted, unweighted, adjustedr2, adjustedrcorr, adjustedr2f).

The rest of the arguments were defined in Section 12.2.

12.4.3.2 Data Analysis and Output

The exploratory plots produced by the macro `%COPULA` are shown in Figure 12.20 (top and bottom panels). For the ovarian cancer study, the surrogacy measures $\widehat{R}^2_{\text{indiv}} = 0.8711$ (0.8596, 0.8826) and $\widehat{R}^2_{\text{trial}} = 0.8733$ (0.7989, 0.9476) indicate that the progression-free survival is a valid surrogate for overall survival at both trial- and individual-level surrogacy. The treatment effects plot in Figure 12.31 can be used to visualize trial-level surrogacy.

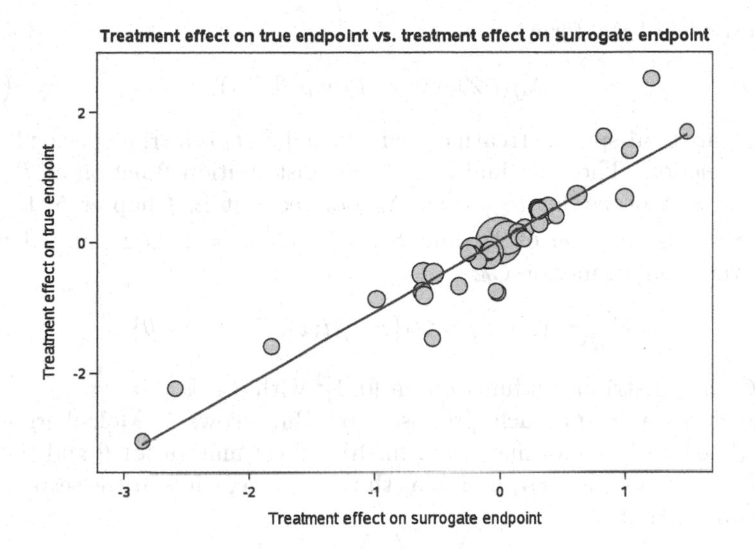

FIGURE 12.31

The Ovarian Cancer Study. Treatment effects on the true endpoints (survival time) versus treatment effects on the surrogate endpoints (progression-free survival). Circle areas are proportional to trial size.

12.5 Validation Using Joint Modeling of a Time-to-Event and a Binary Endpoint

The setting we consider in this section consists of a binary surrogate endpoint and a time-to-event true endpoint. A bivariate copula model, proposed by Burzykowski, Molenberghs, and Buyse (2004), is formulated for the true endpoint T_{ij} and a latent normally distributed variable $\tilde{S}_{ij}$. The binary surrogate is defined by

$$S_{ij} = \begin{cases} 1 & \text{if} \quad \tilde{S}_{ij} > 0, \\ 0 & \text{if} \quad \tilde{S}_{ij} \leq 0. \end{cases} \tag{12.28}$$

For the surrogate endpoint, S_{ij}, a logistic regression model is assumed

$$\text{logit}\{P(S_{ij} = 1|Z_{ij})\} = \gamma_{ij} + \alpha_i Z_{ij}. \tag{12.29}$$

The marginal cumulative distribution function of $\tilde{S}_{ij}$, given $Z_{ij} = z$, is denoted by $F_{\tilde{S}_{ij}}(s; z)$.

To model the effect of treatment on the marginal distribution of T_{ij}, Burzykowski, Molenberghs, and Buyse (2004) proposed to use a proportional hazard model of the form

$$\lambda_{ij}(t|Z_{ij}) = \lambda_i(t)\exp(\beta_i Z_{ij}), \tag{12.30}$$

where β_i are trial-specific treatment effects and $\lambda_i(t)$ is a trial-specific baseline hazard function. The marginal cumulative distribution function of T_{ij}, with $Z_{ij} = z$, is denoted by $F_{T_{ij}}(t;z)$. As pointed out in Chapter 5, the joint cumulative distribution of T_{ij} and $\tilde{S}_{ij}$, given $Z_{ij} = z$, is generated by one parameter copula function C_θ:

$$F_{T_{ij},\tilde{S}_{ij}}(t,s;z) = C_\theta\{F_{T_{ij}}(t;z), F_{\tilde{S}_{ij}}(s;z), \theta\}. \tag{12.31}$$

Here, C_θ is a distribution function on $[0,1]^2$ with $\theta \in \mathbb{R}^1$.

The two-stage approach proposed by Burzykowski, Molenberghs, and Buyse (2004) consists of maximum likelihood estimation for θ and the trial-specific treatment effects α_i and β_i at the first stage, while at the second stage, it is assumed that

$$\begin{pmatrix}\alpha_i\\ \beta_i\end{pmatrix} = \begin{pmatrix}\alpha\\ \beta\end{pmatrix} + \begin{pmatrix}a_i\\ b_i\end{pmatrix}. \tag{12.32}$$

The second term of the right-hand side of (12.32) is assumed to follow a bivariate normal distribution with mean zero and covariance matrix given by

$$D = \begin{pmatrix} d_{aa} & d_{ab} \\ & d_{bb}\end{pmatrix}. \tag{12.33}$$

Hence, similar to Section 4.3.2, trial-level surrogacy is estimated by:

$$R^2_{\text{trial}} = \frac{d^2_{ab}}{d_{aa}d_{bb}}. \tag{12.34}$$

To assess the quality of the surrogate endpoint at the individual level, a measure of association between S_{ij} and T_{ij} is needed. Burzykowski, Molenberghs, and Buyse (2004) proposed to use the bivariate Plackett copula. This particular choice was motivated by the fact that, for the Plackett copula, the association parameter θ takes the form of a (constant) global odds ratio.

$$\theta = \frac{P(T_{ij} > t, S_{ij} > k)P(T_{ij} \le t, S_{ij} \le k)}{P(T_{ij} > t, S_{ij} \le k)P(T_{ij} \le t, S_{ij} > k)}. \tag{12.35}$$

For a binary surrogate, it is just the odds ratio for responders versus non-responders (assuming $k = 2$ indicates the response).

12.5.1 Data Structure

We use the colorectal cancer data for illustration of the analysis for the survival-binary surrogacy setting. The true endpoint is overall survival and

Obs	PATIENTID	SURVIVAL	SURVIND	BINRESP	TREAT	CENTER	TRIAL
1	1	0.94722	1	2	0	1	1
2	2	1.01389	1	1	1	1	1
3	3	1.91667	1	1	1	1	1
4	4	0.60278	1	1	1	1	1
5	5	1.48333	1	1	0	1	1
6	6	0.30278	1	1	0	1	1
7	7	0.20833	0	1	1	1	1
8	8	0.26944	1	1	0	1	1
9	9	1.06389	1	1	1	1	1
10	10	0.08333	1	1	0	1	1
11	11	1.83611	1	2	1	1	1
12	12	0.60000	1	1	0	1	1
13	13	0.67222	1	2	1	1	1
14	14	0.81389	1	1	0	1	1

FIGURE 12.32
Data structure for the survival-binary setting.

the surrogate endpoint is a two-category tumor response: patients with complete or partial response are considered as responders and patients with stable or progressive disease are considered non-responders.

The data for each subject appears in a single line in which time-to-event (`surv`) and censoring status (`survind`) are given to the true endpoint and the response status (`binresp`) is the surrogate endpoint. The unit for the analysis is the `Trial`; see Figure 12.32.

12.5.2 The SAS Macro %SURVBIN

The joint model discussed above is implemented in the macro `%SURVBIN` that, for the colorectal cancer data, is called as follows:

```
%SURVBIN(data=colorectal,true=Surv,trueind=survind,
        surrog=responder,trt=treat,center=center,
        trial=center,vars=,patid=patientid)
```

The macro's arguments were discussed in Section 12.2. The argument `surrog=responder` defines the variable for the surrogate endpoint (2=responder, 1=no-responder) and it is assumed to be a binary variable.

12.5.3 Data Analysis and Output

The `%SURVBIN` macro produces three default exploratory plots shown in Figure 12.33. The Kaplan-Meier curves (by endpoint) in Figure 12.33 (top panel) indicates that there is no difference between the treatment arms across the level of the surrogate endpoint. The box plots for the survival times in Figure 12.33 (middle panel) reveal the same pattern. The number of patients per trial and treatment arm is shown in Figure 12.33 (bottom panel). Individual- and trial-level surrogacy, global odds = 4.9108 (4.15794, 5.6638) and $R^2_{Trial} = 0.4417$ (0.1564, 0.7269), shown in Figure 12.34 indicate that two-category tumor response is a surrogate of moderate value to overall survival for the colorectal cancer data.

Figure 12.35 shows the parameter estimates for the treatment effects for both the surrogate and true endpoints that were used to estimate trial-level surrogacy.

12.5.4 The SAS Macro %SURVCAT

The analysis presented in Section 6.3.1.1 for a categorical (ordinal) and survival endpoint, and in Section 6.3.1.2, for binary tumor response, was conducted using the SAS macro `%SURVCAT`. The macro has the general form:

```
%SURVCAT(data=colorectal,true=Surv,trueind=survind,
   surrog=responder,trt=treat,center=center,trial=center,
vars=,patid=patientid)
```

The macro's arguments are:

- `true`: measurement of the failure-time endpoint.
- `trueind`: censoring indicator (1=event, 0=censoring).
- `surrog`: measurement of the ordinal categorical surrogate (levels $1, 2, \ldots, K$).
- `treat`: treatment indicator (0 or 1).
- `center`: unique id (continuous) for units, for which specific treatment effects are estimated.
- `trial`: unique id (continuous) for groups of the units, for which common "baselines" are to be used.
- `vars`: macro variable containing possible covariates for adjustment of the Weibull and proportional odds models. The names of these covariates have to be passed to the program through the macro variable `vars`.
- `patid`: patient's identification number.

The macro's output is presented in Chapter 6. Note that if the number of categories is 2, the analysis using the macro `%SURVCAT` the macro `%SURVCAT` is identical to the analysis using the macro `%SURVBIN`.

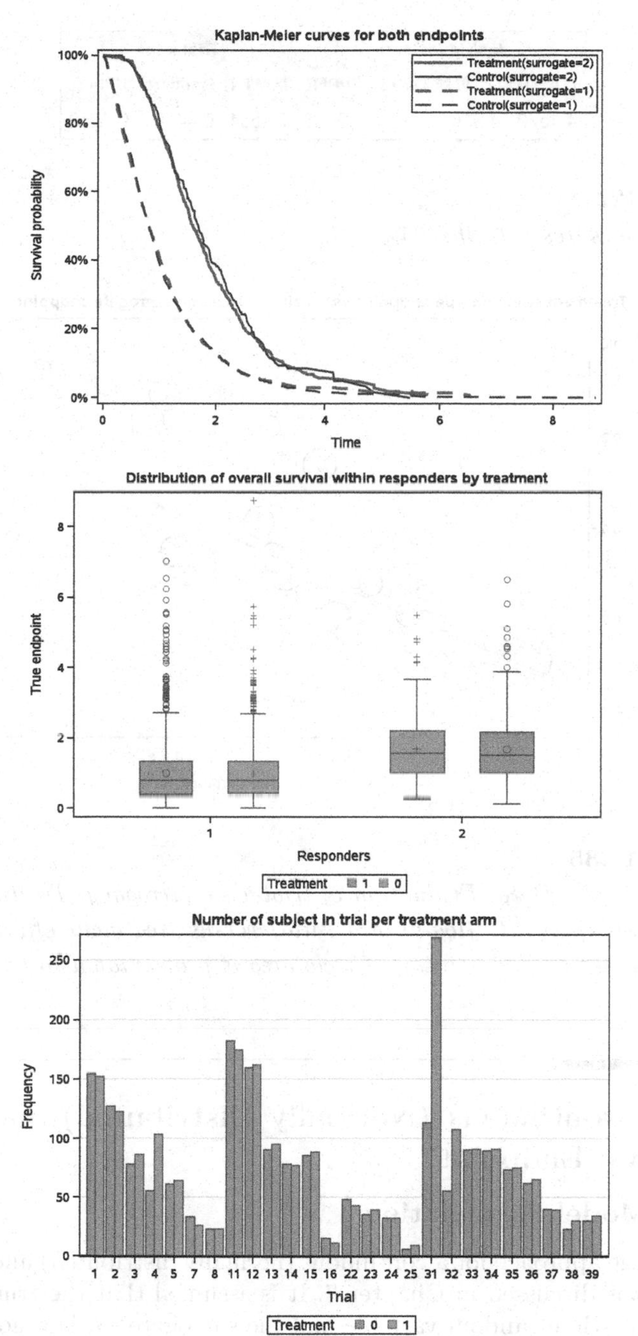

FIGURE 12.33

Colorectal Cancer Data. Descriptive plots. Panel a: KM curves stratified by the binary surrogate endpoint. Panel b: Survival time distribution by treatment arm across the levels of the binary surrogate. Panel c: Distribution of patients by treatment arm.

Individual level			Trial level		
LOWER	GLOBAL ODDS	UPPER	LOWER	R square	UPPER
4.1579	4.9108	5.6638	0.1564	0.4417	0.7269

FIGURE 12.34
Surrogacy measures with the 95% C.I.

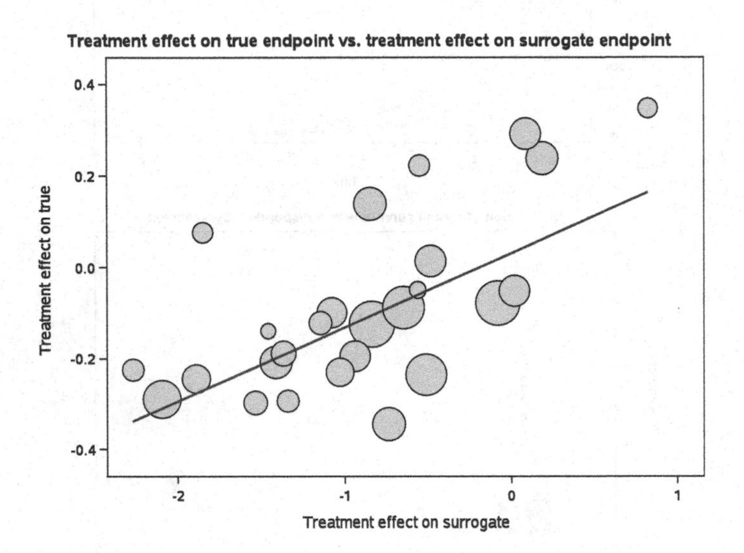

FIGURE 12.35
Colorectal Cancer Data. Evaluation of trial-level surrogacy. Treatment effects upon the true endpoints (log-hazard ratio) versus treatment effects upon the binary surrogate (log-odds ratio). Circle area is proportional to trial size.

12.6 A Continuous (Normally Distributed) and a Survival Endpoint

12.6.1 Model Formulation

The two-stage approach for a continuous (normally distributed) and a survival endpoints was discussed in Chapter 7. It is assumed that the true endpoint, T, is a failure-time random variable and the surrogate, S, is a normally distributed continuous variable.

Briefly, the first stage consists of the classical linear regression model for

Obs	PATIENT	SURV	SURVIND	CONT	TREAT	CENTER
1	2	0.6570841889	1	-3.144152279	1	7
2	3	1.5578370979	1	-3.496507561	1	7
3	4	1.0321697467	1	-5.107156861	1	7
4	5	1.2320328542	0	-3.546739687	0	7
5	7	1.568788501	1	-4.420044702	0	7
6	9	0.9117043121	1	-4.295923936	0	7
7	10	0.6762491444	0	-4.480740108	0	7
8	11	2.6611909651	1	-3.964615456	1	7
9	12	0.9034907598	1	-4.407938016	1	7
10	13	0.5229295003	1	-4.900820428	1	7

FIGURE 12.36
Data structure.

the surrogate given by

$$S_{ij} = \alpha_{0,i} + \alpha_i Z_{ij} + \varepsilon_{ij}, \tag{12.36}$$

where ε_{ij} is normally distributed with mean zero and variance σ_i^2. The proportional hazard model for the true endpoints given by

$$\lambda_{ij}(t|Z_{ij}) = \lambda_i(t)\exp(\beta_i Z_{ij}), \tag{12.37}$$

where β_i are trial-specific effects of treatment Z and $\lambda_i(t)$, is a trial-specific baseline hazard function.

If a parametric (e.g., Weibull-distribution-based) baseline hazard is used in (12.37), the joint distribution function defined by the copula and the marginal models (12.36) and (12.37) allows us to construct the likelihood function for the observed data and obtain estimates of the treatment effects α_i and β_i.

Individual-level surrogacy can be evaluated by using Kendall's τ or Spearman's ρ (see Section 5.2). Trial-level surrogacy is assessed using the correlation coefficient between the estimated treatment effects α_i and β_i.

12.6.2 Data Structure

The advanced prostate cancer data described in Section 7 is used for illustration of the analysis for the survival-normal surrogacy setting. The true endpoint is overall survival time and the surrogate endpoint is the logarithm of prostate-specific antigen (PSA), measured at about 28 days. The data structure for the survival-normal setting is shown in Figure 12.36, in which time-to-event (`surv`) and censoring status (`survind`) are given to the true endpoint and the continuous response (`cont`) is the surrogate endpoint.

12.6.3 The SAS Macro %NORMSURV

The SAS macro %NORMSURV can be used in order to fit the models specified in (12.36)–(12.37). For the prostate data we use:

```
%NORMSURV(data=prostate,true=surv,trueind=survind,surrog=cont,
trt=treat,trial=center,patid=patientId,copula=hougaard,
    adjustement=weighted)
```

The specification of the macro's arguments is the same as the specification presented in Section 5.2.

12.6.4 Data Analysis and Output

The exploratory plots produced by the macro %NORMSURV are shown in Figure 12.37. The histogram in Figure 12.37 (bottom left panel) suggests that the logarithm of PSA at 28 days is normally distributed. The scatter plot for the survival time and the continuous surrogate in Figure 12.37 (bottom right panel) reveal a weak association (ignoring censoring on the true endpoint).

Individual- and trial-level surrogacy, Kendall's $\tau = 0.2763\ (0.2124, 0.3403)$ and $R^2_{\text{trial}} = 0.0066\ (-0.0724, 0.0856)$, shown in Figure 12.38 indicate that the logarithm of PSA after 28 days is a weak surrogate to overall survival time for the prostate cancer data. The Hougaard copula is presented in the output as well.

Figure 12.39 shows the parameter estimates for the treatment effects for both surrogate and true endpoints that were used to estimate trial-level surrogacy.

12.7 Validation Using a Joint Model for Continuous and Binary Endpoints

Similar to the previous section, we assume an underlying latent normally distributed surrogate endpoint, $\tilde{S}_{ij}$, and an observed surrogate given by (Van Sanden et al., 2012):

$$S_{ij} = \begin{cases} 1 & \text{if} \quad \tilde{S}_{ij} > 0, \\ 0 & \text{if} \quad \tilde{S}_{ij} \leq 0. \end{cases} \tag{12.38}$$

A joint model is assumed for the latent surrogate variable $\tilde{S}_{ij}$ and the true endpoint T_{ij},

$$\begin{cases} T_{ij} = \mu_{Ti} + \beta_i Z_{ij} + \varepsilon_{T_{ij}}, \\ \tilde{S}_{ij} = \mu_{Si} + \alpha_i Z_{ij} + \varepsilon_{\tilde{S}_{ij}}, \end{cases} \tag{12.39}$$

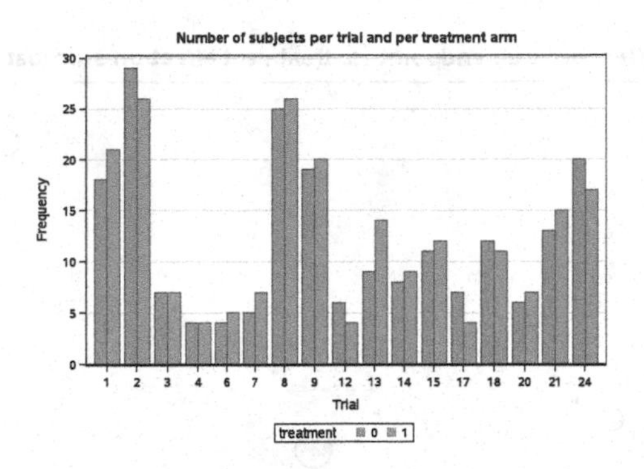

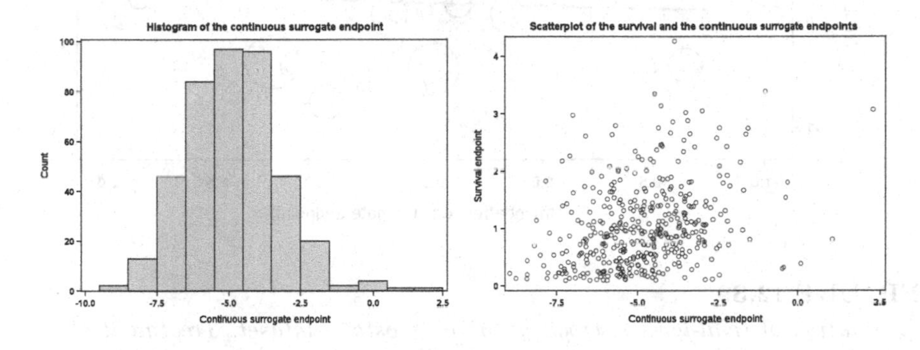

FIGURE 12.37
Descriptive plots for the prostate dataset. Panel a: Patients distribution by treatment arms across trials. Panel b: Histogram for the continuous surrogate endpoint. Panel c: Scatter plot between the survival time (ignoring censoring) true endpoint and the continuous surrogate endpoint.

COPULA PARAMETER			INDIVIDUAL			TRIAL		
LOWER	ALPHA	UPPER	LOWER	TAU	UPPER	LOWER	R square	UPPER
0.6597	0.7237	0.7876	0.2124	0.2763	0.3403	-0.0724	0.0066	0.0856

FIGURE 12.38
Prostate Data. Surrogacy measures.

where

$$\begin{pmatrix} \varepsilon_{T_{ij}} \\ \varepsilon_{\tilde{S}_{ij}} \end{pmatrix} \sim N\left[\begin{pmatrix} 0 \\ 0 \end{pmatrix}, \begin{pmatrix} \sigma_{TT} & \sigma_{ST} \\ & 1 \end{pmatrix}\right]. \tag{12.40}$$

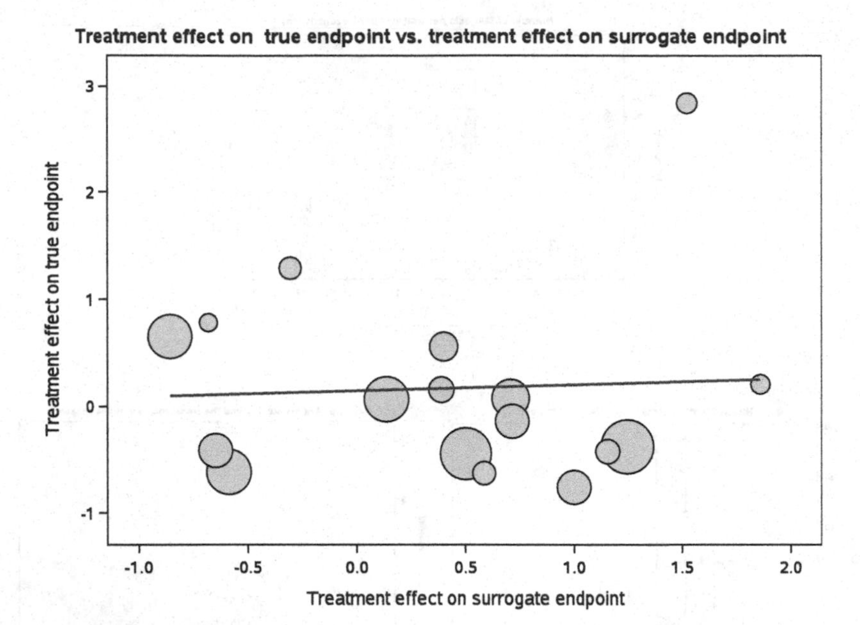

FIGURE 12.39
Evaluation of trial-level surrogacy for the prostate dataset. Treatment effects upon the true endpoints (log-hazard ratio) versus treatment effects upon the continuous surrogate. The size of the circle per trial is proportional to the sample size of the trial.

Model formulation for the observed binary outcome S_{ij} and the T_{ij} are given by

$$\begin{aligned} T_{ij} &= \mu_{Ti} + \beta_i Z_{ij} + \varepsilon_{Tij}, \\ \text{logit}\{P(S_{ij} = 1|Z_{ij})\} &= \mu_{Si} + \alpha_i Z_{ij}. \end{aligned} \tag{12.41}$$

The correlation between the measurement of the response variables can be modeled directly using the covariance matrix of the residuals, specified in (12.40), and a measure for individual-level surrogacy is given by

$$R^2_{\text{indiv}} = \frac{\sigma^2_{ST}}{1 \times \sigma_{TT}}. \tag{12.42}$$

Note that for this surrogacy setting the measure for individual-level surrogacy is the adjusted association between the true endpoint and the latent surrogate endpoint.

Trial-level surrogacy is estimated using a second-stage model for the parameter estimates of the treatment effects for the surrogate and true endpoints (Section 12.3.2).

Obs	patid	trialend	treatn	truend	surrogend
1	121	3	-1	5	1
2	278	3	1	-39	0
3	321	3	1	-17	1
4	541	3	-1	-31	0
5	632	3	1	24	1
6	767	3	1	-46	0
7	902	3	-1	-10	1
8	975	3	1	-11	1
9	1111	3	1	26	1

FIGURE 12.40
Data structure for some selected patients.

12.7.1 Data Structure

For the analysis presented in this section we use the Schizophrenia study (see Section 2.2.2) for illustration. The true endpoint is the PANSS score. For the binary surrogate we use the CGI, score which was dichotomized in the following way:

$$S_{ij} = \begin{cases} 1 & \text{if } \mathrm{CGI}_{ij} \text{ changed 3 points from baseline,} \\ 0 & \text{otherwise.} \end{cases} \tag{12.43}$$

Patient's data appear on a single line. The treatment variable is coded 1 and −1. Note that only trials with at least two patients per treatment arm were included (i.e., data obtained for 99 investigators and 1757 patients); see Figure 12.40.

12.7.2 The SAS Macro %NORMALBIN

The SAS macro `%NORMALBIN` can be used to fit the joint model specified in (12.41). For the Schizophrenia study the macro is called as follows:

```
%NORMALBIN(data=schizo,true=panss,surrog=cgi,trt=trtmnt,
           trial=investid,patid=patientid)
```

The macro's arguments were defined in Sections 12.2.

12.7.3 Data Analysis and Output

Descriptive plots produced by the macro include the distribution of patients by treatment arm (shown in Figure 12.41, top panel) and the distribution of the PANSS score by treatment arm across the levels of the surrogate endpoint in Figure 12.41 (bottom panel).

Individual- and trial-level surrogacy measures are equal to 0.3761 (0.3403, 0.4119) and 0.3747 (0.2216, 0.5279), respectively, implying that CGI is a poor surrogate to the PANSS score. Note that, due to convergence problems, only trials with at least two patients per treatment arm were included in the analysis. The results presented above are slightly different from those presented in Section 13.5.1, in which information theory was used to calculate the surrogacy measures. Figure 12.43 shows a scatter plot of the trial-specific parameter estimates for the treatment effects used in the second-stage model for the evaluation of trial-level surrogacy.

12.7.4 SAS Code for the First-Stage Model

In this section we discuss the implementation of the first-stage model using SAS procedure `GLIMMIX`. Note that the macro `%NORMALBIN` uses the same implementation, although it is not visible for the user. The joint model (12.41) is fitted using the following code:

```
proc glimmix data=norbin;
class patientid endp trial;
model response(event='1') = endp endp*treat*trial /
      noint s dist=byobs(endp) link=byobs(lin) cl;
random _residual_ / subject=patientid type=un cl;
run;
```

It is assumed that there are two records per subject in the input dataset, one corresponding to the surrogate endpoint and the other to the true endpoint.

The `response` variable contains the observed measurements on the continuous true endpoint and the binary surrogate endpoints for each patient. The option `event=1` specifies the event category for the binary surrogate. The probability of the event category (`event=1`) is modeled.

For the mean structure, the variable `endp` allows one to obtain endpoint-specific intercepts (common intercepts), while the interaction term `endp*treat*trial` allows us to obtain trial-specific treatment effects for both surrogate and true endpoints.

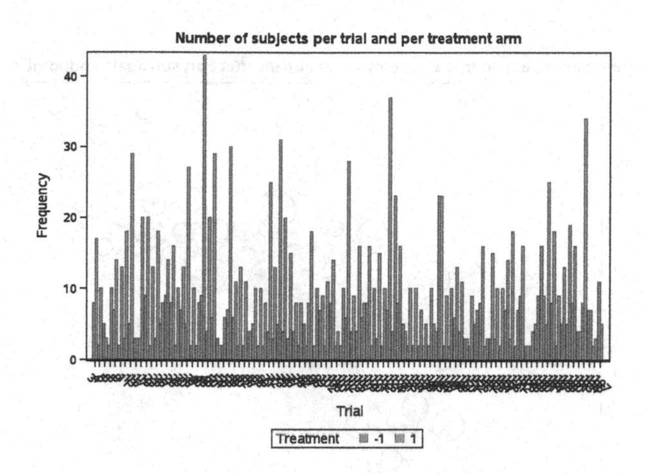

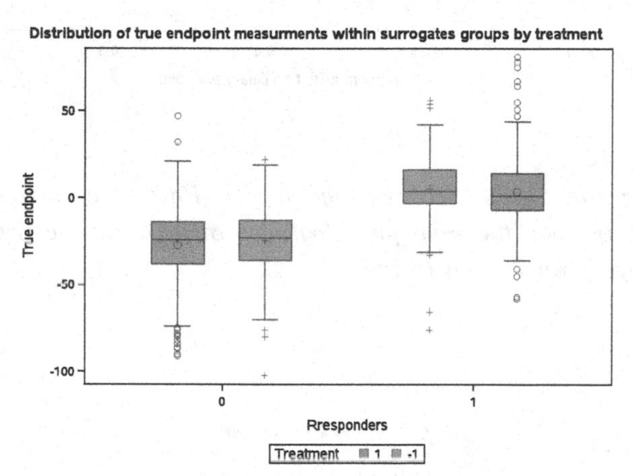

FIGURE 12.41

The Schizophrenia Study. Exploratory plots for a normal-binary surrogacy setting. Panel a: Patients distribution by treatment arm. Panel b: PANSS score distribution by treatment arm across the levels of CGI scores.

INDIVIDUAL			TRIAL		
LOWER	Individual	UPPER	LOWER	R square	UPPER
0.3403	0.3761	0.4119	0.2216	0.3747	0.5279

FIGURE 12.42

Trial- and individual-level surrogacy measures with 95% C.I.

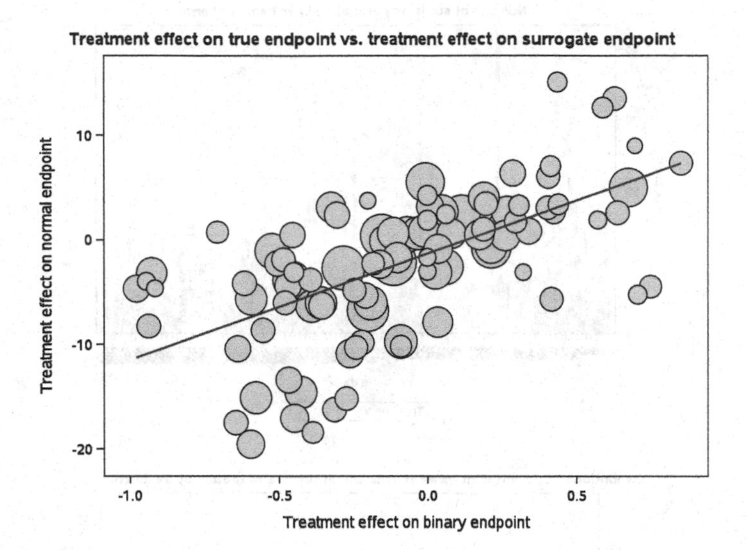

FIGURE 12.43
The Schizophrenia Study. Second-stage model. Parameter estimates for the treatment effects upon the surrogate (log(odds ratio)) and the true endpoints. Circle areas are proportional to trial size.

Covariance Parameter Estimates			
Cov Parm	Subject	Estimate	Standard Error
UN(1,1)	patid	554.85	19.2779
UN(2,1)	patid	15.1447	0.7027
UN(2,2)	patid	1.0602	0.03684

Solutions for Fixed Effects										
Effect	dist	trial	Estimate	Standard Error	DF	t Value	Pr > |t|	Alpha	Lower	Upper
dist	Binary		-0.2840	0.03808	1757	-7.46	<.0001	0.05	-0.3587	-0.2093
dist	Normal		-13.6610	0.6697	1757	-20.40	<.0001	0.05	-14.9745	-12.3475
treat*dist*trial	Binary	3	0.04939	0.2619	1757	0.19	0.8504	0.05	-0.4643	0.5631
treat*dist*trial	Binary	4	0.6277	0.3890	1757	1.61	0.1068	0.05	-0.1352	1.3906
treat*dist*trial	Binary	5	-0.4535	0.4741	1757	-0.96	0.3390	0.05	-1.3834	0.4765
treat*dist*trial	Binary	6	0.4239	0.3799	1757	1.12	0.2646	0.05	-0.3212	1.1689
treat*dist*trial	Binary	8	0.03478	0.2858	1757	0.12	0.9031	0.05	-0.5257	0.5953

FIGURE 12.44
SAS output for selected trials.

The option `noint` requests that no intercept be included in the mean structure (since these are defined by `endp`).

The argument `dist` specifies the built-in (conditional) probability distribution of the data (normal distribution for the true endpoint, and the binomial distribution for the surrogate endpoint). The option `dist=byobs(endp)` designates a variable whose value identifies the distribution to which an observation belongs, while the option `link=byobs(variable)` designates a variable whose values identify the link function associated with each endpoint (i.e., identity link for the continuous endpoint and logit link for the binary endpoint).

The statement and argument `RANDOM _residual_` specify the residual covariance structure. Finally, the `subject` argument identifies the subject for the analysis, while `type` is used to define the covariance matrix (a 2 × 2 matrix in our case). The panel in Figure 12.44 displays the covariance matrix and selected parameter estimates for the fixed effects.

12.8 Validation Using a Joint Model for Two Binary Endpoints

To extend the methodology used for continuous endpoints to the case of binary endpoints, Renard et al. (2002) adopted a latent variable approach, assuming that the observed binary variables (S_{ij}, T_{ij}) are obtained from dichotomizing unobserved continuous variables $(\tilde{S}_{ij}, \tilde{T}_{ij})$. The realized value of S_{ij} (T_{ij}) equals 1 if $\tilde{S}_{ij} > 0$ $(\tilde{T}_{ij} > 0)$, and 0 otherwise. It is assumed that the latent variables, representing the continuous underlying values of the surrogate and the true endpoints for the jth subject in the ith trial, follow a random-effects model at latent scale given by:

$$\begin{cases} \tilde{S}_{ij} = \mu_S + m_{S_i} + (\alpha + a_i)Z_{ij} + \tilde{\varepsilon}_{S_{ij}}, \\ \tilde{T}_{ij} = \mu_T + m_{T_i} + (\beta + b_i)Z_{ij} + \tilde{\varepsilon}_{T_{ij}}. \end{cases} \tag{12.44}$$

Here, μ_s and μ_T are fixed intercepts, α and β are fixed treatment effects, m_{Si} and m_{Ti} are random (i.e., trial-specific) intercepts, a_i and b_i are random treatment effects, and $\tilde{\varepsilon}_{S_{ij}}$ and $\tilde{\varepsilon}_{T_{ij}}$ are error terms. The random effects are zero-mean normally distributed with covariance matrix D. The error terms are assumed to follow a bivariate normal distribution with zero-mean and covariance matrix given by

$$\sum = \begin{pmatrix} 1 & \rho_{ST} \\ & 1 \end{pmatrix}. \tag{12.45}$$

The model formulated in (12.44) leads to a joint probit model:

$$\begin{cases} \Phi^{-1}(P[S_{ij} = 1|Z_{ij}, m_{Si}, a_i, m_{Ti}, b_i]) = \mu_s + m_{Si} + (\alpha + a_i)Z_{ij}, \\ \Phi^{-1}(P[T_{ij} = 1|Z_{ij}, m_{Si}, a_i, m_{Ti}, b_i]) = \mu_T + m_{Ti} + (\beta + b_i)Z_{ij}, \end{cases} \quad (12.46)$$

where Φ denotes the standard normal cumulative distribution function. Similar to the normal-normal setting, a reduced fixed-effects model in which the random intercepts and slopes are excluded and assuming common intercepts can be formulated as

$$\begin{cases} \Phi^{-1}(P[S_{ij} = 1|Z_{ij}]) = \mu_s + \alpha_i Z_{ij}, \\ \Phi^{-1}(P[T_{ij} = 1|Z_{ij}]) = \mu_T + \beta_i Z_{ij}. \end{cases} \quad (12.47)$$

Individual-level surrogacy can be estimated using the adjusted association based on the covariance matrix (12.45). This implies that for the binary-binary setting, this level of surrogacy should be interpreted at the scale of the linear predictors. Trial-specific treatment effects upon the true and the surrogate endpoints can be used in the second stage to fit a linear regression model of the form

$$\widehat{\beta}_i = \gamma_0 + \gamma_1 \widehat{\alpha}_i + \varepsilon_i. \quad (12.48)$$

As in previous sections, the trial sizes are used as weights in order to account for the variability due to difference in sample sizes. The trial-level surrogacy measure is equal to the coefficient of determination for model (12.48).

12.8.1 Data Structure

The schizophrenia study is used for illustration of the binary-binary setting. The true endpoint is based on the PANSS score and the surrogate endpoint is based on the CGI score. The binary endpoints PANSS/CGI reflect the presence or absence of clinically relevant change in schizophrenic symptomatology. Clinically relevant change is defined as a reduction of 20% or more in the PANSS scores, i.e., 20% reduction in post-treatment scores relative to baseline scores, or a change of 3 points in the original CGI scale (Kane et al., 1988; Leucht et al., 2005). Hence, the true and surrogate binary endpoints are defined, respectively, as:

$$T_{ij} = \begin{cases} 1 & \text{if PANSS}_{ij} \text{ reduced in at least 20\% from baseline,} \\ 0 & \text{otherwise,} \end{cases}$$

$$S_{ij} = \begin{cases} 1 & \text{if CGI}_{ij} \text{ changed of 3 points from baseline,} \\ 0 & \text{otherwise.} \end{cases}$$

A partial print of the data is given in Figure 12.45.

Obs	PATIENTID	TRUE	SURROGATE	TREAT	TRIAL
1	121	0	0	-1	3
2	278	1	1	1	3
3	321	0	0	1	3
4	541	1	1	-1	3
5	632	0	0	1	3
6	767	1	1	1	3
7	902	0	0	-1	3
8	975	0	0	1	3
9	1111	0	0	1	3

FIGURE 12.45
Data structure for the binary-binary setting.

INDIVIDUAL			TRIAL		
LOWER	Individual	UPPER	LOWER	R Square	UPPER
0.6852	0.7108	0.7364	0.6227	0.7363	0.8499

FIGURE 12.46
Individual-level and trial-level surrogacy measures with 95% C.I.

12.8.2 The SAS Macro %BINBIN

The reduced fixed-effects model formulated in (12.47) can be fitted using the SAS macro %BINBIN, which has the general form

```
%BINBIN (data=schizo,true=cgi,surrog=panss,trt=trtmnt,
         trial=investid,patid=patientid,looa=1)
```

The macro's arguments were defined in Section 12.2.

12.8.3 Data Analysis and Output

Parameter estimates for individual and trial-level surrogacy (shown below) are equal to 0.7108 (0,6852, 0.7364) and 0.7363 (0.6227, 0.8499), respectively, indicating that PANSS is a surrogate of moderate value for CGI at both surrogacy levels. Figure 12.47 shows the estimated treatment effects upon both endpoints with the fitted regression line.

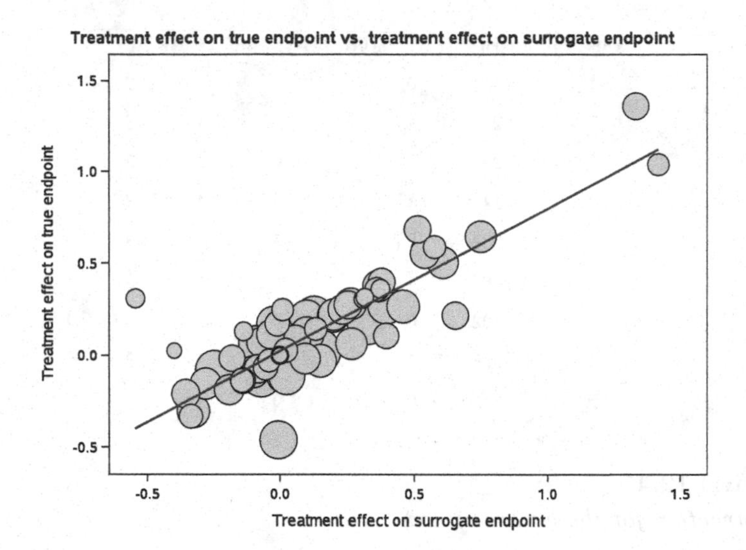

FIGURE 12.47
The Schizophrenia Study. Estimation of trial-level surrogacy. Circle areas are proportional to trial size.

12.8.4 SAS Code for the First-Stage Model

The SAS code to fit the reduced fixed-effects model formulated in (12.44) can be written as follows:

```
proc glimmix data=binbin;
class patientid endp trial;
model response(event='1') = endp endp*treat*trial /
      noint s dist=byobs(endp) link=byobs(lin) cl;
random _residual_ / subject=patientid type=un cl;
run;
```

It is assumed that there are two records per subject in the input dataset, one corresponding to the surrogate endpoint and the other to the true endpoint. A partial print of the data is shown in Figure 12.48. The `response` variable contains the observed categories on both endpoints for each patient. The statement `event=1` specifies the event category for both endpoints. The mean structure, for both endpoints, is similar to the mean structure of the reduced fixed-effects model discussed in Section 12.3.2. The option `dist=byobs(endp)` defines the distribution for each endpoint and the link function to be used is specified by the option `link=byobs(lin)`.

As in the previous section, the statement `RANDOM _residual_` specifies the residual covariance structures from which individual-level surrogacy can be

Obs	PATIENTID	RESPONSE	ENDP	TREAT	TRIAL
1	767	1	1	1	3
2	767	1	-1	1	3
3	1321	0	1	1	3
4	1321	1	-1	1	3
5	1743	1	1	1	17
6	1743	0	-1	1	17
7	2032	1	1	-1	17
8	2032	0	-1	-1	17

FIGURE 12.48
Partial print of the data.

Covariance Parameter Estimates			
Cov Parm	Subject	Estimate	Standard Error
UN(1,1)	patid	1.0000	.
UN(2,1)	patid	0.8431	0.006032
UN(2,2)	patid	1.0000	.

Solutions for Fixed Effects										
Effect	dist	trial	Estimate	Standard Error	DF	t Value	Pr > |t|	Alpha	Lower	Upper
dist	Binary		-0.1814	0.04018	1395	-4.51	<.0001	0.05	-0.2602	-0.1025
dist	binary		-0.1489	0.04029	1395	-3.69	0.0002	0.05	-0.2279	-0.06982
treat*dist*trial	Binary	3	-0.08955	0.2535	1395	-0.35	0.7239	0.05	-0.5867	0.4077
treat*dist*trial	Binary	5	0.3615	0.4338	1395	0.83	0.4049	0.05	-0.4896	1.2125
treat*dist*trial	Binary	8	0.2486	0.2771	1395	0.90	0.3698	0.05	-0.2949	0.7921
treat*dist*trial	Binary	11	0.5702	0.2856	1395	2.00	0.0461	0.05	0.009903	1.1305

FIGURE 12.49
SAS output for selected trials.

derived. The output from the above code is shown in Figure 12.49 for some trials. For the schizophrenia study, the estimated covariance matrix is

$$\widehat{\Sigma} = \begin{pmatrix} 1.0000 & 0.8431 \\ & 1.0000 \end{pmatrix}. \tag{12.49}$$

Hence, individual-level surrogacy is equal to $\widehat{R}^2_{\text{indiv}} = 0.8431^2 = 0.7108$.

12.9 Validation Using the Information-Theory Approach

12.9.1 Individual-Level Surrogacy

The information-theoretic approach for the evaluation of surrogate endpoints (Alonso and Molenberghs, 2007) is discussed in detail in Chapters 8 and 9. Briefly, this approach allows us to evaluate surrogacy at the individual and trial levels in a general surrogacy setting. In this section, we briefly present the setting and illustrate the use of two SAS macros for a normal-normal and survival-binary setting. We consider a multi-trial setting and the following models for the true endpoint:

$$\begin{cases} M_0 : g_T\{E(T_{ij}|Z_{ij})\} = \mu_{T_i} + \beta_i Z_{ij}, \\ M_1 : g_T\{E(T_{ij}|Z_{ij}, S_{ij})\} = \theta_{0_i} + \theta_{1i} Z_{ij} + \theta_{2i} S_{ij}. \end{cases} \tag{12.50}$$

Let G_i^2 be the likelihood ratio test statistic to compare models M_0 and M_1 in (12.50) within the ith trial. The association between both endpoints is quantified using the *likelihood reduction factor* (LRF) given by:

$$LRF = 1 - \frac{1}{N} \sum_i \exp\left(-\frac{G_i^2}{n_i}\right), \tag{12.51}$$

where N is the total number of the trials, and n_i is trial-specific sample size. As pointed out in Chapter 9, the LRF ranges between 0 and 1. The case with LRF=0 indicates that the surrogate and the true endpoint are independent in each trial.

12.9.2 Trial-Level Surrogacy

Trial-level surrogacy can be estimated using a two-stage approach. At the first stage, the following models are formulated for the two endpoints:

$$\begin{cases} g_T\{E(S_{ij}|Z_{ij})\} = \mu_{S_i} + \alpha_i Z_{ij}, \\ g_T\{E(T_{ij}|Z_{ij})\} = \mu_{T_i} + \beta_i Z_{ij}. \end{cases} \tag{12.52}$$

Here, μ_{T_i} and μ_{S_i} are trial-specific intercepts and α_i and β_i are trial-specific treatment effects. Note that the models can be fitted with common intercepts (i.e., reduced fixed-effects models). At the second stage, the parameter estimates obtained from (12.52) are used to fit two linear regression models given by

$$\begin{cases} M_0 : \widehat{\beta}_i = \gamma_0 + \varepsilon_{0i}, \\ M_1 : \widehat{\beta}_i = \gamma_0 + \gamma_1 \widehat{\mu}_{si} + \gamma \widehat{\alpha}_i + \varepsilon_{1i}, \end{cases} \tag{12.53}$$

where the error terms ε_{0i} and ε_{1i} are normally distributed with zero mean and constant variance σ_0^2 and σ_1^2, respectively. When the reduced fixed-effects models are used in (12.52), $\widehat{\mu}_{S_i}$ is dropped in (12.53). The trial-level surrogacy is estimated by:

$$R^2_{ht} = 1 - \exp\left(-\frac{G^2}{N}\right), \tag{12.54}$$

where G^2 is the likelihood ratio test statistic comparing the two models in (12.53).

12.9.3 Evaluation of Surrogate Endpoint for Two Continuous Endpoints

We use the age-related macular degeneration data for illustration of the analysis for the normal-normal surrogacy setting with the information-theoretic approach. As before, the true endpoint is visual acuity 52 weeks after the start of the treatment (`Diff52`) and the surrogate endpoint is the visual acuity 24 weeks after the start of treatment (`Diff24`).

The data structure for the normal-normal setting is shown in Section 12.2.

12.9.3.1 The SAS Macro %NORMNORMINFO

The models for two normally distributed endpoints can be fitted using the SAS macro `%NORMNORMINFO`. The macro fits the models formulated in (12.52)–(12.53), to estimate both individual-level and trial-level surrogacy. The call takes the form:

```
%NORMNORMINFO(data=ARMD,true=Diff54,surrog=Diff24,
   treat=treat,trial=center,patid=patientid,weighted=1,
   model="full",boot=10)
```

Arguments specific for the `%NORMNORMINFO` are:

- `model`: the model used in (12.52) and (12.53) ("reduced" or "full").
- `boot`: the number of bootstrap samples used to construct the confidence intervals for the parameter estimates of the surrogacy measures.

Other arguments have been defined in Sections 12.2 and 12.4.1.

12.9.3.2 Data Analysis and Output

The `%NORMNORMINFO` macro produces exploratory plots, displaying the distribution of the patients per trial (see, for example, Figure 12.3, left panel). Parameter estimates for the LRF and trial-level surrogacy are shown in Figure 12.52.

The estimated individual- and trial-level surrogacy are equal to $\widehat{R}^2_h = 0.5297$ (0.3785, 0.6809), and $\widehat{R}^2_{ht} = 0.7119$ (0.5074, 0.8550), respectively. Both surrogacy measures indicate that visual acuity, 24 weeks after the start of

Individual level (LRF)			Trial level		
Lower	Estimate	Upper	Lower	Estimate	Upper
0.3785	0.5297	0.6809	0.5074	0.7119	0.8550

FIGURE 12.50
Individual-level surrogacy and trial-level surrogacy measures with 95% C.I.

treatment, is a moderate surrogate for visual acuity 52 weeks after the start of the treatment.

As a sensitivity analysis, the trial-specific likelihood reduction factor is presented in Figure 12.53.

Note that the macro `%NORMNORMINFO` uses the same model formulation as the R function `FixedContContIT` (i.e., fixed-effects models for two continuous endpoints).

12.9.4 Evaluation of Surrogacy for Survival and Binary Endpoints

We use the colorectal cancer study to illustrate the analysis for the survival-binary surrogacy setting using the information-theoretic approach. The true endpoint is overall survival and the surrogate endpoint is a two-category tumor response: patients with complete or partial response are considered as responders and patients with stable or progressive disease are considered non-responders. The data structure for the survival-binary setting is shown in Section 12.5.

12.9.4.1 The SAS Macro %SURVBININFO

The information-theoretic approach discussed above can be used to evaluate surrogacy in different settings. In this section, we present the results for the survival-binary setting using the SAS macro `%SURVBININFO`. The macro fits logistic regression and the Cox proportional hazards model for a binary and survival endpoint, respectively, and uses the models formulated in (12.53) to estimate trial-level surrogacy:

```
%SURVBININFO(data=colo,true=Surv,trueind=survind,
             surrog=responder,treat=treat,trial=center,
             patid=patientid,weighted=1,
             model="reduced",boot=10)
```

Arguments specific to the `%SURVBININFO` are:

- `model`: the model used in (12.52) and (12.53) (`"Reduced"` or `"Full"`).

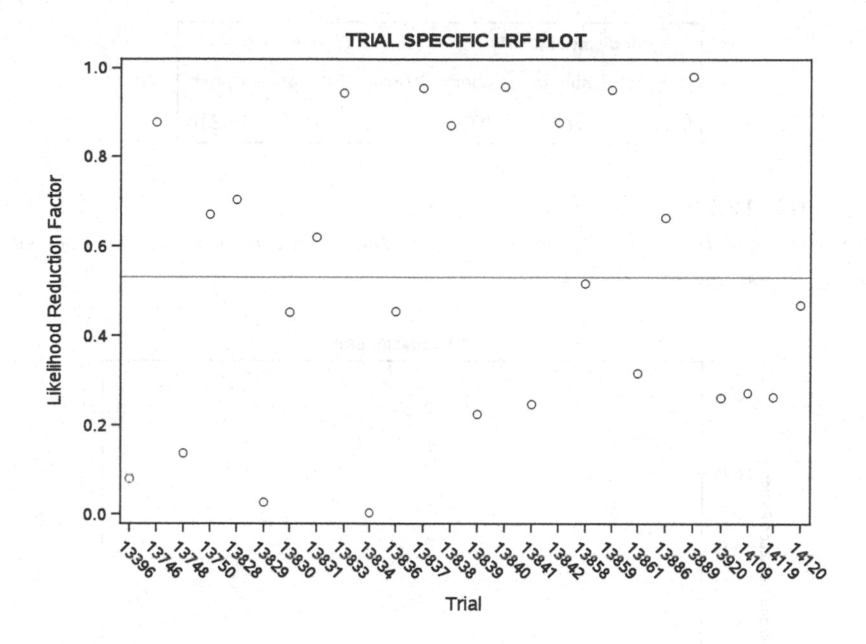

FIGURE 12.51
Trial-specific likelihood reduction factor (horizontal line: the overall LRF).

TABLE 12.3
SAS macros available for analyses using the information-theoretic approach.

Surrogacy Setting	SAS Macro	Data structure
Normal-Normal	`%NORMNORMINFO`	12.3.1
Normal-Binary	`%NORMBININFO`	12.7
Survival-Survival	`%SURVSURVINFO`	12.4
Survival-Binary	`%SURVBININFO`	12.5
Binary-Binary	`%BINBININFO`	12.8

- `boot`: the number of bootstrap samples used to construct the confidence intervals for the parameter estimates of the surrogacy measures.

Other arguments were defined in Sections 12.2.

12.9.4.2 Data Analysis and Output

The `%SURVBININFO` macro produces exploratory plots displaying the distribution of the patients per trial (see, for example, Figure 12.33, bottom panel). Estimates for the LRF and trial-level surrogacy are shown in Figure 12.52. For the colorectal study, the estimated individual- and trial-level surrogacy mea-

Individual level			Trial level		
Lower	Estimate	Upper	Lower	Estimate	Upper
0.0561	0.0797	0.1033	0.1096	0.3559	0.6216

FIGURE 12.52
The estimated likelihood reduction factor. Individual-level and trial-level surrogacy measures with 95% C.I.

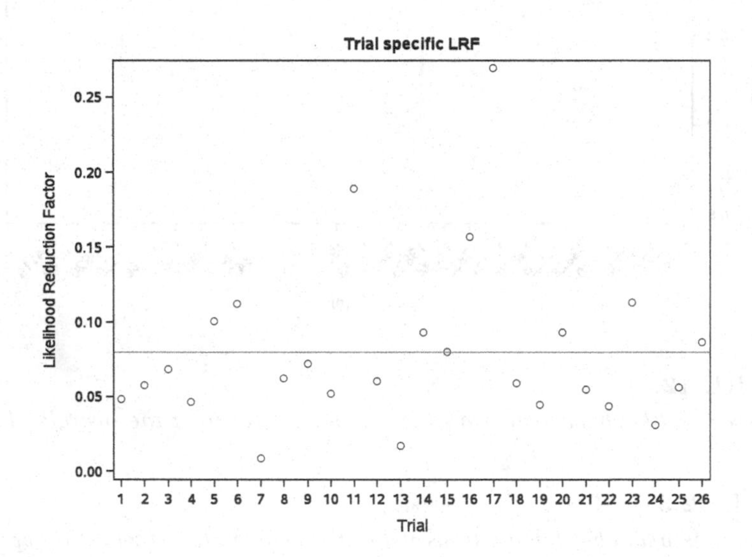

FIGURE 12.53
The Colorectal Cancer Study. Trial-specific and overall LRF (horizontal line).

sures are equal to $\widehat{R}^2_h = 0.0797$ (0.0561, 0.1033), and $\widehat{R}^2_{ht} = 0.3559$ (0.1096, 0.6216), respectively. Both surrogacy measures indicate that the binary tumor response is a poor surrogate for the overall survival. As a sensitivity analysis, trial-specific LRF is presented in Figure 12.53.

12.9.5 Other Surrogacy Settings

SAS macros that were developed for the evaluation of surrogacy using the information-theoretic approach are presented in Table 12.3. Note that, as discussed in previous sections in the chapter, the data structure depends on the surrogacy setting.

13

The R Package Surrogate

Wim Van der Elst
Hasselt University and Janssen Pharmaceutica, Belgium

Ariel Alonso Abad
KU Leuven, Belgium

Geert Molenberghs
Hasselt University and KU Leuven, Belgium

CONTENTS

13.1 Introduction

This chapter explains how the case studies that were considered in the earlier chapters can be analyzed using the R package *Surrogate*. It is assumed that a recent version of the *Surrogate* package is installed (at least version 0.1-7.3). The package can be installed by entering the command `install.packages("Surrogate")` in R. In the current chapter, only a part of the available functions in the *Surrogate* package are illustrated. A comprehensive listing of all available functions, their arguments, and output components is available in the package manual which can be downloaded at the CRAN (via `https://cran.r-project.org/web/packages/Surrogate/Surrogate.pdf`).

Loading the package and the datasets

In the analyses below, the surrogate methodology is illustrated based on the `ARMD`, `Schizo` and `Ovarian` datasets (for details, see Chapter 2.1). These datasets are included in the *Surrogate* package. The following commands can be used to load the *Surrogate* package and the datasets into memory:

```
> library(Surrogate)  # load the Surrogate library
> data(ARMD)          # load the ARMD dataset
> data(Schizo)        # load the Schizophrenia dataset
> data (Ovarian)      # load the ovarian cancer dataset

# Have a look at the first observations of the ARMD dataset:
> head(ARMD)

# Generated output:
  Id Center Treat Diff24 Diff52
1  1  13395     1      0    -10
2  2  13395    -1     -3      1
3  3  13396     1     -6    -17
4  4  13396    -1      8      1
5  5  13396    -1     -2     -2
6  6  13396     1     -5     -1
```

13.2 Two Normally Distributed Endpoints

13.2.1 The Meta-Analytic Framework

In the *Surrogate* package, there are four main functions that can be used to evaluate the appropriateness of a candidate surrogate endpoint based on the meta-analytic framework in the setting where both endpoints are normally distributed variables: the functions `BimixedContCont()`, `UnimixedContCont()`, `BifixedContCont()`, and `UnifixedContCont()`. The first part of the function name refers to the endpoint dimension of the model, i.e., whether a Univariate or a Bivariate modeling approach is used (for details, see Section 4.3.3). The second part of the function name refers to the trial dimension, i.e., whether a fixed- or mixed-effects model should be fitted (for details, see Section 4.3.1). The third part of the function name refers to the fact that both S and T are assumed to be normally distributed Continuous endpoints. Further, the arguments `Model="Full"` or `Model="Reduced"` can be used in the function call to specify whether a full or a reduced model should be fitted, respectively (for details, see Section 4.3.2). Finally, the arguments `Weighted=TRUE` or `Weighted=FALSE` can be used in the function call to specify whether measurement error should be accounted for or not, respectively (for details, see 4.3.4). Note that the latter argument is not used in the `BimixedContCont()` function because it is irrelevant when the bivariate mixed-effects (hierarchical) approach is used, i.e., measurement error is automatically accounted for in that approach. A summary of the different models that can be fitted using the `BimixedContCont()`, `UnimixedContCont()`, `BifixedContCont()`, and `UnifixedContCont()` functions is provided in Table 13.1.

Main function arguments

The functions

- `BimixedContCont()`,
- `UnimixedContCont()`,
- `BifixedContCont()`, and
- `UnifixedContCont()`

require the following arguments:

- `Dataset=`: The name of a `data.frame` that should consist of one line per patient. Each line should contain (at least) a surrogate value, a true endpoint value, a treatment indicator, a patient ID, and a trial ID.
- `Surr=, True=, Trial.ID=, Pat.ID=`: The names of the variables in the dataset that contain the surrogate and true endpoint values, the trial indicator, and the patient indicator, respectively.
- `Treat=`: The name of the variable in the dataset that contains the treatment indicator. The treatment indicator should be coded as 1 for the experimental

TABLE 13.1

Surrogate *package. Overview of the functions that can be used to evaluate surrogacy in the meta-analytic framework when both* S *and* T *are normally distributed endpoints.*

Note. *The indicator* `(...)` *refers to a number of required function arguments; for details see Section 13.2.1.*

	Full		Reduced	
	Mixed-effects approach			
	(Un)weighted		(Un)weighted	
Bivariate	`BimixedContCont(..., Model="Full")`		`BimixedContCont(..., Model="Reduced")`	
	Unweighted	Weighted	Unweighted	Weighted
Univariate	`UnimixedContCont(..., Model="Full", Weighted=FALSE)`	`UnimixedContCont(..., Model="Full", Weighted=TRUE)`	`UnimixedContCont(..., Model="Reduced", Weighted=FALSE)`	`UnimixedContCont(..., Model="Reduced", Weighted=TRUE)`
	Fixed-effects approach			
	Unweighted	Weighted	Unweighted	Weighted
Bivariate	`BifixedContCont(..., Model="Full", Weighted=FALSE)`	`BifixedContCont(..., Model="Full", Weighted=TRUE)`	`BifixedContCont(..., Model="Reduced", Weighted=FALSE)`	`BifixedContCont(..., Model="Reduced", Weighted=TRUE)`
	Unweighted	Weighted	Unweighted	Weighted
Univariate	`UnifixedContCont(..., Model="Full", Weighted=FALSE)`	`UnifixedContCont(..., Model="Full", Weighted=TRUE)`	`UnifixedContCont(..., Model="Reduced", Weighted=FALSE)`	`UnifixedContCont(..., Model="Reduced", Weighted=TRUE)`

group or −1 for the control group, or as 1 for the experimental group or 0 for the control group. Notice that the choice for a 0/1 or −1/1 coding of treatment is relevant and may impact the results when a hierarchical (bivariate mixed-effects) modeling strategy is used (see Section 4.4).

- `Model=`: The type of model that should be fitted, i.e., `Model=c("Full")` or `Model=c("Reduced")`. For details, see Section 4.3.2. If `Model=` is not specified, `Model=c("Full")` is used by default.

- `Weighted=`: A logical indicator that specifies whether a weighted (argument `Weighted=TRUE`) or unweighted (argument `Weighted=FALSE`) model should be fitted in Stage 2 (for details, see Section 4.3.4). Weighting accounts for the heterogeneity in information content between the different trial-level contributions. It is mainly relevant to take this heterogeneity into account when there are large differences in the number of patients in the different trials. If the argument `Weighted=` is not specified, by default `Weighted=TRUE` is used. Note that the `Weighted=` argument is only used in the `UnimixedContCont()`, `BifixedContCont()`, and `UnifixedContCont()` functions, because the heterogeneity in information content is automatically accounted for when the bivariate mixed-effects approach (implemented in the `BimixedContCont()` function) is used.

- `Alpha=`: The α-level that should be used to establish confidence intervals around R^2_{trial} and R^2_{indiv}. When this argument is not specified, `Alpha=0.05` is used by default.

- `Min.Trial.Size=`: The minimum number of patients that a trial-level unit should contain in order to be included in the analysis. If the number of patients in a trial is smaller than the value specified by `Min.Trial.Size=`, the data of the trial are excluded from the analysis. When this argument is not specified, `Min.Trial.Size=2` is used by default.

Depending on the function at hand, additional arguments can be used. For example, the functions `UnimixedContCont()` and `UnifixedContCont()` use bootstrapping to establish a confidence interval around R^2_{indiv}. In these functions, the argument `Number.Bootstraps=` can be used to specify the number of bootstrap samples that should be used (by default `Number.Bootstraps=500` is used) and the argument `Seed=` can be used to specify a seed (for reproducibility of the results). Full details with respect to the arguments that can be used in the different functions are provided in the *Surrogate* manual.

13.2.1.1 Analyzing the Age-Related Macular Degeneration Dataset

The bivariate mixed-effects (hierarchical) approach

After the *Surrogate* package and the ARMD dataset are loaded in memory (see Section 13.1), the following commands can be used to evaluate whether the change in visual acuity after 24 weeks (coded as `Diff24` in the `ARMD` dataset) is an appropriate surrogate for the change in visual acuity after 52 weeks (coded as `Diff52`) using the full and the reduced bivariate mixed-effects (hierarchical) approaches (for details see Chapter 4):

```
# Fit full bivariate mixed-effects model
> BimixedContCont(Dataset = ARMD, Surr = Diff24, True = Diff52,
Treat = Treat, Trial.ID = Center, Pat.ID = Id, Model = "Full")

# Fit reduced bivariate mixed-effects model
> BimixedContCont(Dataset = ARMD, Surr = Diff24, True = Diff52,
Treat = Treat, Trial.ID = Center, Pat.ID = Id,
Model = "Reduced")
```

When these commands are run, error messages are given that indicate that the (full and reduced) bivariate mixed-effects models failed to converge. For example, R gives the following error messages when the reduced hierarchical model is fitted:

```
Error in lme.formula(outcome ~ -1 + as.factor(endpoint):Treat +
as.factor(endpoint),  :
  nlminb problem, convergence error code = 1
  message = singular convergence (7)
```

As was noted in Section 4.3, such model convergence issues often occur when the hierarchical modeling approach is used in real-life datasets. When such problems occur, the simplified modeling strategies (detailed in 4.3) can be used. This is illustrated below.

The bivariate fixed-effects approach

The function `BifixedContCont()` uses a two-stage approach to evaluate surrogacy. In Stage 1, the bivariate model (4.10) is fitted, and in Stage 2, the trial-specific treatment effects on T are regressed on the trial-specific treatment effects on S (when a reduced model is fitted) or on the trial-specific intercepts and treatment effects on S (when a full model is fitted). In Stage 2, a weighted or unweighted model can be fitted. Thus, four different bivariate fixed-effect models can be fitted, i.e., a full weighted, full unweighted, reduced weighted, and reduced unweighted bivariate fixed-effect model. By means of illustration, a reduced weighted bivariate fixed-effects model is used here. Such a model can be specified by using the arguments `Weighted = TRUE` and `Model = "Reduced"` in the function call:

```
> ARMD_Bifixed_Fit <- BifixedContCont(Dataset = ARMD,
Surr = Diff24, True = Diff52, Treat = Treat,
Trial.ID = Center, Pat.ID = Id, Model = "Reduced",
Weighted = TRUE)
```

The fitted object ARMD_Bifixed_Fit (of class BifixedContCont) is placed in the R workspace and can subsequently be examined. For example, the summary() function can be applied to the fitted object ARMD_Bifixed_Fit to explore the results:

```
> summary(ARMD_Bifixed_Fit)

# Generated output:

Function call:

BifixedContCont(Dataset = ARMD, Surr = Diff24, True = Diff52,
    Treat = Treat, Trial.ID = Center, Pat.ID = Id,
    Model = "Reduced", Weighted = TRUE)


# Data summary and descriptives
#~~~~~~~~~~~~~~~~~~~~~~~~~~~~~~~~~~~~~~~~~~~~~~~~~~~~~~~~~~


Total number of trials:  36
Total number of patients:  181
M(SD) patients per trial: 5.0278 (2.9129)  [min: 2; max: 18]
Total number of patients in experimental treatment group:  84
Total number of patients in control treatment group:  97

Mean surrogate and true endpoint values
in each treatment group:

              Control.Treatment Experimental.treatment
Surrogate               -6.0309                -7.8095
True endpoint          -11.7423               -14.6548


Var surrogate and true endpoint values
in each treatment group:

              Control.Treatment Experimental.treatment
Surrogate              188.9261               132.6380
True endpoint          264.7975               231.7709


Correlations between the true and surrogate endpoints
```

```
in the control (r_T0S0) and the experimental treatment
groups (r_T1S1):

        Estimate Standard Error CI lower limit CI upper limit
r_T0S0    0.7693          0.0478         0.7022         0.8228
r_T1S1    0.7118          0.0525         0.6315         0.7770


# Meta-analytic results summary
#~~~~~~~~~~~~~~~~~~~~~~~~~~~~~~~~~~~~~~~~~~~~~~~~~~~~~~~~~~~~~~

  R2 Trial Standard Error CI lower limit CI upper limit
    0.6585         0.0965         0.4695         0.8476

  R2 Indiv Standard Error CI lower limit CI upper limit
    0.5318         0.0512         0.4315         0.6321

  R Trial Standard Error CI lower limit CI upper limit
   0.8115         0.1002         0.6585         0.9001

  R Indiv Standard Error CI lower limit CI upper limit
   0.7293         0.0511         0.5270         0.8533
```

The first part of the output shows descriptives like the number of trials in the data, the number of patients per treatment condition, and the correlations between S and T in both treatment conditions. The second part of the output is of main interest, as it provides the estimates of R^2_{trial} and R^2_{indiv}, their standard errors, and their $(1-\alpha)\%$ confidence intervals. As can be seen, $\widehat{R}^2_{\text{trial}} = 0.6585$ with 95% confidence interval [0.4695; 0.8476], and $\widehat{R}^2_{\text{indiv}} = 0.5318$ with 95% confidence interval [0.4315; 0.6321] (see also Table 4.2). To depict the results graphically, the `plot()` function can be applied to the fitted object `ARMD_Bifixed_Fit`.

```
# Plot of trial-level surrogacy
> plot(ARMD_Bifixed_Fit, Trial.Level = TRUE,
Indiv.Level = FALSE)

# Generated output:
```

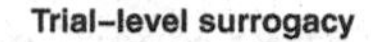

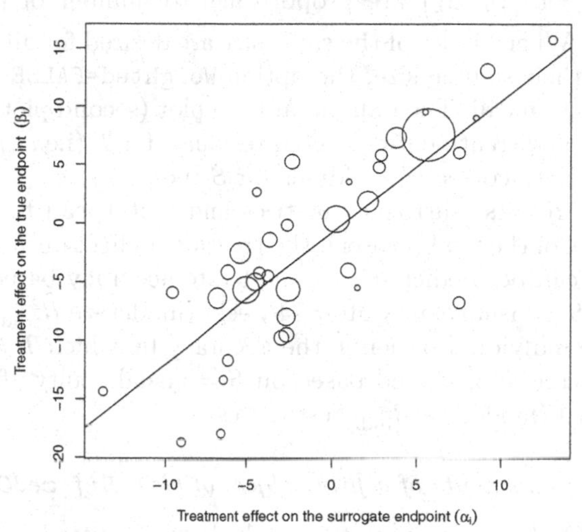


```
# Plot of individual-level surrogacy
> plot(ARMD_Bifixed_Fit, Trial.Level = FALSE,
Indiv.Level = TRUE)

# Generated output:
```

Individual-level surrogacy

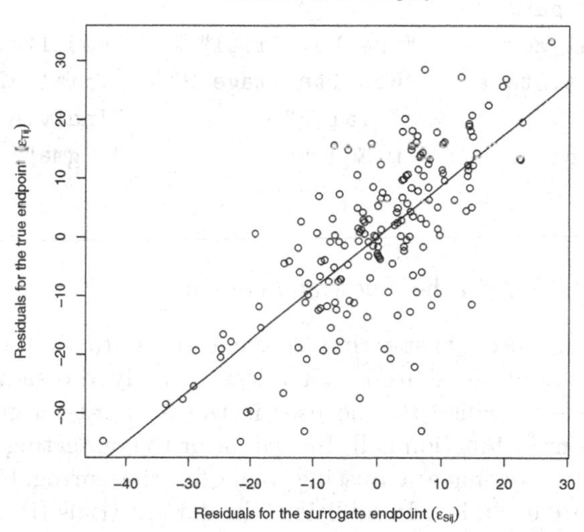

The trial-level plot (first plot in the output) shows the estimated trial-specific (here: center-specific) treatment effects on T = visual acuity after 52 weeks (i.e., $\widehat{\beta}_i$) against the estimated trial-specific (center-specific) treatment effects on S = visual acuity after 24 weeks (i.e., $\widehat{\alpha}_i$). By default, the sizes of the circles that depict $\left(\widehat{\beta}_i, \widehat{\alpha}_i\right)$ are proportional to number of patients in the trials (centers). When circles of the same size are desired for all trials (centers) irrespective of their sample size, the option `Weighted=FALSE` can be used in the `plot()` function call. The individual-level plot (second plot in the output) shows the trial- and treatment-corrected residuals for T (i.e., ε_{Tij}) against the trial- and treatment-corrected residuals for S (i.e., ε_{Sij}).

Overall, the results (surrogacy metrics and plots) lead to the conclusion that, at the level of the trial (center), the treatment effect on T = visual acuity after 52 weeks can be predicted with moderate accuracy based on the treatment effect on S = visual acuity after 24 weeks (moderate $\widehat{R}^2_{\text{trial}}$ estimates). At the level of the individual patients, the accuracy by which T = visual acuity after 52 weeks can be predicted based on S = visual acuity after 24 weeks is moderate as well (moderate $\widehat{R}^2_{\text{indiv}}$ estimates).

Examining the components of a fitted object of class `BifixedContCont()`

The `summary()` function can be applied to a fitted object of class `BifixedContCont` to obtain a summary of the most relevant results (see previous paragraph). The different components of a fitted object can also be examined in more detail. When the function `names()` is applied to the fitted object, an overview of the components that can be accessed is provided:

```
> names(ARMD_Bifixed_Fit)


# Generated output:
 [1] "Data.Analyze"       "Obs.Per.Trial"      "Results.Stage.1"
 [4] "Residuals.Stage.1" "Results.Stage.2"    "Trial.R2"
 [7] "Indiv.R2"           "Trial.R"            "Indiv.R"
[10] "Cor.Endpoints"      "D.Equiv"            "Sigma"
[13] "Call"
```

These components contain the following information:

- `Data.Analyze`: A `data.frame` that contains the data that were actually included in the analysis. This is not always exactly the same dataset as the one that was specified by the user in the `Dataset=` argument of the `BifixedContCont()` function call. Indeed, prior to conducting the analysis, data of patients who have a missing value for the surrogate and/or the true endpoint are excluded. In addition, the data of trials (i) in which only one type of the treatment was administered (i.e., all patients within a trial received the control treatment or all patients within the trial received the experimental treatment), and (ii) in which either the surrogate or the true endpoint was a constant (i.e., all patients within a trial had exactly the same surrogate and/or true endpoint value) are excluded. The user can also specify the minimum number of patients that a trial should contain in order to be included in the analysis (using the `Min.Trial.Size=` argument in the function call). If the number of patients in a particular trial is smaller than the value specified by `Min.Trial.Size`, the data of the trial are excluded as well.

- `Obs.Per.Trial`: A `data.frame` that contains the total number of patients per trial and the number of patients who were administered the control treatment and the experimental treatment in each of the trials.
- `Results.Stage.1`: The results of Stage 1 of the two-stage model-fitting approach, i.e., a `data.frame` that contains the trial-specific intercepts and treatment effects for S and T.
- `Residuals.Stage.1`: A `data.frame` that contains the residuals for S and T that are obtained in Stage 1 of the analysis, i.e., ε_{Sij} and ε_{Tij}.
- `Results.Stage.2`: An object of class `lm` (linear model) that contains the parameter estimates of the regression model that is fitted in Stage 2 of the analysis.
- `Trial.R2`: A `data.frame` that contains the trial-level coefficient of determination (R^2_{trial}), its standard error, and confidence interval.
- `Indiv.R2`: A `data.frame` that contains the individual-level coefficient of determination (R^2_{indiv}), its standard error, and confidence interval.
- `Trial.R`: A `data.frame` that contains the trial-level correlation coefficient (R_{trial}), its standard error, and confidence interval.
- `Indiv.R`: A `data.frame` that contains the individual-level correlation coefficient (R_{indiv}), its standard error, and confidence interval.
- `Cor.Endpoints`: A `data.frame` that contains the correlations between S and T in the control treatment group and in the experimental treatment group, their standard errors, and their confidence intervals.
- `D.Equiv`: The variance-covariance matrix of the trial-specific intercept and treatment effects for S and T. The name `D.Equiv` refers to the fact that the matrix is similar to the **D** matrix that is obtained when the hierarchical (bivariate mixed-effects) approach is used.
- `Sigma`: The 2-by-2 variance-covariance matrix of the residuals (ε_{Sij} and ε_{Tij}).
- `Call`: The function call that was specified by the user.

These components can be accessed using the `[Name_Fitted_Object]$[Component_Name]` command. For example, the trial-specific intercepts and treatment effects on S and T can be obtained using the following command:

```
# Request trial-specific results for first 5 trials (centers)
> ARMD_Bifixed_Fit$Results.Stage.1[1:5,]

# Generated output:
  Trial Obs.per.trial Treatment.S Treatment.T
1 13395             2    1.500000   -5.500000
2 13396             4   -4.250000   -4.250000
3 13745             3   -4.417648    2.626629
4 13746             7    2.106722    1.839984
5 13748             5    0.949411   -4.024023
```

The output shows that, for example, in the first trial (center) (coded as Trial ID = 13395 in the ARMD dataset) there were 2 patients and the estimated treatment effects on S and T in this center equaled $\alpha_1 = 1.5$ and $\beta_1 = -5.5$, respectively. As another example, the results of the Stage 2 analysis can be obtained by the command:

```
# Request Stage 2 model results
> ARMD_Bifixed_Fit$Results.Stage.2

# Generated output:
Call:
lm(formula = Treatment.T ~ Treatment.S, data = Results.Stage.1,
    weights = Results.Stage.1$Obs.per.trial)

Coefficients:
(Intercept)  Treatment.S
    -0.4467       1.1252
```

Thus, when the Stage 2 model $\widehat{\beta}_i = \lambda_0 + \lambda_1 \widehat{\alpha}_i + \varepsilon_i$ is fitted based on the Stage 1 results, it is obtained that $\widehat{\lambda}_0 = -0.4467$ and $\widehat{\lambda}_1 = 1.1252$. As noted above, `ARMD_Bifixed_Fit$Results.Stage.2` is a fitted object of class `lm` and thus it can be explored in a straightforward way using the available functions for this class. For example, diagnostic plots of model fit (e.g., a normal Q-Q plot) can be obtained by applying the `plot()` function, or more details regarding the fitted model (e.g., the standard errors of the parameter estimates) can be obtained by using the `summary()` function. By means of illustration, the `summary()` function is applied here:

```
> summary(ARMD_Bifixed_Fit$Results.Stage.2)

# Generated output:
Call:
lm(formula = Treatment.T ~ Treatment.S, data = Results.Stage.1,
```

```
    weights = Results.Stage.1$Obs.per.trial)

Weighted Residuals:
    Min      1Q  Median      3Q     Max
-29.485  -8.913   1.746   6.538  18.591

Coefficients:
            Estimate Std. Error t value Pr(>|t|)
(Intercept)  -0.4467     0.7666  -0.583    0.564
Treatment.S   1.1252     0.1390   8.098 1.92e-09 ***
---
Signif. codes:  0 '***' 0.001 '**' 0.01 '*' 0.05 '.' 0.1 ' ' 1

Residual standard error: 10.18 on 34 degrees of freedom
Multiple R-squared:  0.6585,Adjusted R-squared:  0.6485
F-statistic: 65.57 on 1 and 34 DF,  p-value: 1.925e-09
```

Notice that the `Multiple R-squared: 0.6585` component toward the end of the output corresponds to the estimated R^2_{trial}.

The expected treatment effect on T in a new trial

The main motivation to evaluate a candidate surrogate endpoint is to be able to predict the treatment effect on T based on the estimated treatment effect on S in a new trial $i = 0$. For example, suppose that a new clinical trial is conducted using the same treatments as the ones that were used in the ARMD trial in a similar patient population. In this new trial, visual acuity is only measured after 24 weeks but not after 52 weeks. Interest is in the prediction of the expected treatment effect on visual acuity after 52 weeks, based on the treatment effect on visual acuity after 24 weeks. Suppose that $\widehat{\alpha}_0 = -1$, i.e., the estimated treatment effect on visual acuity after 24 weeks in the new trial, equals -1. Based on this estimate and using the results of the bivariate weighted reduced fixed-effects model that was fitted above, the expected treatment effect on T, i.e., $E\left(\beta + b_0 \mid a_0 = -1\right)$, can be obtained using the following commands:

```
# Compute expected treatment effect on T in new trial
# i = 0 where alpha_0 = -1
> ExpTreatT <- Pred.TrialT.ContCont(ARMD_Bifixed_Fit,
alpha_0 = -1)
```

The results can be explored by applying the `summary()` and `plot()` functions to the fitted `ExpTreatT` object:

```
# Request summary of the results:
```

```
> summary(ExpTreatT)

# Generated output:
Function call:
Pred.TrialT.ContCont(Object = Reduced_Weighted, alpha_0 = -1)

Results:
--------
Expected treatment effect (variance) on T (beta_0) = -1.9324
 (25.1379)  95% CI: [-11.7592; 7.8944]


# Plot the results
> plot(ExpTreatT)

# Generated output:
```

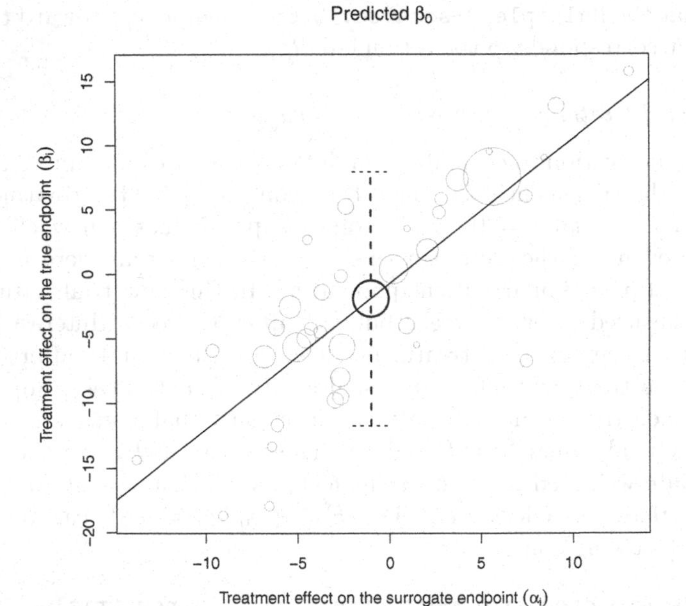

The plot shows the trial-specific treatment effects on T and S that were obtained in the ARMD dataset using the weighted reduced bivariate fixed-effects model (gray circles), the expected treatment effect on T in the hypothetical new trial $i = 0$ (black circle), and the 95% confidence interval around the expected treatment effect on T in the new trial (black dashed line).

The output of the summary() function shows that the expected treatment effect on T given $\widehat{\alpha}_0 = -1$ equals $E\left(\beta + b_0 \mid a_0 = -1\right) = -1.9324$, with 95% confidence interval $[-11.7592; 7.8944]$. The confidence interval around the expected treatment effect on T is thus wide, as could be expected given the fact that the trial-level surrogacy coefficient was moderate (i.e., $\widehat{R}^2_{\text{trial}} = 0.6585$).

The univariate mixed- and fixed-effects approaches

Similar to what was the case with the BifixedContCont() function, the functions UnimixedContCont() and UnifixedContCont() use a two-stage approach to assess surrogacy. In Stage 1, two univariate mixed- or fixed-effects models are fitted. In Stage 2, the trial-specific treatment effects on T are regressed on the trial-specific treatment effects on S (when a reduced model is fitted) or on both the trial-specific intercepts and treatment effects on S (when a full model is fitted). In Stage 2, one can opt again for a weighted or an unweighted analysis.

For example, suppose that we want to use a reduced weighted univariate mixed-effects model to evaluate surrogacy in the ARMD dataset. Such a model can be specified by the following command:

```
# Fit the model
> ARMD_Unimixed_Fit <- UnimixedContCont(Dataset = ARMD,
Surr = Diff24, True = Diff52, Treat = Treat,
Trial.ID = Center, Pat.ID = Id, Model = "Reduced",
Weighted = TRUE)
```

Similar to what was done above, the output can be examined by applying the summary() and plot() functions or by directly accessing components in the fitted object ARMD_Unimixed_Fit using the ARMD_Unimixed_Fit$[Name_Component] command.

13.2.2 The Information-Theoretic Framework

When both S and T are normally distributed (continuous) endpoints, two functions can be used to estimate the individual- and trial-levels of surrogacy based on the information-theoretic approach: MixedContContIT() and FixedContContIT(). The first part of the function names refer to the endpoint dimension of the model, i.e., whether a Fixed- or Mixed-effects model is fitted to estimate the trial-specific parameters (for details, see Section 4.3.1). The second part of the function name refers to the fact that both S and T should be normally distributed Continuous endpoints. The last part of the function name indicates that the Information-Theoretic (IT) approach is used. Further, the arguments Model="Full" or Model="Reduced" can be used in the function call to specify whether a full or a reduced model should be fitted (for details, see Section 4.3.2). Finally, the arguments Weighted=TRUE and

Weighted=FALSE can be used in the function call to specify whether measurement error should be accounted for or not, respectively (for details, see 4.3.4). A summary of the different models that can be fitted is shown in Table 13.2.

Main function arguments

The main arguments of the MixedContContIT() and FixedContContIT() functions are identical to those of the functions BimixedContCont(), BifixedContCont(), UnimixedContCont() and UnifixedContCont(), detailed in Section 13.2.1.

13.2.2.1 Analyzing the Age-Related Macular Degeneration Dataset

The following command can be used to evaluate whether the change in visual acuity after 24 weeks is a good surrogate for the change in visual acuity after 52 weeks, as evaluated based on a reduced weighted mixed-effects approach in the information-theoretic framework:

```
> ARMD_Mixed_Fit_IT <- MixedContContIT(Dataset = ARMD,
Surr = Diff24, True = Diff52, Treat = Treat,
Trial.ID = Center, Pat.ID = Id, Model = "Reduced",
Weighted = TRUE)
```

Applying the summary() function to the fitted object ARMD_Mixed_Fit_IT provides the following output:

```
> summary(ARMD_Mixed_Fit_IT)

# Generated output:
Function call:

MixedContContIT(Dataset = ARMD, Surr = Diff24, True = Diff52,
    Treat = Treat, Trial.ID = Center, Pat.ID = Id,
    Model = "Reduced", Weighted = TRUE)


# Data summary and descriptives
#~~~~~~~~~~~~~~~~~~~~~~~~~~~~~~~~~~~~~~~~~~~~~~~~~~~~~~~~~~~~

Total number of trials:  36
Total number of patients:  181
M(SD) patients per trial: 5.0278 (2.9129)  [min: 2; max: 18]
Total number of patients in experimental treatment group:  84
Total number of patients in control treatment group:  97
```

TABLE 13.2
Surrogate *package. Overview of the functions that can be used to evaluate surrogacy in the information-theoretic framework when both S and T are normally distributed endpoints.*
Note. *The indicator `(...)` refers to a number of required function arguments; for details see Section 13.2.2.*

	Full	
	Unweighted	Weighted
Mixed-effects	`MixedContContIT(..., Model="Full", Weighted=FALSE)`	`MixedContContIT(..., Model="Full", Weighted=TRUE)`
Fixed-effects	`FixedContContIT(..., Model="Full", Weighted=FALSE)`	`FixedContContIT(..., Model="Full", Weighted=TRUE)`
	Reduced	
	Unweighted	Weighted
Mixed-effects	`MixedContContIT(..., Model="Reduced", Weighted=FALSE)`	`MixedContContIT(..., Model="Reduced", Weighted=TRUE)`
Fixed-effects	`FixedContContIT(..., Model="Reduced", Weighted=FALSE)`	`FixedContContIT(..., Model="Reduced", Weighted=TRUE)`

```
Mean surrogate and true endpoint values in each treatment
group:

              Control.Treatment Experimental.treatment
Surrogate               -6.0309                -7.8095
True endpoint          -11.7423               -14.6548


Var surrogate and true endpoint values in each treatment
group:

              Control.Treatment Experimental.treatment
Surrogate              188.9261               132.6380
True endpoint          264.7975               231.7709


Correlations between the true and surrogate endpoints in the
control (r_T0S0) and the experimental treatment groups
(r_T1S1):

       Estimate Standard Error CI lower limit CI upper limit
r_T0S0   0.7693         0.0478         0.7022         0.8228
r_T1S1   0.7118         0.0525         0.6315         0.7770



# Information-theoretic surrogacy estimates summary
#~~~~~~~~~~~~~~~~~~~~~~~~~~~~~~~~~~~~~~~~~~~~~~~~~~~~~~~~~~

Trial-level surrogacy (R2_ht):
    R2ht CI lower limit CI upper limit
  0.6864         0.4750         0.8388

Individual-level surrogacy (R2_hind):
  R2h.ind CI lower limit CI upper limit
   0.5339         0.4315         0.6292
```

The first part of the output shows descriptives like the number of trials (here: centers) in the data, the means (variances) of S and T in the different treatment groups, and so on. The last part of the output provides the estimates of trial- and individual-level surrogacy. As can be seen, $\widehat{R}^2_{ht} = 0.6864$ with 95% confidence interval [0.4750; 0.8388], and $\widehat{R}^2_{h\text{indiv}} = 0.5339$ with 95% confidence interval [0.4315; 0.6292] (the same results as in Section 10.2.1). These results thus indicate (i) that the uncertainty about the treatment effect on T that is reduced when the treatment effect on S becomes known (trial-level surrogacy) is moderate, and (ii) that the uncertainty about T that is reduced when S becomes known (individual-level surrogacy) is moderate as well.

The results can be further explored by applying the `plot()` function and by directly accessing the components in the fitted `ARMD_Mixed_Fit_IT` object in the same way as was illustrated in Section 13.2.1.

13.3 Two Time-to-Event Endpoints

In the *Surrogate* package, the function `SurvSurv()` can be used to evaluate the appropriateness of a candidate surrogate when both the surrogate and the true endpoints are time-to-event (Survival time) endpoints.

The function `SurvSurv()` implements the information-theoretic approach to estimate individual-level surrogacy (see Section 10). Trial-level surrogacy (R^2_{trial}) is estimated using a two-stage approach proposed by Buyse et al. (2011). In particular, the following trial-specific Cox proportional hazard models are fitted in Stage 1:

$$\begin{aligned} S_{ij}(t) &= S_{i0}(t)\exp(\alpha_i Z_{ij}), \\ T_{ij}(t) &= T_{i0}(t)\exp(\beta_i Z_{ij}), \end{aligned}$$

where $S_{i0}(t)$, $T_{i0}(t)$ are the trial-specific baseline hazard functions, Z_{ij} is the treatment indicator for subject j in trial i, and α_i, β_i are the trial-specific treatment effects on S and T, respectively. In Stage 2, the following model is fitted:

$$\widehat{\beta}_i = \lambda_0 + \lambda_1 \widehat{\alpha}_i + \varepsilon_i, \tag{13.1}$$

where the parameter estimates for β_i and α_i are based on the model that was fitted in Stage 1. The classical coefficient of determination of the fitted Stage 2 model provides an estimate of R^2_{trial}.

Main function arguments

The function `SurvSurv()` requires the following arguments:

- `Dataset=, Surr=, True=, Trial.ID=, Pat.ID=`: The name of the dataset and the names of the variables in the dataset that contain the surrogate and true endpoint values, the trial indicator, and the patient indicator, respectively.

- `SurrCens=, TrueCens=`: The names of the variables in the dataset that contain the censoring indicators for the surrogate and the true endpoints, respectively. These censoring indicators should be coded as 1 = event and 0 = censored.

- `Weighted=`: A logical argument. If `TRUE`, then a weighted regression analysis is conducted at Stage 2 of the two-stage approach. If `FALSE`, then an unweighted regression analysis is conducted at Stage 2. Default `Weighted=TRUE`.
- `Alpha=`: The α-level that is used to determine the confidence intervals around R^2_{trial}, LRF, and LRF_a. Default `Alpha=0.05`.

13.3.1 Analyzing the Ovarian Cancer Dataset

After the *Surrogate* package and the Ovarian dataset are loaded into memory (see Section 13.1), the following command can be used to examine whether progression-free survival (PFS) is an appropriate surrogate for overall survival (OS):

```
> Ovarian_SurvSurv <- SurvSurv(Dataset = Ovarian, Surr = Pfs,
SurrCens = PfsInd, True = Surv, TrueCens = SurvInd,
Treat = Treat, Trial.ID = Center)

# Generated output:
Note. The trial with ID 28 did not have >=3 observations in
each treatment arm and was excluded from the trial-level
analyses (estimation of R2_ht) due to estimability
constraints.

                              (...)

Note. The trial with ID 66 did not have >=3 observations in
each treatment arm and was excluded from the trial-level
analyses (estimation of R2_ht) due to estimability
constraints.
```

Note that trials (clusters) with less than 3 observations are not considered in the analyses due to estimability constraints (Burzykowski et al., 2001). When such trials (clusters) are present in the dataset, the user is warned that these will not be considered in the analysis.

The fitted object `Ovarian_SurvSurv` (of class `SurvSurv`) is placed in the R workspace and it can subsequently be examined. To explore the results, the `summary()` function can be applied:

```
> summary(Ovarian_SurvSurv)
```

```
# Generated output:

Function call:

SurvSurv(Dataset = Ovarian, Surr = Pfs, SurrCens = PfsInd,
True = Surv, TrueCens = SurvInd, Treat = Treat,
Trial.ID = Center)


# R^2_trial results
#~~~~~~~~~~~~~~~~~~~~~~~~~~~~~~~~~~~~~~~~~~~~~~~~~~~~~~~~~~~~
  R2_trial Standard Error CI lower limit CI upper limit
    0.9184         0.0261         0.8674         0.9695


# R^2_{h.ind} (LRF) results
#~~~~~~~~~~~~~~~~~~~~~~~~~~~~~~~~~~~~~~~~~~~~~~~~~~~~~~~~~~~~
Overall R^2_{h.ind} (LRF):

  R2h.ind CI lower limit CI upper limit
   0.7446         0.7152         0.7720


# R^2_{h.ind.QF} (LRF_a; O'Quinly and Flandre, 2006) results
#~~~~~~~~~~~~~~~~~~~~~~~~~~~~~~~~~~~~~~~~~~~~~~~~~~~~~~~~~~~~
Overall R^2_{h.ind.QF} (LRF_a):

  R2h.ind.QF CI lower limit CI upper limit
      0.8193         0.7928         0.8433


R^2_{h.ind.QF} (LRF_a) per trial:

    TrialID R2h.ind R2h_low R2h_up
1   -4.0000  0.8408  0.7555 0.9021
2   -3.0000  0.7279  0.6578 0.7884
3    2.0000  0.7847  0.3171 0.9687
                 (...)
```

```
4    3.0000  0.8313  0.5220 0.9621
42 109.0000  0.9757  0.8185 0.9985
43 111.0000  0.8048  0.5635 0.9334
```

The top of the output shows that $\widehat{R}^2_{\text{trial}} = 0.9184$, with 95% confidence interval [0.8674; 0.9695]. This result thus indicates that PFS is a good surrogate for OS at the level of the trial (cluster), i.e., the treatment effect on OS can be predicted with a high level of accuracy based on the predicted treatment effect on PFS.

The individual-level results are shown below the trial-level results. As can be seen, the estimated $LRF = 0.7446$ with 95% confidence interval [0.7152; 0.7720], and $LRF_a = 0.8193$ with 95% confidence interval [0.7928; 0.8433]. Thus, the amount of uncertainty in $T =$ OS that is removed when the value of $S =$ PFS becomes known is quite high as well. Overall, the results indicate that PFS is a good surrogate for OS at both the levels of the individual patients and the trials (clusters).

At the end of the output, estimates of LRF_a (and their 95% confidence intervals) are provided for each of the trials (clusters) separately. For example, when attention is restricted to the first trial (cluster) in the dataset (coded as `TrialID = -4` in the `Ovarian` dataset), it is obtained that $\widehat{LRF}_{a_1} = 0.8408$ with 95% confidence interval [0.7555; 0.9021].

The results can be graphically explored by applying the `plot()` function to the fitted `Ovarian_SurvSurv` object:

```
# Plot of trial-level surrogacy
> plot(Ovarian_SurvSurv, Indiv.Level.By.Trial = FALSE,
Trial.Level = TRUE)

# Generated output:
```

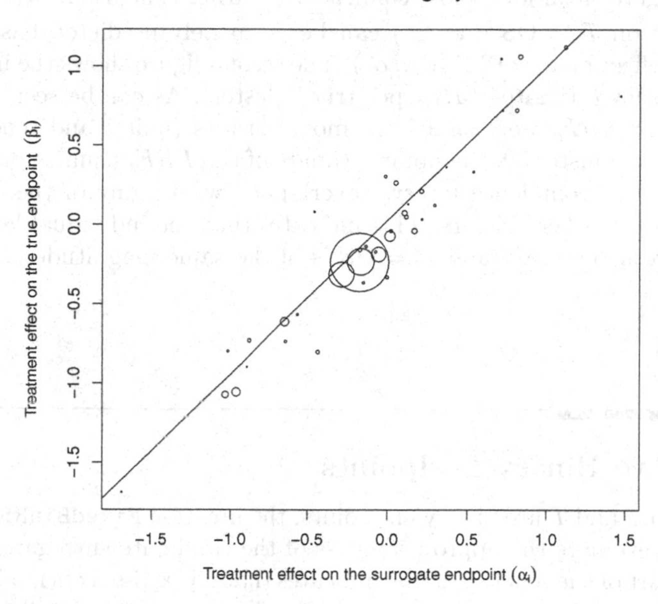


```
# Plot of individual-level surrogacy (per cluster)
> plot(Ovarian_SurvSurv, Indiv.Level.By.Trial = TRUE,
Trial.Level = FALSE)

# Generated output:
```

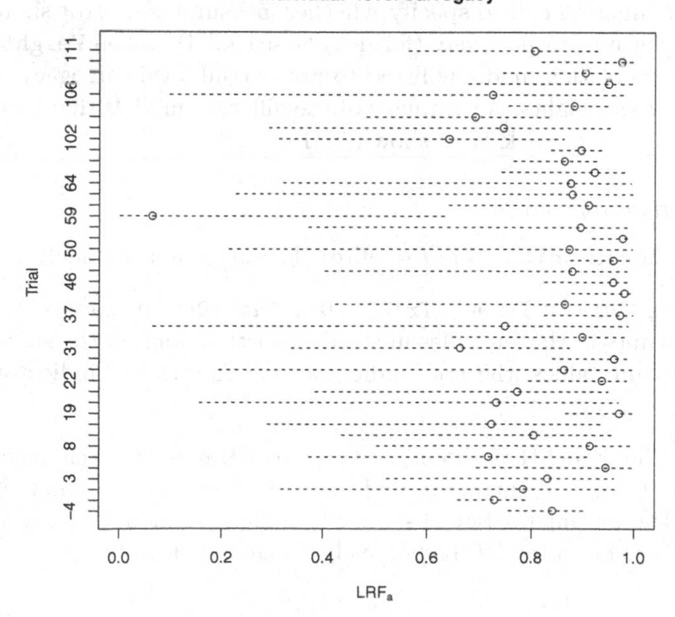

The first figure (trial-level plot) confirms the earlier conclusion that the treatment effect on T = OS (i.e., $\widehat{\beta}_i$) can be accurately predicted based on the treatment effect on S = PFS (i.e., $\widehat{\alpha}_i$). The second figure shows the individual-level surrogacy estimates LRF_a per trial (cluster). As can be seen, the point estimates for LRF_a were similar in most clusters (units) and tended to be above 0.65. In cluster 59, the point estimate of the LRF_a equaled only 0.0639, though its 95% confidence interval overlapped with many of the confidence intervals of the other clusters. This indicates that the individual-level association between S = PFS and T = OS is of the same magnitude across trials (centers).

13.4 Two Binary Endpoints

When both S and T are binary endpoints, the function `FixedBinBinIT()` can be used to evaluate the appropriateness of the candidate surrogate endpoint. The first part of the function name indicates that a Fixed-effects model is fitted to estimate the trial-specific treatment effects α_i and β_i (for details, see Chapter 9). The second and third parts of the function name indicate that both S and T should be Binary endpoints and that the Information-Theoretic (IT) approach is used. Further, the arguments `Model="Full"` or `Model="Reduced"` can be used in the function call to specify whether a full or a reduced model should be fitted to obtain estimates for α_i and β_i (for details, see Section 4.3.2). Finally, the arguments `Weighted=TRUE` and `Weighted=FALSE` can be used in the function call to specify whether measurement error should be accounted for or not, respectively (for details, see 4.3.4). When `Weighted=TRUE`, a weighted regression model is fitted to assess trial-level surrogacy, with trial (cluster) size as weights. A summary of the different models that can be fitted using the *Surrogate* package is shown in Table 13.3.

Main function arguments

The function `FixedBinBinIT()` requires the following arguments:

- `Dataset=, Surr=, True=, Trial.ID=, Pat.ID=`: The name of the dataset and the names of the variables in the dataset that contain the surrogate and true endpoint values, the trial indicator, and the patient indicator, respectively.

- `Model=`: The model that should be fitted to estimate the trial-specific treatment effects on the surrogate and the true endpoints (α_i and β_i, respectively). The arguments `Model="Full"` or `Model="Reduced"` are used to fit a full or a reduced model, respectively. Default `Model="Full"`.

- `Weighted=`: A logical argument. If `TRUE`, then a weighted regression analysis is used to estimate trial-level surrogacy. If `FALSE`, then an unweighted regression analysis is used. Default `Weighted=TRUE`.
- `Alpha=`: The α-level that is used to determine the confidence intervals around the estimates of trial- and individual-level surrogacy. Default 0.05.
- `Number.Bootstraps=`: The standard errors and confidence intervals for the individual-level surrogacy estimates are determined based on a bootstrap. `Number.Bootstraps=` specifies the number of bootstrap samples that are used. Default `Number.Bootstraps=50`.

13.4.1 Analyzing the Data of Five Clinical Trials in Schizophrenia

Here, it is examined whether the dichotomized BPRS score (1 = clinically relevant change on the BPRS at the end of the treatment; 0 = no clinically relevant change at the end of the treatment) is an appropriate surrogate for the dichotomized PANSS score (1 = clinically relevant change on PANSS at the end of the treatment; 0 = no clinically relevant change at the end of the treatment) using the data of the five clinical trials in schizophrenia (for details, see Section 2.2.2). The data of only five trials were available, which is insufficient to use clinical trial as the cluster-level unit (see Section 4.4). In the different trials, information was also available regarding the psychiatrists who treated the patients. Hence, treating physician was used as the clustering unit in the analysis below.

After the *Surrogate* package and the `Schizo` dataset are loaded in memory (see Section 13.1), the function `FixedBinBinIT()` is called to conduct the analysis. Different models can be fitted (see Table 13.3). By means of illustration, a full weighted model is requested here:

```
> Schizo_BinBin <- FixedBinBinIT(Dataset = Schizo,
Surr = BPRS_Bin, True = PANSS_Bin, Treat = Treat,
Model = "Full", Weighted = TRUE, Trial.ID = InvestId,
Pat.ID = Id, Seed = 1) # Seed used for reproducibility
```

Applying the `summary()` function to the fitted object `Schizo_BinBin` provides the following output:

```
> summary(Schizo_BinBin)

# Generated output:
Function call:

FixedBinBinIT(Dataset = Schizo, Surr = BPRS_Bin,
```

TABLE 13.3
Surrogate *package. Overview of the functions that can be used to evaluate surrogacy in the information-theoretic framework when both S and T are binary endpoints.*
Note. *The indicator* `(...)` *refers to a number of required function arguments; for details see Section 13.4.*

	Unweighted	Weighted
Full model	`FixedBinBinIT(..., Model="Full", Weighted=FALSE)`	`FixedBinBinIT(..., Model="Full", Weighted=TRUE)`
Reduced model	`FixedBinBinIT(..., Model="Reduced", Weighted=FALSE)`	`FixedBinBinIT(..., Model="Reduced", Weighted=TRUE)`

```
True = PANSS_Bin, Treat = Treat, Trial.ID = InvestId,
Pat.ID = Id, Model = "Full", Weighted = TRUE, Seed = 1)


# Data summary and descriptives
#~~~~~~~~~~~~~~~~~~~~~~~~~~~~~~~~~~~~~~~~~~~~~~~~~~~~~~~~~~~~~~~~~~~~~~~


Total number of trials:  144
Total number of patients:  1988
M(SD) patients per trial: 13.8056 (10.1522)  [min: 2; max: 52]
Total number of patients in experimental treatment group: 1472
Total number of patients in control treatment group:  516


# Information-theoretic surrogacy estimates summary
#~~~~~~~~~~~~~~~~~~~~~~~~~~~~~~~~~~~~~~~~~~~~~~~~~~~~~~~~~~~~~~~~~~~~~~~


Trial-level surrogacy (R2_ht):
    R2ht CI lower limit CI upper limit
  0.7414          0.6510         0.8155

Individual-level surrogacy (R2_h.ind):
  R2h.ind CI lower limit CI upper limit
   0.5392          0.5089         0.5688
```

The first part of the output shows descriptives like the number of trials in the data and the number of patients in the different treatment groups. Note that a total of 2128 patients participated in the five clinical trials, though the output shows that the data of only 1988 patients were actually included in the analyses.

The reason for this is that, prior to conducting the surrogacy analysis, data of patients who have a missing value for the surrogate and/or the true endpoint are excluded. In addition, the data of trials (or: clusters, treating physicians, ...) (i) in which only one type of the treatment was administered (i.e., all patients received the experimental treatment or all patients received the control treatment), and (ii) in which either the surrogate or the true endpoint was a constant (i.e., all patients within a trial had exactly the same surrogate and/or true endpoint value) are excluded because trial-specific treatment effects cannot be estimated in such trials (clusters). The subset of the dataset that was included in the analysis can be obtained by using the `Schizo_BinBin$Data.Analyze` command.

The second part of the output provides the estimates of trial- and individual-level surrogacy. The $\widehat{R}^2_{ht} = 0.7414$ with 95% confidence interval

[0.6510; 0.8155], indicating that the uncertainty about the treatment effect on T = clinically relevant change on the PANSS that is reduced when the treatment effect on S = clinically relevant change on the BPRS becomes known (trial-level surrogacy) is relatively high. The individual-level surrogacy estimate equaled $\widehat{R}^2_{h\text{indiv}} = 0.5392$ with 95% confidence interval [0.5089; 0.5688] (see also the results in Section 10.7). These results thus indicate that the uncertainty about T that is reduced when S becomes known (individual-level surrogacy) is moderate. Overall, it can be concluded that clinically relevant change on the BPRS is a moderately good surrogate for clinically relevant change on the PANSS.

The results can be further graphically explored by applying the `plot()` function to the fitted `Schizo_BinBin` object. For example, a plot of the individual-level surrogacy estimates for each cluster can be obtained using the command:

```
# Plot of individual-level surrogacy (per cluster)
> plot(Schizo_BinBin, Indiv.Level.By.Trial = TRUE,
Trial.Level = FALSE)

# Generated output:
```

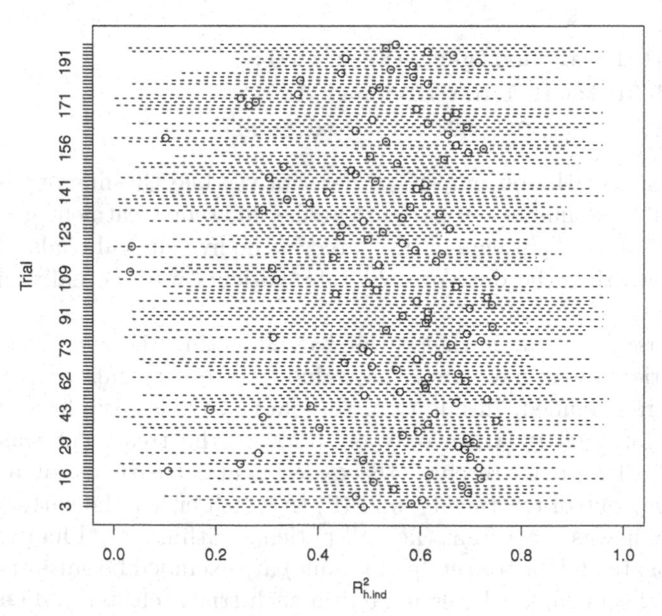

The figure shows the individual-level surrogacy estimates $\widehat{R}^2_{h\text{indiv}}$ per cluster (treating physician). As can be seen, there was substantial variability in the point estimates for $R^2_{h\text{ind}}$ across clusters. Nonetheless, the 95% confidence intervals largely overlapped, indicating that the individual-level surrogacy estimates were of similar magnitude across trials.

13.5 A Binary and a Normally Distributed Endpoint

When T is a normally distributed endpoint and S is a binary endpoint, the function `FixedContBinIT()` can be used to evaluate the appropriateness of the candidate surrogate endpoint. Similarly, when T is a binary endpoint and S is a normally distributed endpoint, the function `FixedBinContIT()` can be used. The first part of these function names indicate that a Fixed-effects model is fitted to estimate the trial-specific treatment effects α_i and β_i (for details, see Chapter 9). The second part of the function names indicate whether T is a binary endpoint (function `FixedBinContIT()`) or a normally distributed (continuous) endpoint (function `FixedContBinIT()`). Similarly, the third part of the function names indicate whether S is a binary or normally distributed endpoint (functions `FixedContBinIT()` and `FixedBinContIT()`, respectively). The last part of the function names indicate that the Information-Theoretic (IT) approach is used. In addition, the arguments `Model="Full"` or `Model="Reduced"` can be used in the function call to specify whether a full or a reduced model should be fitted (to obtain estimates for α_i and β_i; for details, see Section 4.3.2). Finally, the arguments `Weighted=TRUE` and `Weighted=FALSE` can be used to specify whether measurement error should be accounted for or not (for details, see 4.3.4). The different models that can be fitted using the *Surrogate* package are identical to those shown in Table 13.3, where `FixedBinBinIT()` is replaced by `FixedBinContIT()` or `FixedContBinIT()`.

Main function arguments

The functions `FixedContBinIT()` and `FixedBinContIT()` require the same arguments as those of the function `FixedBinBinIT()`. For details, see Section 13.4.

13.5.1 Analyzing the Data of Five Clinical Trials in Schizophrenia

It is examined here whether the dichotomized BPRS score (1 = clinically relevant change on the BPRS at the end of the treatment; 0 = no clinically relevant change) is an appropriate surrogate for the (non-dichotomized, normally distributed) PANSS score using the `Schizo` dataset described in more detail in Section 2.2.2. In this analysis, treating physician is used as the clustering unit.

After loading the *Surrogate* package and the Schizo dataset in memory (see Section 13.1), the function FixedContBinIT() can be used to conduct the analysis. Here, a full weighted model is requested:

```
> Schizo_ContBin <- FixedContBinIT(Dataset = Schizo,
Surr = CGI_Bin, True = PANSS, Treat = Treat,
Model = "Full", Weighted = TRUE, Trial.ID = InvestId,
Pat.ID = Id, Seed = 1) # Seed used for reproducibility
```

When the summary() function is applied to the fitted object Schizo_ContBin, the following output is obtained:

```
> summary(Schizo_ContBin)

Function call:

FixedContBinIT(Dataset = Schizo, Surr = CGI_Bin, True = PANSS,
    Treat = Treat, Trial.ID = InvestId, Pat.ID = Id,
    Model = "Full", Weighted = TRUE, Seed = 1)


# Data summary and descriptives
#~~~~~~~~~~~~~~~~~~~~~~~~~~~~~~~~~~~~~~~~~~~~~~~~~~~~~~~~~


Total number of trials:  140
Total number of patients:  1967
M(SD) patients per trial: 14.0500 (10.1502)  [min: 2; max: 52]
Total number of patients in experimental treatment group:  1464
Total number of patients in control treatment group:  503


# Information-theoretic surrogacy estimates summary
#~~~~~~~~~~~~~~~~~~~~~~~~~~~~~~~~~~~~~~~~~~~~~~~~~~~~~~~~~


Trial-level surrogacy (R2_ht):
    R2ht CI lower limit CI upper limit
  0.5296         0.4126          0.6376

Individual-level surrogacy (R2_h.ind):
  R2h.ind CI lower limit CI upper limit
   0.4545         0.4229          0.4859
```

The first part of the output shows descriptives like the number of trials in the data and the number of patients in the different treatment groups. Notice that a total of 2128 patients participated in the five studies, but the output shows that the data of only 1967 patients were actually included in the analyses. The reason for this is that, prior to conducting the surrogacy analysis, data of patients who have a missing value for the surrogate and/or the true endpoint are excluded. In addition, the data of trials (clusters/treating physicians) (i) in which only one type of the treatment was administered (i.e., all patients received the experimental treatment or all patients received the control treatment), and (ii) in which either the surrogate or the true endpoint was a constant (i.e., all patients within a trial had exactly the same surrogate and/or true endpoint value) are excluded because trial-specific treatment effects cannot be estimated in such trials (clusters). The subset of the dataset that was included in the analysis can be obtained by using the `[name_of_fitted_object]$Data.Analyze` command (e.g., `Schizo_ContBin$Data.Analyze`).

The second part of the output provides the estimates of trial- and individual-level surrogacy. As can be seen, $\widehat{R}^2_{ht} = 0.5296$ with 95% confidence interval [0.4126; 0.6376]. This result indicates that the uncertainty about the treatment effect on T = change on the PANSS that is reduced when the treatment effect on S = clinically relevant change on the CGI becomes known (trial-level surrogacy) is moderate. Further, the output shows that $\widehat{R}^2_{h\text{indiv}} = 0.4545$ with 95% confidence interval [0.4229; 0.4859] (see also the results in Section 10.7). The latter result indicates that the uncertainty about T that is reduced when S becomes known (individual-level surrogacy) is moderate. Overall, it can be concluded that clinically relevant change on the CGI is a moderately good surrogate for change on the PANSS.

Note that, at first, the results look different from those obtained with the SAS macro (Section 12.7.3). Indeed, there, a value of 0.37, with confidence interval [0.22,0.52] was obtained. However, in Section 12.7.3, only trials with at least two patients per treatment arm were included. At this point, the inclusion criterion was trials with at least 3 patients. When the SAS macro is run with the same data, then a value of 0.4482 is obtained, sufficiently close to the value obtained with R.

The results can be further graphically explored by applying the `plot()` function to the fitted `Schizo_ContBin` object. For example, a plot of the individual-level surrogacy estimates for each cluster can be obtained using the command:

```
# Plot of individual-level surrogacy (per cluster)
> plot(Schizo_ContBin, Indiv.Level.By.Trial = TRUE,
Trial.Level = FALSE)

# Generated output:
```

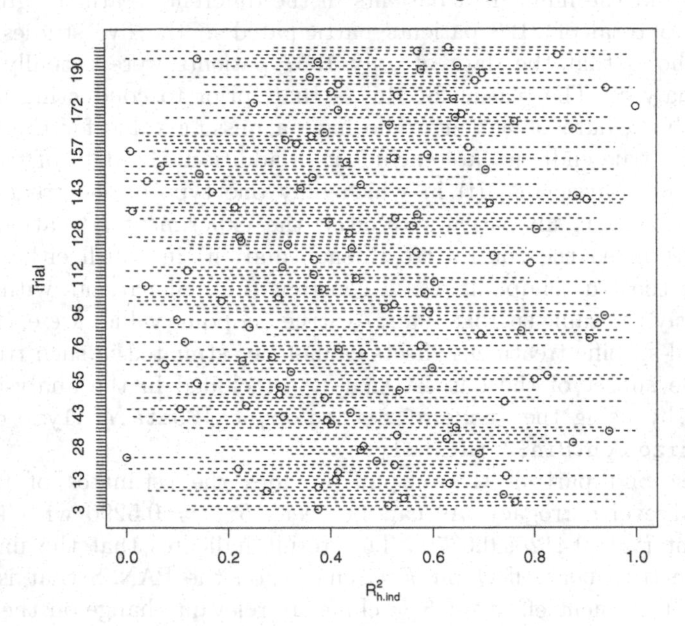

The figure shows that there was substantial variability in the cluster-specific $\widehat{R}^2_{hindiv}$, though the confidence intervals largely overlapped, indicating that individual-level surrogacy across clusters were of similar magnitude.

13.6 Estimation of Trial-Level Surrogacy When Only Trial-Level Data Are Available

In some settings, one may merely have access to trial-level data (i.e., the estimated treatment effects on S and T, respectively), but not to the individual-level data. Obviously, based on such data, it will only be possible to estimate R^2_{trial} (and not R^2_{indiv}). The function `TrialLevelMA()` allows for estimating R^2_{trial} using the meta-analytic framework.

Main function arguments

The function `TrialLevelMA()` requires the following arguments:

- `Alpha.Vector=, Beta.Vector=`: The vectors of the estimated treatment effects on S ($\widehat{\alpha}_i$) and T ($\widehat{\beta}_i$) in the different studies, respectively.

- `N.Vector=`: The vector of the sample sizes in the different studies.

- `Weighted=`: A logical indicator that indicates whether a weighted (argument

`Weighted=TRUE`) or unweighted (argument `Weighted=FALSE`) model should be fitted (stage 2 model). Weighting accounts for the heterogeneity in information content between the different trial-level contributions and is mainly important when there are large differences in the number of patients in the different studies that are considered. Default `Weighted=TRUE`).

- `Alpha=`: The α-level that is used to determine the confidence intervals around R^2_{trial}. Default `Alpha=0.05`.

13.6.1 Analyzing Ten Hypothetical Trials

Suppose that 10 estimates for the treatment effects on S and T are available in the published literature, as well as the sample sizes on which these estimates were based. Using this information, an estimate of R^2_{trial} can be obtained using the following command:

```
# Fit the model

> Trial_Fit <-  TrialLevelMA(
Alpha.Vector=c(4.7, 4.9, 5.2, 5.7, 5.1, 5.8, 6.0, 5.8, 5.9,
5.4), Beta.Vector=c(13.6, 15.3, 15.9, 16.4, 16.1, 18.5, 17.3,
18.2, 17.7, 16.4), N.Vector=c(130, 140, 150, 200, 210, 240,
300, 350, 350, 400))
```

The fitted object `Trial_Fit` of class `TrialLevelMA` can subsequently be examined by applying the `summary()` and `plot()` functions:

```
# Obtain summary of the results:

> summary(Trial_Fit)

Function call:

TrialLevelMA(Alpha.Vector = c(4.7, 4.9, 5.2, 5.7, 5.1, 5.8, 6,
    5.8, 5.9, 5.4), Beta.Vector = c(13.6, 15.3, 15.9, 16.4,
    16.1,18.5, 17.3, 18.2, 17.7, 16.4), N.Vector = c(130,
    140, 150, 200, 210, 240, 300, 350, 350, 400))


# Data summary and descriptives
#~~~~~~~~~~~~~~~~~~~~~~~~~~~~~~~~~~~~~~~~~~~~~~~~~~~~~~~~~~~~~~~~

Total number of trials:  10
```

```
# Meta-analytic results summary
#~~~~~~~~~~~~~~~~~~~~~~~~~~~~~~~~~~~~~~~~~~~~~~~~~~~~~

  R2 Trial Standard Error CI lower limit CI upper limit
    0.7608           0.1577          0.4517         1.0000

  R Trial Standard Error CI lower limit CI upper limit
   0.8722           0.1729          0.5382         0.9695


# Obtain plot of the (trial-level) results
> plot(Trial_Fit)

# Generated output:
```

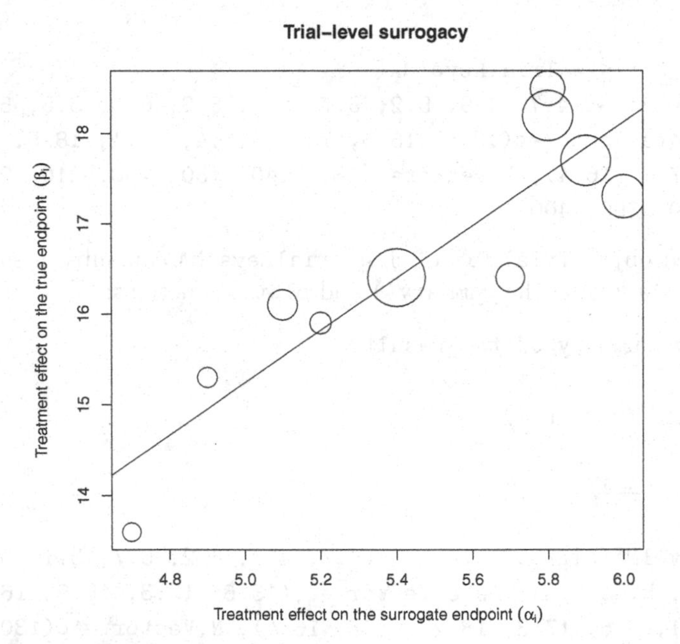

The output shows that the treatment effect on T can be predicted with moderate accuracy based on the treatment effect on S, i.e., $\widehat{R}^2_{\text{trial}} = 0.7608$ with 95% confidence interval [0.4517; 1.000]. Notice that the confidence interval around $\widehat{R}^2_{\text{trial}}$ is wide, which could be expected given the small number of clustering units (trials) that were available for analysis.

14

Cloud Computing

Theophile Bigirumurame

Hasselt University, Belgium

Ziv Shkedy

Hasselt University, Belgium

CONTENTS

14.1 The `Surrogate` Shiny App

Shiny is an R package (available on CRAN) developed by RStudio that allows us to create web-based applications from R-code. The Surrogate Shiny App was developed as an online shiny application for the evaluation of surrogate endpoints in randomized clinical trials and has the same capacity, in terms of the methods implemented in the App, as the `Surrogate` R package discussed in Chapter 13.

The Surrogate Shiny App can be used on a local computer or online using the shiny cloud platform. Other cloud platforms, such as Amazon Web Service or Google Cloud platform can be used as well. In contrast with the `Surrogate` R package, the user does not need to install R in order to conduct the analysis. The Surrogate Shiny App is a graphical user interface (GUI) and the user is not exposed to the R code behind the analysis.

The Surrogate Shiny App can be found on the Shiny Cloud at:

`https://uhasselt.shinyapps.io/surrogate`

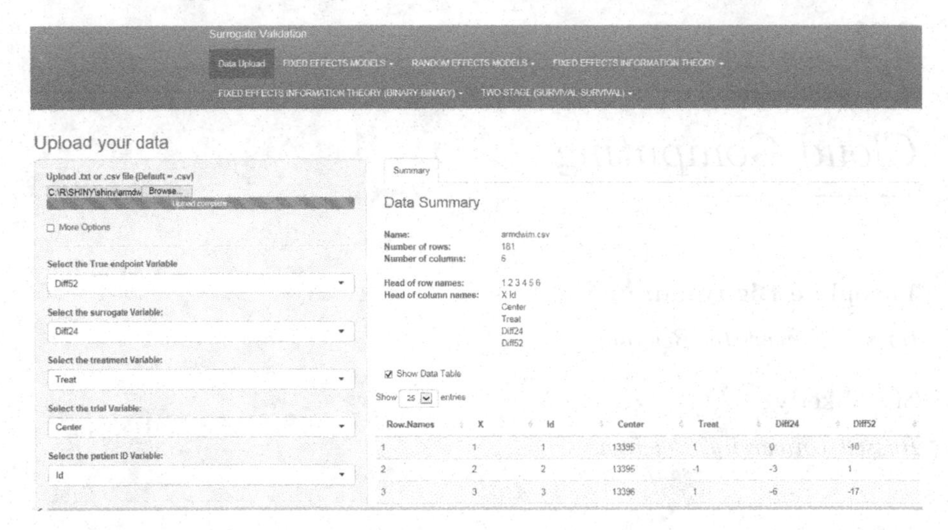

FIGURE 14.1
The Age-Related Macular Degeneration Data and variables for the analysis are specified in the left panel. A short summary of the data and a partial print are shown in the right panel.

In addition, the app is available as a stand-alone version in a `SurrShiny.zip` file that can be downloaded from

`http://ibiostat.be/online-resources`.

In this chapter, we briefly illustrate the capacity of Surrogate Shiny App for selected methods that were discussed in previous chapters. For each method, we present the GUI screen that can be used to conduct the analysis and the corresponding R code of the `Surrogate` package to perform an identical analysis. The code is presented only for clarity and it is not needed for the Surrogate Shiny App. The capacity of the Surrogate Shiny App is illustrated using case studies for three surrogacy settings: two continuous endpoints (Section 12.3.1, 12.3.2, and 13.2), two survival endpoints (Section 12.4 and 13.3), and two binary endpoints (Section 12.8 and 13.4).

The first step of the analysis requires uploading the data to the app. Figure 14.1 shows the data loading screen for the age-related macular degeneration data. Similar to Chapter 12, we need to specify the true and surrogate endpoints (`Diff52` and `Diff24`, respectively), the treatment (`Treat`), the unit for which R^2_{trial} will be calculated (`center`), and the patient's identification number (`Id`).

14.2 Two Continuous Endpoints: The Reduced Fixed-Effects Model

In Chapter 4, we discussed the reduced fixed-effects model for two continuous endpoints. The model can be formulated as:

$$\begin{cases} S_{ij} = \mu_S + \alpha_i Z_{ij} + \varepsilon_{Sij}, \\ T_{ij} = \mu_T + \beta_i Z_{ij} + \varepsilon_{Tij}. \end{cases} \tag{14.1}$$

For the reduced fixed-effect model, trial-level surrogacy is assessed using the coefficient of determination obtained by fitting a linear regression model of the form:

$$\widehat{\beta}_i = \lambda_0 + \lambda_1 \widehat{\alpha}_i + \varepsilon_i, \tag{14.2}$$

where $\widehat{\beta}_i$ and $\widehat{\alpha}_i$ are the trial-specific estimated treatment effects upon T_{ij} and S_{ij}, respectively. The error terms, ε_i, are normally distributed with mean zero and a constant variance. Individual-level surrogacy is assessed by the squared correlation between S and T after adjusting for trial-specific treatment effects and is given by:

$$R^2_{\text{indiv}} = \frac{\sigma^2_{ST}}{\sigma_{SS}\sigma_{TT}}. \tag{14.3}$$

Once the variables specification is complete (see the left panel in Figure 14.1), one can choose the model to be fitted using the command bar in the upper part in Figure 14.1. The Surrogate Shiny App produces a default output shown in Figure 14.2. For the ARMD study, $\widehat{R}^2_{\text{indiv}} = 0.5318$ (0.4315, 0.6321) and $\widehat{R}^2_{\text{trial}} = 0.6585$ (0.4695, 0.8476). If other statistics are of interest, one can use the R package `Surrogate` to produce them.

The reduced fixed-effects model specified in (14.1) and in the Surrogate Shiny App in Figure 14.1 is identical to the model fitted using the function `BifixedContCont` below:

```
Sur<-BifixedContCont(Dataset=ARMD, Surr=Diff24, True=Diff52,
                     Treat=Treat, Trial.ID=Center,
                     Pat.ID=Id,Model="Reduced", Weighted=TRUE)
```

14.3 Two Time-to-Event Endpoints: A Two-Stage Approach

The analysis for the surrogacy setting of two time-to-event endpoints was discussed in Chapters 5 and 12, where a joint model and a two-stage approach

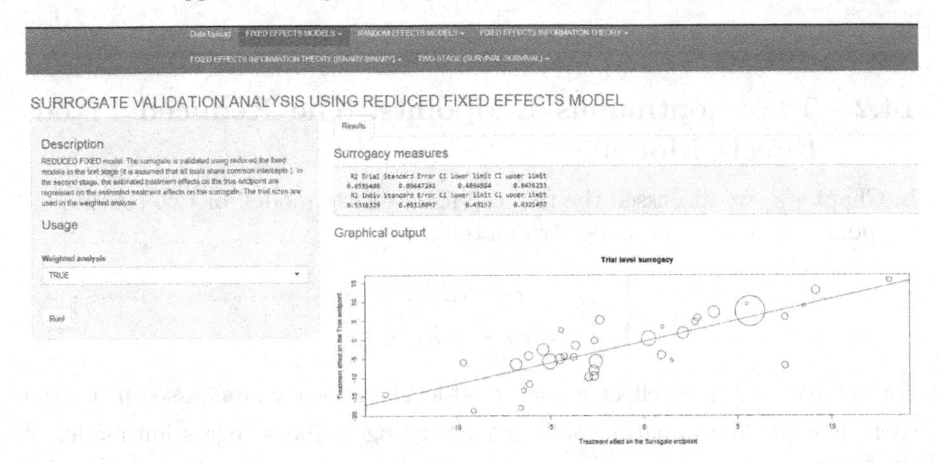

FIGURE 14.2
Age-Related Macular Degeneration Trial. Default output for the reduced fixed-effects model.

was used to estimate individual- and trial-level surrogacy. The two-stage approach is implemented in the Surrogate Shiny App. We use the ovarian cancer study (see Section 2.2.3) for illustration. The specification of the data is shown in Figure 14.3. In the same screen, we select the tab *Two-stage (Survival-Survival)* to perform the analysis, to select the censoring indicators and to determine the model's type for the second stage (weighted or unweighted). The output is presented in Figure 14.4. The estimated trial-level surrogacy is equal to $\widehat{R}^2_{\text{trial}} = 0.9184$ (0.8674, 0.9695). For the ovarian cancer dataset, the two-stage model discussed above is identical to the model specified in the function `TwoStageSurvSurv`:

```
Sur<-TwoStageSurvSurv(Dataset=ovarian, Surr=pfs,
SurrCens=PfsInd,True=surv,TrueCens=SurvInd,
Treat=Treat,Trial.ID=Center)
```

14.4 Information-Theoretic Approach

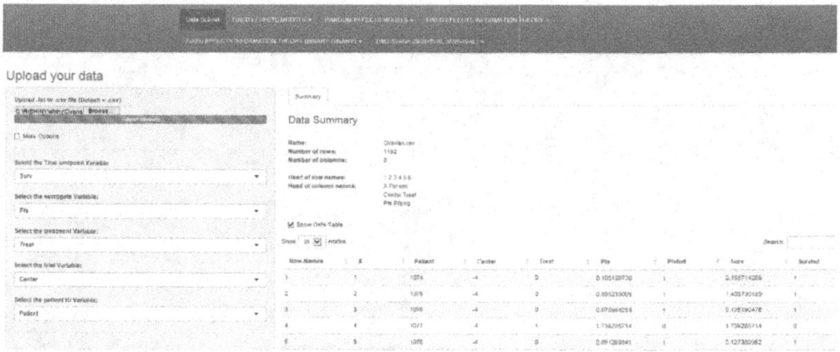

FIGURE 14.3

Ovarian Cancer Data. Evaluation of trial-level surrogacy (using a two-stage model) for a surrogacy setting with two time-to-event endpoints. True endpoint: overall survival. Surrogate endpoint: progression-free survival.

14.4.1 Individual- and Trial-Level Surrogacy

The information-theoretic approach was discussed in Chapters 9 and 10. For a multi-trial setting, we consider two models for the true endpoint T_{ij}:

$$\begin{cases} M_0 : g\{E(T_{ij}|Z_{ij})\} = \mu_{T_i} + \beta_i Z_{ij}, \\ M_1 : g\{E(T_{ij}|Z_{ij}, S_{ij})\} = \delta_{0_i} + \delta_{1i} Z_{ij} + \delta_{2i} S_{ij} \end{cases} \tag{14.4}$$

Here, g is an appropriate link function. For the remainder of this section, we briefly discuss the surrogacy measures implemented in the Surrogate Shiny App. For an elaborate discussion about the modeling approach and the derivation of the surrogacy measures we refer to Chapter 9. An information-theoretic measure for individual-level surrogacy for a multi-trial setting is given by

$$R_h^2 = 1 - \frac{1}{N} \sum_{i=1}^{N} \exp\left(\frac{L_{0_i} - L_{1_i}}{n_i}\right),$$

where L_{k_i} is the -2 log likelihood of model M_k, $k = 0, 1$ defined in (14.4), and n_i is the sample size of the ith trial. For a single trial setting (i.e., $N = 1$) the surrogacy measure is reduced to

$$R_h^2 = 1 - \exp\left(\frac{L_0 - L_1}{n}\right).$$

To estimate the trial-level surrogacy measure, the following models are fitted:

$$\begin{cases} g\{E(S_{ij}|Z_{ij})\} = \mu_{S_i} + \alpha_i Z_{ij}, \\ g\{E(T_{ij}|Z_{ij})\} = \mu_{T_i} + \beta_i Z_{ij}. \end{cases} \tag{14.5}$$

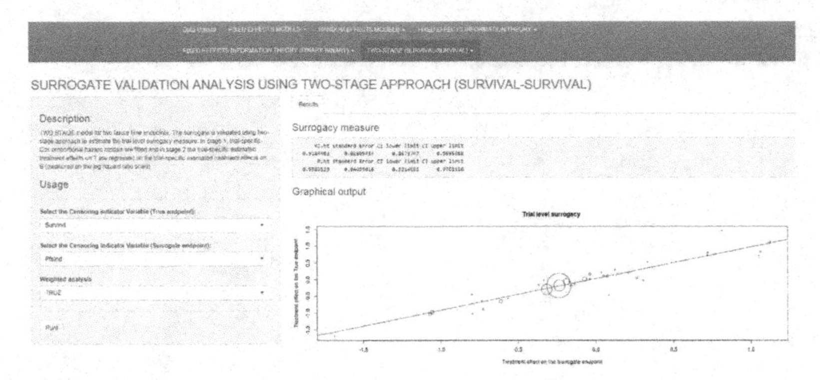

FIGURE 14.4
Ovarian Cancer Data. Evaluation of trial-level surrogacy (using a two-stage model) for a surrogacy setting with two time-to-event endpoints. Estimation of trial-level surrogacy.

At the second stage, the trial-specific parameter estimates obtained from generalized linear models defined in (14.5) are used to fit two linear regression models:

$$\begin{cases} M_0 : \widehat{\beta}_i = \gamma_0 + \varepsilon_i, \\ M_1 : \widehat{\beta}_i = \gamma_0 + \gamma_1 \widehat{\mu}_{S_i} + \gamma_2 \widehat{\alpha}_i + \varepsilon_i. \end{cases} \tag{14.6}$$

A trial-level surrogacy measure is given by

$$R^2_{ht} = \exp\left(-\frac{G^2}{N}\right), \tag{14.7}$$

where G^2 is the likelihood ratio test statistic comparing the models M_0 and M_1 in (14.6) and N is the number of trials.

14.4.2 Information-Theoretic Approach for Two Continuous Endpoints

The information-theoretic approach for two continuous endpoints was applied to the ARMD data in Section 2.2.1. The function `FixedContContIT` was used to estimate both individual- and trial-level surrogacy in the following way:

```
Sur<-FixedContContIT(Dataset=ARMD, Surr=Diff24,
                     True=Diff52, Treat=Treat,
                     Trial.ID=Center, Weighted=TRUE,
                     Pat.ID=Id, Model="Reduced",
                     Number.Bootstraps=500,Seed=1)
```

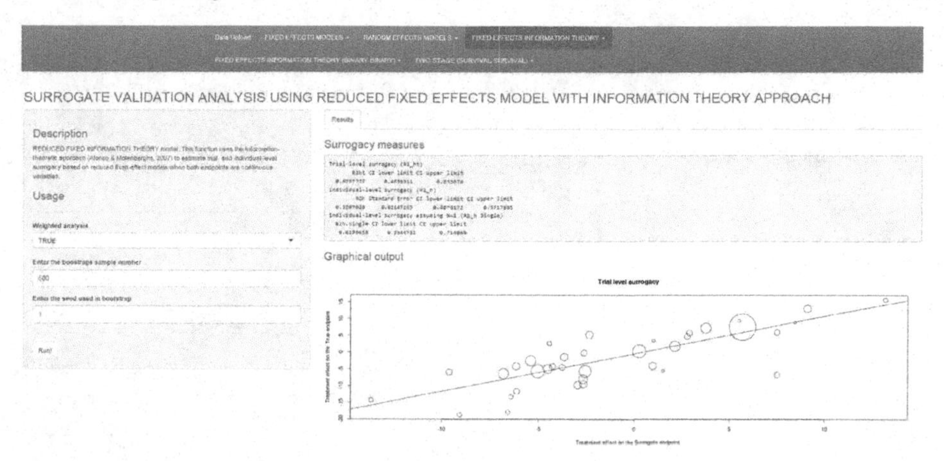

FIGURE 14.5
Age-Related Macular Degeneration Trial. Analysis using the information-theoretic approach for two continuous endpoints.

An identical model can be fitted using the Surrogate Shiny App. Figure 14.1 shows the specification of the variables for the ARMD data in the data loading screen of the surrogate app. Note that this specification is identical to the one used in the previous section because both examples use the same data. Figure 14.5 presents the output. The number of bootstrap samples (`Number.Bootstraps=500`) and the seed (`Seed=1`) are specified in the left panel in Figure 14.5. As shown in Chapter 10, for the ARMD data, trial-level surrogacy and individual-level surrogacy measures are equal to $\widehat{R}^2_{ht} = 0.6788$ (0.4655-0.8338) and $\widehat{R}^2_h = 0.5297$ (0.4876-0.5718), respectively.

14.4.3 Information-Theoretic Approach for Two Binary Endpoints

For the Schizophrenia study, presented in Section 2.2.2 (see also Chapters 12 and 13 for a similar analysis in R and SAS, respectively), the two binary endpoints are defined as:

$$T_{ij} = \begin{cases} 1 & \text{PANSS reduction (at least } -20\%), \\ 0 & \text{otherwise,} \end{cases}$$

$$S_{ij} = \begin{cases} 1 & \text{CGI change of 3 points,} \\ 0 & \text{otherwise.} \end{cases}$$

In R, using the `Surrogate` package, for a multi-trial setting with two binary endpoints, the function `FixedBinBintIT` can be used to estimate both

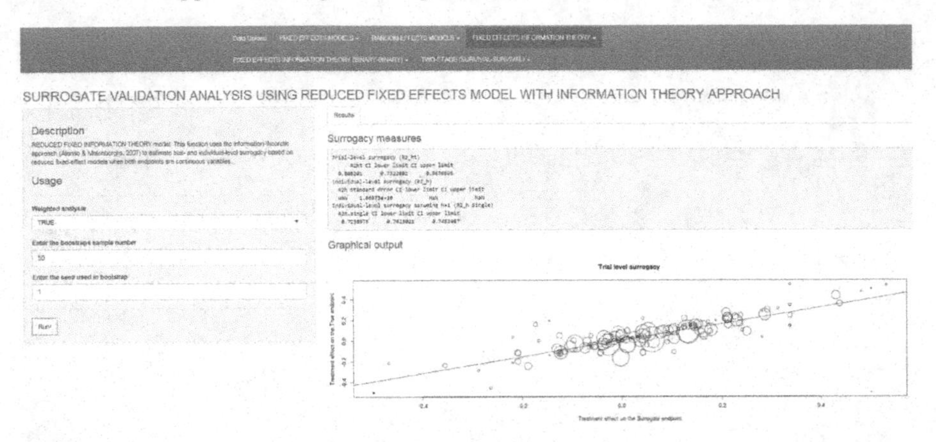

FIGURE 14.6
Schizophrenia Study. Analysis using the information-theoretic approach for two binary endpoints.

individual-level and trial-level surrogacy measures. For the schizophrenia study, the function is called in the following way:

```
Sur<-FixedBinBinIT(Dataset=Schizo, Surr=Panss_Bin,
                   True=CGI_Bin, Treat=Treat,
                   Trial.ID=InvestId, Weighted=TRUE,
                   Pat.ID=Id, Model="Reduced",
                   Number.Bootstraps=500,Seed=1)
```

In the Surrogate Shiny App, the following specifications should be used in the data loading screen in Figure 14.1: the true (`CGI bin`) and the surrogate endpoints (`PANSS bin`), the treatment variable (`Treat`), the unit for which R^2_{ht} will be calculated (`InvestId`), and the patient's identification number (`Id`). In the same screen, the tab *Fixed effects information theory (Binary-Binary)* is selected in order to perform the analysis. The number of bootstrap samples (`Number.Bootstraps=500`) and the seed (`Seed=1`) are specified in the left panel in Figure 14.6. For the schizophrenia study, trial and individual-level surrogacy measures are equal to $\widehat{R}^2_{ht} = 0.8213$ (0.7469, 0.87864) and $\widehat{R}^2_h = 0.3305$ (0.2992, 0.3623), respectively.

Part IV

Additional Considerations and Further Topics

15

Surrogate Endpoints in Rare Diseases

Wim Van der Elst

Hasselt University and Janssen Pharmaceutica, Belgium

Geert Molenberghs

Hasselt University nad KU Leuven, Belgium

CONTENTS

15.1 Introduction

Evaluating a surrogate endpoint typically requires a large amount of data, and this is particularly so when the contemporary multiple-trial surrogate endpoint evaluation methods are used. The need for a large sample size is an issue in all clinical trials (e.g., an increased study duration and cost, a higher probability of missing values due to study drop-out, and so on), and it is particularly problematic in clinical trials in rare diseases (or in clinical trials in small patient subgroups that are identified within the context of a common disease). Indeed, in rare diseases the number of patients that are available for study participation is typically substantially smaller compared to what is the case in non-rare disease clinical trials. Yet, surrogate endpoints may be particularly useful in rare disease clinical trials (Korn et al., 2013). Indeed, the use of a surrogate endpoint may result in a smaller sample size that is needed to show the effectiveness of a new treatment, because (i) the surrogate endpoint may be an event that occurs more frequently than the true endpoint, and/or because (ii) the treatment effect on the surrogate endpoint may be larger compared to the treatment effect on the true endpoint (in particular when the surrogate endpoint is closer to the treatment in terms of time and the biological mechanism that is being targeted (Korn et al., 2013).

As detailed in Part II, the contemporary multiple-trial surrogate evaluation methods usually involve the fitting of complex hierarchical models. For example, when both S and T are normally distributed endpoints, a linear mixed-effects model (see Eq. (4.1)) is fitted to estimate the trial- and individual-level surrogacy coefficients. When the number of available patients is small, fitting such linear mixed-effects models is often problematic. Indeed, when the data are sparse, the Newton-Raphson (or quasi-Newton)-based iterative process that is typically used to fit the model (i) may not converge at all, or (ii) may converge to values that are close to or outside the boundary of the parameter space. In the latter case, the estimated variance components are close to zero or negative, which may lead to a non-positive-definite variance-covariance matrix of the random effects D (see (4.2)). A non-positive-definite D matrix is not an issue when one is merely interested in the fixed-effect components, because the marginal model can still be used to make valid inferences regarding the fixed-effect parameters as long as the overall V matrix is positive-definite (with $V_i = Z_i D Z_i^{'} + \Sigma_i$, where Z_i are matrices of known covariates associated with the random effects (Verbeke and Molenberghs, 2000; West et al., 2007)). However, in a surrogate evaluation context, interest is in the random effects rather than in the fixed effects. In the latter setting, it is paramount that D is positive-definite, as this condition will guarantee that $\widehat{R}^2_{\text{trial}}$ is within the unit interval.

The remainder of this chapter is organized in the following way. In Section 15.2, a simulation study is conducted to examine which factors affect convergence of linear mixed-effects models. Based on the results of these simulations, a multiple imputation (MI)-based strategy that can be used to overcome model convergence problems is detailed in Section 15.3. As an alternative to overcome model convergence issues, a two-stage model-fitting approach can be used (for details, see Section 4.3). Section 15.4 provides a formal basis for the latter approach. Notice that the current chapter focuses on the setting where both S and T are normally distributed endpoints, but similar strategies are conceivable in other settings as well.

15.2 Convergence Problems in Fitting Linear Mixed-Effects Models

In a surrogate evaluation context, the (S, T) endpoints (level 1) are nested within patients (level 2), and the patients are nested within clinical trials (or other relevant clustering units; level 3). Given the complex hierarchical structure of the data, it is hardly surprising that convergence problems are frequently encountered in a surrogate evaluation context. To gain more insight into the factors that affect the convergence of hierarchical models, simulations can be useful.

15.2.1 A Simulation Study

Simulation scenarios

Consider the following mixed-effects model that is typically fitted to evaluate surrogacy in the setting when both S and T are normally distributed endpoints (see also Chapter 4):

$$\begin{cases} S_{ij} = \mu_S + m_{Si} + (\alpha + a_i)\, Z_{ij} + \varepsilon_{Sij}, \\ T_{ij} = \mu_T + m_{Ti} + (\beta + b_i)\, Z_{ij} + \varepsilon_{Tij}, \end{cases} \tag{15.1}$$

where μ_S, μ_T are the fixed intercepts for S and T, m_{Si}, m_{Ti} are the corresponding random intercepts, α, β are the fixed treatment effects for S and T, and a_i, b_i are the corresponding random treatment effects. Further, $(m_{Si},\, m_{Ti},\, a_i,\, b_i) \sim N(\mathbf{0},\, D)$, with D an unstructured variance-covariance matrix of the random effects, and $(\varepsilon_{Sij}, \varepsilon_{Tij}) \sim N(\mathbf{0},\, \Sigma)$ with Σ an unstructured variance-covariance matrix of the residuals.

Using Model (15.1), data were simulated. In all simulations, $\mu_S = 450$, $\mu_T = 500$, $\alpha = 300$, $\beta = 500$, and

$$\Sigma = \begin{pmatrix} 300 & 212.132 \\ 212.132 & 300 \end{pmatrix},$$

yielding $R^2_{\text{indiv}} = \text{corr}\,(\varepsilon_{Sij},\, \varepsilon_{Tij})^2 = 0.5$. Three conditions were varied in the simulations. First, the number of clusters $N = \{5,\, 10,\, 20,\, 50\}$. Second, the between-cluster variability (D), which is either large ($\gamma = 1$) or small ($\gamma = 0.1$) relative to the residual variability (Σ):

$$D = \gamma \begin{pmatrix} 1000 & 400 & 0 & 0 \\ 400 & 1000 & 0 & 0 \\ 0 & 0 & 1000 & 707.107 \\ 0 & 0 & 707.107 & 1000 \end{pmatrix},$$

yielding $R^2_{\text{trial}} = \text{corr}\,(a_i,\, b_i)^2 = 0.5$. Third, the level of imbalance in the cluster sizes n_i (the rationale to consider this factor is described in more detail in the next paragraph). In the balanced scenario, all cluster sizes were equal, i.e., $n_i = n = 20$. In the two unbalanced scenarios, $\widetilde{n}_i$ was determined based on a draw from a normal distribution and rounded to the nearest integer (i.e., $n_i = \text{round}(\widetilde{n}_i)$). In the low-imbalance scenario, $\widetilde{n}_i \sim N(20, 2.5^2)$. In the high-imbalance scenario, $\widetilde{n}_i \sim N(20, 5^2)$. In the balanced scenario, treatment (Z) is also balanced within a cluster. In the unbalanced scenarios, treatment allocation is determined based on a binomial distribution with success probability 0.50.

Balance in cluster size

To understand why balance in cluster size may be a relevant factor to consider in fitting linear mixed-effects models, recall that the key computational difficulty in fitting mixed-effects models is in the estimation of the covariance parameters (Verbeke and Molenberghs, 2000). Iterative numerical optimization of the log-likelihood functions using (RE)ML estimation is conducted, subject to constraints that are imposed on the model parameters to ensure positive-definiteness of the D and $V_i = Z_i D Z_i^{'} + \Sigma_i$ matrices (where Z_i are matrices of known covariates associated with the random effects). To maximize complicated likelihoods or to find good starting values that can subsequently be used in the Newton-Raphson algorithm, the Expectation Maximization (EM) algorithm is often used (Dempster et al., 1977). When *unbalanced* data are considered, the E-step involves, at least conceptually, the creation of a "balanced" dataset (or a "complete" dataset in a missing data context (Molenberghs and Kenward, 2007), based on a hypothetical scenario where it is assumed that data have been obtained from a balanced design (or from a study in which there were no missing values in a missing data context (West et al., 2007). Based on the "balanced" data, an objective function is constructed and maximized in the M-step, and the parameter estimates are subsequently iteratively updated. In essence, the underlying assumption behind the EM algorithm is that the optimization of the balanced (complete) data log-likelihood function is easier than the optimization of the unbalanced (observed) data log-likelihood (West et al., 2007). In the same spirit, it can be expected that model convergence issues will occur more frequently when the actually observed data are unbalanced in cluster size, compared to the setting where the actually observed data are balanced.

Outcomes of interest

A total of 1000 datasets were generated for each of the 24 settings. The generated data were subsequently analyzed by fitting Model (15.1) in SAS. Two different parameterizations for the D matrix were considered. First, a completely general (unstructured; UN) D matrix that is parameterized directly in terms of variances and covariances. Second, a non-diagonal factor-analytic structure with 4 factors (FA0(4)). The latter structure specifies a Cholesky root parameterization for the 4×4 unstructured blocks in D. This leads to a substantial simplification of the optimization problem, i.e., the problem now changes from a constrained one to an unconstrained one. The FA0(4) structure has $\frac{q}{2}(2t - q + 1)$ covariance parameters, where q refers to the number of factors and t is the dimension of the matrix. In the present setting, the FA0(4) structure thus has a total of 10 parameters. These parameters are used to compute the components in D, i.e., the $(i,\ j)^{th}$ element of D is computed as $\Sigma_{k=1}^{\min(i,j,k)} \lambda_{ik}\lambda_{jk}$. The Cholesky root parameterization ensures that D (and V_i) is positive-definite during the entire estimation process (West et al., 2007).

The key outcome of interest in the simulations was model convergence. Three model convergence categories were distinguished: (i) proper convergence, i.e., the model converged and the variance-covariance matrix of the random effects (D) and the final Hessian (H), used to compute the standard errors of the covariance parameters, were positive-definite (PD); (ii) the model converged but D or H was not PD; and finally, (iii) divergence.

Results

Table 15.1 summarizes the results. As can be seen, a larger number of clusters (N) and a larger between-cluster variability relative to the residual variability (larger γ) were associated with higher rates of proper and overall convergence. When an unstructured (UN) D matrix was used, overall convergence exceeded 99.7% when the cluster sizes were balanced. The overall convergence rates were, however, substantially lower in the unbalanced scenarios, in particular when N and γ were small. For example, when $N = 5$ and $\gamma = 0.1$, the model divergence rates were as high as 65.5% and 77.3% in the small and large imbalance scenarios, respectively (compared to only 0.3% in the balanced scenario). At the same time, the impact of level of imbalance on *proper* convergence was small, i.e., proper convergence rates were quite similar in all scenarios irrespective of the level of imbalance in the data. When a non-diagonal factor analytic structure with 4 factors (FA0(4)) was used for the D matrix, the rates of proper convergence exceeded 71.0% in all scenarios (see Table 15.1). Thus, proper convergence rates were substantially higher in the FA0(4) scenario compared to those that were observed in the UN scenario.

The results thus indicate that model convergence problems decrease as a function of (i) the number of available clusters, (ii) the size of the between-cluster variability relative to the residual variability, and (iii) the level of balance in cluster sizes. Other simulations (not discussed here) showed that factors such as the normality assumption for S and T, or the strength of the correlation between the random treatment effects do not affect model convergence (for details, see Buyse et al., 2000 and Renard et al., 2002).

TABLE 15.1

Simulation Results. Convergence rates for the UN (unstructured) and FA0(4) (factor analytic) models as a function of balance of n_i, the number of clusters (5, 10, 20, 50) and the between-cluster variability.

Model	Convergence category	Between-cluster variability γ	Balanced (equal n_i) Number of clusters 5	10	20	50	Small imbalance $\widetilde{n}_i \sim N(20, 2.5^2)$ Number of clusters 5	10	20	50	Large imbalance $\widetilde{n}_i \sim N(20, 5^2)$ Number of clusters 5	10	20	50
UN	Proper convergence	Small (0.1)	0.112	0.826	0.999	1	0.090	0.816	1	1	0.091	0.800	0.999	1
		Large (1)	0.555	0.998	1	1	0.566	0.999	1	1	0.540	0.996	1	1
	Convergence but non-PD D/H matrix	Small (0.1)	0.885	0.174	0.001	0	0.255	0.171	0	0	0.136	0.155	0.001	0
		Large (1)	0.444	0.002	0	0	0.163	0.001	0	0	0.119	0.001	0	0
	Divergence	Small (0.1)	0.003	0	0	0	0.655	0.013	0	0	0.773	0.045	0	0
		Large (1)	0.001	0	0	0	0.271	0	0	0	0.341	0.003	0	0
FA0(4)	Proper convergence	Small (0.1)	0.745	0.984	1	1	0.717	0.976	1	1	0.710	0.976	0.999	1
		Large (1)	0.931	1	1	1	0.931	0.994	0.997	0.998	0.935	0.992	0.998	0.999
	Convergence but non-PD D/H matrix	Small (0.1)	0.068	0.007	0	0	0.054	0.016	0	0	0.044	0.015	0	0
		Large (1)	0.030	0	0	0	0.027	0.001	0.002	0	0.018	0.004	0.001	0.001
	Divergence	Small (0.1)	0.187	0.009	0	0	0.229	0.008	0	0	0.246	0.009	0.001	0
		Large (1)	0.039	0	0	0	0.042	0.005	0.001	0.002	0.047	0.004	0.001	0

TABLE 15.2
Hypothetical Dataset. Number of observations per cluster as a function of treatment (Z), before and after imputation.

	Before imputation		After imputation	
Cluster	$Z = -1$	$Z = 1$	$Z = -1$	$Z = 1$
1	5	11	18	18
2	13	8	18	18
3	10	18	18	18
4	9	5	18	18
5	9	11	18	18

15.3 Model Convergence Issues and Multiple Imputation

In the simulation study detailed in Section 15.2.1, it was observed that model convergence problems were more prevalent when cluster sizes were unbalanced, in particular when the number of clusters was small (which is usually the case in rare disease clinical trials) and when γ was small (which is the case in nearly all clinical trials). Based on this observation, it can hypothesized that model convergence problems can be reduced by using multiple imputation (MI) to make an unbalanced dataset "balanced" (in terms of cluster size and treatment allocation). As an example of what is meant by this, consider the hypothetical dataset with 5 clusters that is shown in Table 15.2. As can be seen, the maximum number of patients for each of the cluster by treatment (Z) groups is 18. Thus for all cluster $\times$ treatment groups having less than 18 observations, MI is used to restore balance. For example, in cluster 1 there were 5 observations for S and T in treatment group $Z = -1$ and 11 observations in treatment group $Z = 1$. Thus, the data of 13 and 7 patients are imputed in cluster 1 for $Z = -1$ and $Z = 1$, respectively.

To examine the impact of making unbalanced datasets "balanced" on model convergence, a simulation study can again be useful.

15.3.1 A Simulation Study

The same unbalanced datasets that were used in Section 15.2.1 are considered here. Multiple imputation (MI) was used to introduce balance in terms of cluster size and treatment allocation (Z). Proper multivariate imputations were conducted using the default Markov chain Monte Carlo method (Schafer, 1997) in SAS with a non-informative prior (Jeffreys). This imputation model included S, T, and Z. The imputation model was run "by cluster." A total of 200 burn-in iterations were used, and the number of iterations equaled 100.

The "balanced" data were subsequently analyzed by fitting Model (15.1) using the UN and FA0(4) parameterizations for the D matrix (see Section 15.2.1). The outcome of interest was again model convergence. In addition, the bias, efficiency (standard deviation of the estimate), and Mean Squared Errors of the estimates of the R^2_{trial} and R^2_{indiv} metrics were evaluated.

Results

Table 15.3 shows the convergence rates for the MI UN and MI FA0(4) models. Compared to the case for the models in the unbalanced non-MI scenarios (see Table 15.1), the rates of proper convergence were substantially higher in both the MI UN and MI FA0(4) scenarios — and this was particularly so when N was small. The use of MI to make the unbalanced data "balanced" was thus a successful strategy to improve proper convergence.

Tables 15.4 and 15.5 show the bias, efficiency, and MSE of the estimates of R^2_{indiv} and R^2_{trial}, respectively, in the non-MI and MI settings that properly converged. As expected, the bias, efficiency, and MSE in the estimation of both R^2_{indiv} and R^2_{trial} improved when the number of clusters increased. With respect to the estimation of R^2_{indiv}, the bias was low in all scenarios but the efficiency and MSE were poorer in the MI scenarios compared to the non-MI scenarios (see Table 15.4). In contrast to R^2_{indiv}, the bias, efficiency and MSE in R^2_{trial} were of similar magnitude in the MI and non-MI scenarios (see Table 15.5). Only when $N = 5$ did the bias in the estimation of R^2_{trial} tend to be substantially higher in the MI scenario compared to the non-MI scenario. Note that the bias was negative in all scenarios, indicating that the true R^2_{trial} tends to be underestimated. Further, the bias and MSE in the estimation of R^2_{indiv} was smaller compared to what was observed for R^2_{trial}, and the efficiency somewhat lower, because there is less replication than for the individual-level quantity.

15.3.2 Case Studies

15.3.2.1 The Age-Related Macular Degeneration Trial

The results in Section 15.3.1 indicate that the use of MI to balance an unbalanced dataset prior to fitting Model (15.1) reduces model convergence issues. In this section, this method is applied to estimate surrogacy in the ARMD trial. In particular, it will be examined whether the change in visual acuity after 24 weeks is an appropriate surrogate for the change in visual acuity after 52 weeks. As was detailed in Section 2.2.1, the ARMD trial is a multicenter study that enrolled a total of 181 patients from 36 centers. Here, the clustering variable is center (rather than trial). Centers that enrolled less than 5 patients were discarded from the analyses to avoid problems during the MI phase (recall that the imputations are conducted for each center separately, and thus a

TABLE 15.3
Convergence rates for the surrogate MI UN (unstructured) and MI FA0(4) (factor analytic) models as a function of balance of n_i, the number of clusters (5, 10, 20, 50), and the between-cluster variability.

Model			Small imbalance $\widetilde{n}_i \sim N\left(20, 2.5^2\right)$				Large imbalance $\widetilde{n}_i \sim N\left(20, 5^2\right)$			
	Convergence category	Between-cluster variability γ	Number of clusters 5	10	20	50	Number of clusters 5	10	20	50
MI UN	Proper convergence	Small (.1)	.164	.941	1	1	.189	.946	.999	.999
		Large (1)	.617	.999	1	1	.616	.999	.999	1
	Convergence but non-PD D/H matrix	Small (.1)	.811	.059	0	0	.770	.054	.001	.001
		Large (1)	.365	.001	0	0	.343	.001	.001	0
	Divergence	Small (.1)	.025	0	0	0	.042	0	0	0
		Large (1)	.018	0	0	0	.041	0	0	0
MI FA0(4)	Proper convergence	Small (.1)	.813	.998	1	1	.817	.996	.999	.999
		Large (1)	.954	.999	1	1	.950	1	.999	1
	Convergence but non-PD D/H matrix	Small (.1)	.077	.002	0	0	.072	.003	0	0
		Large (1)	.012	.001	0	0	.022	0	.001	0
	Divergence	Small (.1)	.109	.002	0	0	.111	.001	.001	0
		Large (1)	.029	.001	0	0	.028	0	0	0

TABLE 15.4

Bias, efficiency, and MSE of the estimates of R^2_{indiv} in the non-MI and MI surrogate evaluation models that properly converged as a function of balance of n_i, the number of clusters (5, 10, 20, 50), and the between-cluster variability.

Model			Balanced (equal n_i)				Small imbalance $\widetilde{n}_i \sim N\left(20,\ 2.5^2\right)$				Large imbalance $\widetilde{n}_i \sim N\left(20,\ 5^2\right)$			
	Measure	Between-cluster variability (γ)	Number of clusters				Number of clusters				Number of clusters			
			5	10	20	50	5	10	20	50	5	10	20	50
Non-MI, UN	Bias	Small (.1)	−.001	−.001	−.002	.001	−.014	.001	−.001	.001	.009	.001	−.002	.001
		Large (1)	−.005	−.001	−.001	−.001	−.009	−.001	.001	−.001	−.009	−.001	.001	−.001
	Efficiency	Small (.1)	.080	.052	.037	.023	.072	.053	.037	.023	.067	.052	.038	.023
		Large (1)	.072	.053	.037	.024	.071	.052	.037	.024	.073	.052	.037	.024
	MSE	Small (.1)	.006	.003	.001	.001	.005	.003	.001	.001	.004	.003	.001	.001
		Large (1)	.005	.003	.001	.001	.005	.003	.001	.001	.005	.003	.001	.001
Non-MI, FA0(4)	Bias	Small (.1)	−.001	−.009	−.002	.001	−.001	.001	−.001	.001	−.001	.001	−.002	.001
		Large (1)	−.006	−.001	−.001	−.001	−.007	−.001	.001	−.001	−.007	−.001	.001	−.001
	Efficiency	Small (.1)	.074	.052	.037	.023	.076	.053	.037	.023	.072	.051	.038	.023
		Large (1)	.073	.053	.037	.024	.072	.053	.037	.026	.074	.052	.038	.027
	MSE	Small (.1)	.006	.003	.001	.001	.006	.003	.001	.001	.005	.003	.001	.001
		Large (1)	.005	.003	.001	.001	.005	.003	.001	.001	.006	.003	.001	.001
MI, UN	Bias	Small (.1)	–	–	–	–	−.005	.001	−.001	.003	.008	.004	−.001	.004
		Large (1)	–	–	–	–	−.005	.002	.002	.001	−.005	.001	.004	.001
	Efficiency	Small (.1)	–	–	–	–	.089	.066	.047	.030	.095	.074	.057	.040
		Large (1)	–	–	–	–	.087	.065	.047	.031	.098	.076	.057	.043
	MSE	Small (.1)	–	–	–	–	.008	.004	.002	.001	.009	.005	.003	.002
		Large (1)	–	–	–	–	.008	.004	.002	.001	.010	.006	.003	.002
MI, FA0(4)	Bias	Small (.1)	–	–	–	–	−.001	.001	−.001	.003	.003	.003	−.001	.004
		Large (1)	–	–	–	–	−.005	.002	.002	.001	−.005	.001	.004	.001
	Efficiency	Small (.1)	–	–	–	–	.090	.066	.047	.030	.097	.074	.057	.040
		Large (1)	–	–	–	–	.097	.065	.047	.031	.099	.076	.057	.043
	MSE	Small (.1)	–	–	–	–	.008	.004	.002	.001	.009	.006	.003	.002
		Large (1)	–	–	–	–	.008	.004	.002	.001	.010	.006	.003	.002

Note. UN = unstructured; FA0(4) = factor analytic.

TABLE 15.5

Bias, efficiency, and MSE of the estimates of R^2_{trial} in the non-MI and MI surrogate evaluation models that properly converged as a function of balance of n_i, the number of clusters (5, 10, 20, 50), and the between-cluster variability.

Model	Measure	Between-cluster variability (γ)	Balanced (equal n_i) Number of clusters 5	10	20	50	Small imbalance $\tilde{n}_i \sim N(20, 2.5^2)$ Number of clusters 5	10	20	50	Large imbalance $\tilde{n}_i \sim N(20, 5^2)$ Number of clusters 5	10	20	50
Non-MI, UN	Bias	Small (.1)	−.152	−.097	−.041	−.019	−.168	−.093	−.036	−.016	−.174	−.094	−.034	−.002
		Large (1)	−.168	−.075	−.031	−.013	−.170	−.074	−.031	−.012	−.152	−.074	−.029	−.009
	Efficiency	Small (.1)	.254	.224	.182	.111	.246	.229	.184	.112	.280	.232	.187	.114
		Large (1)	.248	.219	.158	.095	.239	.222	.157	.096	.248	.221	.157	.095
	MSE	Small (.1)	.087	.059	.035	.013	.088	.061	.035	.013	.108	.063	.036	.013
		Large (1)	.089	.053	.026	.009	.086	.055	.026	.009	.084	.054	.025	.009
Non-MI, FA0(4)	Bias	Small (.1)	−.139	−.090	−.071	−.035	−.157	−.088	−.061	−.032	−.151	−.082	−.057	−.018
		Large (1)	−.099	−.077	−.060	−.024	−.109	−.073	−.063	−.024	−.076	−.071	−.058	−.020
	Efficiency	Small (.1)	.267	.233	.203	.121	.269	.238	.197	.122	.273	.237	.201	.125
		Large (1)	.272	.232	.178	.101	.269	.236	.179	.100	.266	.234	.177	.101
	MSE	Small (.1)	.090	.062	.046	.016	.096	.064	.043	.016	.097	.063	.044	.016
		Large (1)	.084	.060	.035	.011	.084	.061	.036	.011	.076	.060	.035	.011
MI, UN	Bias	Small (.1)	–	–	–	–	−.186	−.080	−.034	−.016	−.193	−.087	−.036	−.022
		Large (1)	–	–	–	–	−.165	−.071	−.031	−.012	−.163	−.072	−.032	−.018
	Efficiency	Small (.1)	–	–	–	–	.255	.226	.172	.105	.257	.229	.174	.128
		Large (1)	–	–	–	–	.244	.221	.155	.095	.254	.222	.160	.108
	MSE	Small (.1)	–	–	–	–	.099	.057	.031	.011	.103	.060	.031	.017
		Large (1)	–	–	–	–	.087	.054	.025	.009	.091	.054	.027	.012
MI, FA0(4)	Bias	Small (.1)	–	–	–	–	−.258	−.088	−.034	−.016	−.266	−.094	−.036	−.022
		Large (1)	–	–	–	–	−.193	−.071	−.031	−.012	−.193	−.072	−.032	−.018
	Efficiency	Small (.1)	–	–	–	–	.251	.228	.172	.105	.251	.233	.174	.128
		Large (1)	–	–	–	–	.253	.221	.155	.095	.261	.222	.160	.108
	MSE	Small (.1)	–	–	–	–	.130	.060	.031	.011	.134	.063	.031	.017
		Large (1)	–	–	–	–	.101	.054	.025	.009	.106	.054	.027	.011

Note. UN = unstructured; FA0(4) = factor analytic.

TABLE 15.6
Convergence rates for the Age-Related Macular Degeneration Trial using MI UN (unstructured) and MI FA0(4) (factor analytic) to restore "balance" in cluster sizes.

	MI UN	MI FA0(4)
Proper convergence	0.701	0.944
Convergence but non-PD D/H matrix	0.299	0.015
Divergence	0	0.041

sufficient number of observations should be available in a center). The dataset that was analyzed contained 119 patients from 17 centers. The center that had the largest sample size included 18 patients, of whom 9 patients received placebo and 9 patients received the experimental treatment. The same procedure that was described in Section 15.3 to obtain "balanced" datasets (using MI) was employed here. Thus, in all center-by-treatment groups that had less than 9 patients, data were imputed to achieve balance. The imputations were conducted for each of the centers separately, using change in visual acuity after 24 weeks as S, change in visual acuity after 52 weeks as T, as well as treatment Z in the imputation model. A total of 1000 imputations were conducted. For each of the imputed datasets, Model (15.1) was fitted. Both the FA0(4) and UN covariance parameterizations for D were used.

Results

When Model (15.1) was fitted to the non-imputed data of the case study, convergence issues occurred. In particular, the models that used the UN parameterization for the D matrix did not converge and the models that used the FA0(4) parameterization converged to a non-PD D/H matrix.

Table 15.6 shows the convergence rates that were obtained when the MI-based approaches were used. Overall convergence was high and equaled 100% and 96.9% in the MI UN and MI FA0(4) scenarios, respectively. The use of the MI FA0(4) strategy led to higher rates of proper convergence compared to the MI UN strategy (94.4% versus 70.1%, respectively).

The mean $\widehat{R}^2_{\text{trial}}$ of the properly converged results and their $CI_{95\%}$ for the MI UN and FA0(4) models equaled 0.573 [0.078; 0.941] and 0.597 [0.069; 0.985], respectively. The mean $\widehat{R}^2_{\text{indiv}}$ and their $CI_{95\%}$ were 0.453 [0.192; 0.673] and 0.431 [0.079; 0.696] for the MI UN and FA0(4) models, respectively.

To establish a frame of reference against which these estimates can be compared, the non-imputed ARMD data were analyzed using a two-stage approach (a full bivariate weighted fixed-effect model was used; for details see Chapter 4). This analysis yielded $\widehat{R}^2_{\text{trial}} = 0.729$ with $CI_{95\%} = [0.487; 0.972]$ and $\widehat{R}^2_{\text{indiv}} = 0.512$ with $CI_{95\%} = [0.384; 0.639]$.

The results indicate that there was an acceptable level of agreement between the trial- and individual-level surrogacy estimates that were obtained in the MI-based and non-MI-based approaches. Both analyses lead to the conclusion that, at the level of the trial (center), the treatment effect on T = visual acuity after 52 weeks can be predicted with moderate accuracy based on the treatment effect on S = visual acuity after 24 weeks (moderate $\widehat{R}^2_{\text{trial}}$ estimates). At the level of the individual patients, the accuracy by which T = visual acuity after 52 weeks can be predicted based on S = visual acuity after 24 weeks is moderate as well (moderate $\widehat{R}^2_{\text{indiv}}$ estimates).

The 95% confidence intervals ($CI_{95\%}$) of the MI-based $\widehat{R}^2_{\text{trial}}$ and $\widehat{R}^2_{\text{indiv}}$ were wide, but it should be kept in mind that the number of clusters and patients were relatively small. In addition, there were large imbalances in the cluster sizes in the ARMD dataset. For example, 7 out of the 17 centers that were available for analysis had only 5 patients and thus the ratio of the available data relative to the data that had to be imputed in these centers was small (available: 5 patients, to be imputed: 13 patients). In the next section, another case study is considered where the number of clusters and the number of patients is higher.

15.3.2.2 Five Clinical Trials in Schizophrenia

The combined data of five clinical trials in schizophrenia (for details, see Section 2.2.2) are considered here. It will be examined whether the Brief Psychiatric Rating Scale (BPRS) is an appropriate surrogate for the Positive and Negative Syndrome Scale (PANSS) using the MI-based approach detailed in Section 15.3 to obtain "balanced" datasets. Treating physician is used as the clustering unit in the analyses. The largest cluster size in the dataset was 52, of whom 9 patients received an active control and 43 patients received the experimental treatment. Thus, in all cluster-by-treatment groups that had less than 43 patients, data were imputed to achieve balance. Clusters which contained less than 10 patients were discarded from the analyses (to avoid problems during the MI phase). The imputations were conducted for each of the clusters separately, using $S =$ BPRS, $T =$ PANSS, and $Z =$ treatment in the imputation model. A total of 1000 imputations were conducted, and for each of the imputed datasets, Model (15.1) was fitted (using both the FA0(4) and UN covariance parameterizations for D).

Results

When Model (15.1) was fitted to the non-imputed data, convergence issues occurred. Both the models that used the UN and FA0(4) parameterization for the D matrix converged to a non-PD D/H matrix.

When the MI-based approaches were used, there was 100% proper convergence in both the MI UN and MI FA0(4) scenarios. The mean $\widehat{R}^2_{\text{trial}}$ of the properly converged results and their $CI_{95\%}$ for the MI UN and FA0(4) models both equaled 0.920 [0.875; 0.955]. The mean $\widehat{R}^2_{\text{indiv}}$ and their $CI_{95\%}$ for the MI UN and FA0(4) models were identical and equaled 0.923 [0.913; 0.933].

To establish a frame of reference against which these estimates can be compared, the non-imputed dataset was analyzed using a two-stage approach (a full bivariate weighted fixed-effect model was used; for details see Chapter 4). This analysis yielded $\widehat{R}^2_{\text{trial}} = 0.913$ with $CI_{95\%} = [0.877; 0.949]$ and $\widehat{R}^2_{\text{indiv}} = 0.920$ with $CI_{95\%} = [0.912; 0.927]$.

Overall, the results indicate that there was a good agreement between the trial- and individual-level surrogacy estimates that were obtained in the MI-based and non-MI-based approaches. Both analyses lead to the conclusion that $S =$BPRS is a good surrogate for $T =$PANSS at both the level of the trial (treating physician) and the individual. Thus, the treatment effect on T can be predicted with high accuracy based on the treatment effect on S (high $\widehat{R}^2_{\text{trial}}$), and T can be predicted with high accuracy based on S (high $\widehat{R}^2_{\text{indiv}}$).

15.4 A Formal Basis for the Two-Stage Approach

As was explained in Section 4.3, an alternative strategy (not based on MI) that can be used to avoid the computational problems that arise in the estimation of the variance components of Model (15.1), consists of replacing the mixed-effects model representation by its fixed-effects (two-stage) counterpart (Tibaldi et al., 2003). The two-stage approach is based on the original paper by Laird and Ware (1982). Details can be found in Verbeke and Molenberghs (2000). Tibaldi et al. (2003) obtained very good results with the two-stage approach, confirmed in various chapters of this text. Of course, the question remains as to whether the method is formally valid, i.e., whether it leads to a consistent estimator.

A first observation is that the two-stage approach is consistent when the number of patients per trial approaches infinity, whereas the number of trials is either bounded, or increases sufficiently slowly. A first observation is that the two-stage approach is consistent when the number of patients per trial approaches infinity, whereas the number of trials is either bounded, or increases sufficiently slowly.

Second, as shown in Hermans et al. (2015), with a compound-symmetry structure, or one related to it (i.e., where patients within a trial are exchangeable), weights that are proportional to the trial size can be used, while equal weights may not perform too badly, either. This is because there is a so-called finite information limit in compound-symmetry-type structures (Nassiri, Molenberghs, and Verbeke, 2016).

Third, it is technically possible to derive a closed-form estimator for each of the trials separately, which implies that the weighted two-stage approach can be constructed with high computational efficiency, even in a big-data context.

16

High-Dimensional Biomarkers in Drug Discovery: The QSTAR Framework

Nolen Joy Perulila, Ziv Shkedy, Rudradev Sengupta, Theophile Bigirumurame

Hasselt University, Belgium

Luc Bijnens, Willem Talloen, Bie Verbist, Hinrich W.H. Göhlmann

Janssen Pharmaceutica, Belgium

Adetayo Kasim

Durham University, United Kingdom

QSTAR Consortium

CONTENTS

16.1 Introduction: From a Single Trial to a High-Dimensional Setting

In contrast with the analysis presented in previous chapters, which was focused on data obtained from clinical trials, this chapter focuses on drug discovery experiments. Our aim is to find genetic biomarkers for phenotypic data for a set of compounds under development. The data for the analysis consists of (1) a $m \times n$ gene expression matrix (X) that contains gene expression measurements of m genes for n compounds, (2) a $n \times 1$ vector of phenotypic data ($\mathbf{Y}$), and (3) a $n \times 1$ vector of chemical structure ($\mathbf{Z}$). Figure 16.1 illustrates the relationship between the three variables. Our goal is to model the relationship between the gene expression and the phenotypic data, taking into account that the chemical structure of the compound may (or may not) influence both variables. This modeling approach is called QSTAR, Quantitative Structure-Transcription-Assay Relationship, and it is further discussed in Section 16.2. The connection between the QSTAR framework and the surrogacy framework is illustrated in Section 16.4.

Although the experimental setting that we consider in this chapter is different from the clinical trials setting, the experimental unit, per gene, (X_{ij}, Y_i, Z_i), is similar to the single-trial setting discussed in Chapter 4. The main difference is that, in contrast to a single-trial setting where we have one dataset with one surrogate and one true endpoint, in the current setting, we have a high-dimensional dataset in which there are m candidates (genes) from which we need to select biomarkers for the phenotypic data. Due to the fact that, for a specific gene, the observation unit and the association structure between the three variables are similar to the single trial setting, in this chapter, we proposed to use a joint model for transcriptomic and phenotypic data, conditioned on the chemical structure, as a fundamental modeling tool for data integration within the QSTAR modeling framework. We elaborate on the high dimensionality of the data in Section 16.3.

The joint modeling approach can be used to uncover, for a given set of compounds, the association between gene expression and biological activity (i.e., the phenotypic variable, for example, the half maximal inhibitory concentration, IC50, the negative 10-logarithm of this quantity, pIC50, etc.) taking into account the influence of the chemical structure of the compound on both variables. The model allows us to detect genes that are associated with the bioactivity data, hence facilitating the identification of potential genomic biomarkers for the compound's efficacy. In addition, the effect of every

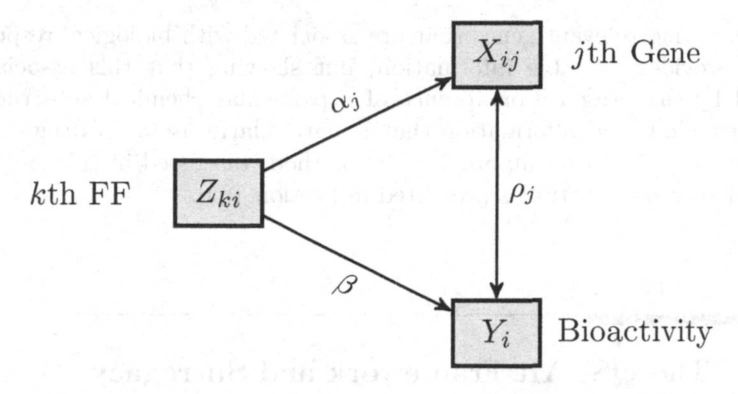

FIGURE 16.1
Relationship between gene expression (for a specific gene X_{ij}, $i = 1, \ldots, n$, $j = 1 \ldots, m$), chemical structures (FF-fingerprint feature), and phenotypic data (i.e., bioactivity data) within the QSTAR framework. The relationship and association structure are similar to the single-trial setting discussed in Chapter 4. In surrogacy terminology, X_{ij} represents the "surrogate" endpoint, Y_i represents the "true" endpoint, and Z_i represents the treatment variable.

chemical structural feature on both gene expression and pIC50 and their associations can be simultaneously investigated. The joint model is presented in Section 16.5.

Biomarker identification is a major application of microarray experiments in early drug development, which often parallels and facilitates compound selection. Many studies have been devoted to identifying genes that are correlated to a biological activity of interest, for instance, the inhibition of a certain enzyme. It is also equally important to detect toxicity at the early stages of development. Reliable biomarkers for toxicity can be very helpful in this respect as it allows cost-effective testing of other drug candidates in compound series under investigation. For example, Lin et al. (2010) and Tilahun et al. (2010) identified gene-specific biomarkers for continuous outcomes (the distance traveled by rats under treatment and the Hamilton Depression (HAMD) scores for psychiatric patients). Van Sanden et al. (2012) identified gene-specific biomarkers for toxicity data presented as a binary response. The joint modeling framework (Lin et al., 2010; Tilahun et al., 2010) that we present in this chapter allows us to: (1) identify gene signatures of activity for directing chemistry, (2) determine chemical substructures (called fingerprint features, FF) of compounds that are associated with the bioassay data for a biological target(s) of interest, and (3) investigate whether the association between the compounds and the bioassay can be confirmed by the gene expression changes (either on- or off-target related).

Identifying relevant genes that are associated with biological response already provides valuable information, but showing that this association is caused by the presence or absence of a particular chemical substructure(s) provides additional information that is particularly useful in drug design to improve or prioritize compounds. The methods discussed in this chapter are applied to two case studies presented in Section 16.6.

16.2 The QSTAR Framework and Surrogacy

Early drug discovery research and the development process involve a range of technologies for measuring the chemical and biological effects of compounds at the molecular level in order to make a decision about the development of a new drug. Consequently, this process generates multiple sources of high-dimensional data which include high-throughput screening (HTS), chemical structures, gene expression, image-based high-content screening (HCS), among others. High-dimensional data are characterized as having an enormous number of features (variables) and relatively few compounds (samples). This leads us to the problem of data integration and opens up a challenging venue for methodological development and application to extract relevant information from the intersection of biology and chemistry. An integrative method that allows us to detect the relationship of all these features can be very relevant to evaluate compound efficacy and safety as lead compounds progress through lead optimization.

In drug discovery, scientists work together and start to identify a potential biomolecular "*target*," which is usually a single molecule, typically a protein, that is involved in a particular disease. This target should be drugable, that is, it can interact with and be affected by a molecule. After the identification and validation of the target, the process of discovering promising compounds that could ultimately turn into a medicine for a particular disease follows. The discovery, therefore, starts with either creating a new molecule or repurposing an existing molecule. At this point, thousands of candidate molecules could be screened against the target for activity using HTS assays and then optimized through structure modification for better activity.

Over several decades, Quantitative Structure-Activity Relationship (QSAR) modeling techniques (Nantasenamat et al., 2009) have been extensively used to quantify the relationship between chemical structure and activity to gain understanding of how the chemical substructures affect the biological activity of a compound and then use this understanding to design compounds with improved activity either relating to greater efficacy or lesser toxicity (Dearden, 2003; Martin, Kofron, and Traphagen, 2002; Bruce et al., 2008). The fundamental principle underlying the QSTAR approach is based on the observation that chemicals of similar structures frequently share simi-

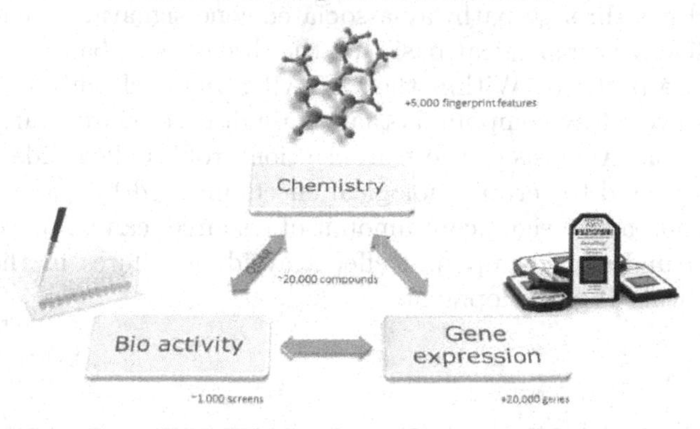

FIGURE 16.2
The QSTAR framework. The integration of 3 high-dimensional datatypes: gene-expression, fingerprints features (FFs representing the chemical structures), and bioassay data (phenotype).

lar physiochemical properties and biological activities (Johnson and Maggiora, 1990; Verma, Khedkhar, and Coutinho, 2010).

The Quantitative Structure-Transcription-Assay Relationship (QSTAR, Verbist et al., 2015) modeling framework is an extension of the QSAR approach (Figure 16.2). Here, transcriptional data are integrated with structural compound information as well as experimental bioactivity data in order to analyze compound effects in biological systems from different angles to elucidate the mechanism of action of compounds (MoA). This could provide insight into inadvertent phenotypic effects, which can greatly help in early-stage pharmaceutical decision-making.

Although the bioactivity data, which is typically measured per target assay, is key in the optimization process of chemically designing compounds, it does not provide much insight in the underlying biological mechanisms. In contrast to the bioassay data that capture single biological effects, the gene expression data, as a multi-dimensional assay, measure a wide diversity of biological effects of a compound on a whole genome transcriptional level, and thereby provide an information-rich snapshot of the biological state of a cell (Göhlmann and Talloen, 2009; Amaratunga, Cabrera, and Shkedy, 2014). Transcriptomic changes following compound administration can also be measured in high throughput, allowing screening of many compounds in multiple cell lines at low cost. It has also been observed that transcriptomic data mostly detect biologically relevant signals and are often able to help in prioritizing compounds beyond conventional target-based assays (Verbist et al., 2015). Applications using gene expression profiles to observe several genes and signaling pathways concurrently enrich the understanding of underlying mechanisms. Moreover, this enables us to investigate downstream effects of candidate drugs through pathway-associated gene signatures. This offers the chance of finding a biological basis for the disease and biomarkers involved in the disease pathway. Within the QSTAR framework, mRNA biomarkers may be discovered by compounds that cause disease-related variation of the gene expression. Analysis of the transcription profiles allows identifying new biomarkers related to certain biological effects induced by these compounds. With this approach, a significant amount of resources can be saved with identification of undesired compound effects avoiding failures in the late-stage pharmaceutical drug development.

16.3 Data

16.3.1 The ROS1 Project

ROS1 (reactive oxygen species) is a proto-oncogene that is highly expressed in a variety of tumor cell lines and belongs to the sevenless subfamily of tyrosine kinase insulin receptor genes. Aberrant expression and oncogenic fusions resulting from chromosomal rearrangement occur in lung cancer, cholangiocarcinoma, and glioblastoma. Aberrant expression is also detected in a variety of other cancer types. ROS1 inhibition is expected to have anti-tumoral effects in cells where ROS1 is activated (Acquaviva, Wong, and Charest, 2009; Charest et al., 2006).

This project sought to develop compounds that inhibit ROS1. The ROS1 dataset consists of eighty-nine (89) compounds tested for target inhibition. A total of 1289 differentially expressed genes were retained after pre-processing. For this project, a total of 312 unique profiles of fingerprint features was generated from the 89 compounds.

16.3.2 The EGFR Project

The EGFR project focuses on inhibition of the epidermal growth factor receptor (Woodburn, 1999). Thirty-five compounds with a macrocycle structure were profiled in order to identify compounds with biological effects, similar to those of the current EGFR inhibitors, Gefitinib and Erlotinib, serving as the reference compounds. Gene expression profiles are available for 3595 genes after all the filtering steps. Moreover, a total of 138 unique profiles of chemical substructures were identified for this compound set.

16.4 Graphical Interpretation (I): The Association between a Gene and Bioactivity Accounting for the Effect of a Fingerprint Feature

Several association patterns between gene expression and a phenotypic variable accounting for the effect of a fingerprint feature can be discovered by using the joint model. The different patterns of association are presented in Figure 16.3 using hypothetical data. Each point in the plot represents a compound and the solid ones are compounds having the fingerprint feature.

For this application, the interest lies only in the fingerprint feature that shows differential effects on the bioactivity, the response in this case; thus the four possible scenarios between the gene and response presented in the upper panels of Figure 16.3 (a)–(d). The lower panels (e)–(h) display the same data with their respective upper panels adjusted for fingerprint feature effect for both the response and the gene expression.

In panel (a) the gene is not differentially expressed and has a linear association with the response irrespective of the presence or absence of the fingerprint feature. Note that the linear pattern remains after adjusting for the fingerprint feature as shown in panel (e). Panel (b) shows an example in which the gene is differentially expressed, the clouds of points are clearly separated in both dimensions. Moreover, it can be observed that within the group, the association between the gene expression and the response does not have a linear pattern, which is evident in panel (f) after the adjustment.

Panel (c) shows a combination of the previous two patterns. Both the gene expression and the response are differentially expressed, that is, compounds having the fingerprint feature induce higher activity than those that do not have the fingerprint feature. In this setting, the association between the gene expression and the response can be summarized by a straight line; this can be clearly seen from panel (g), which shows the same example after adjusting for fingerprint feature.

Lastly, most genes are expected to be uncorrelated with the bioassay data as depicted by panel (d). Within each group of compounds (with and without the fingerprint feature), a linear pattern is not evident; thus, adjusting for this effect also provides a random scattering of points (panel (h)).

The joint modeling framework is useful for identifying genes that can predict compound activity, measured by pIC50, and can therefore serve as genetic biomarkers for a compound's efficacy. On top of this, the effect of a particular chemical substructure on the expression level of each gene and/or its influence on the observed transcriptomic-phenotypic association can be estimated.

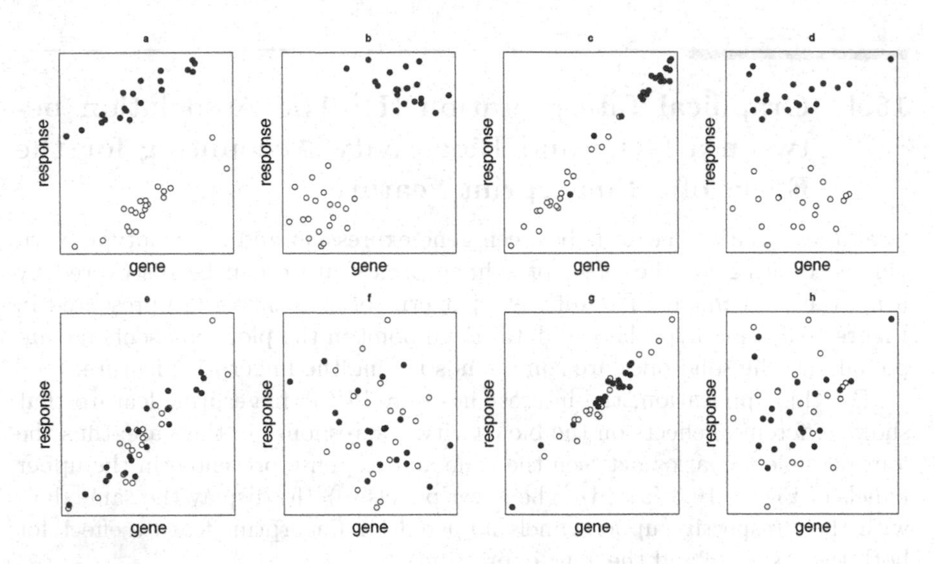

FIGURE 16.3
Hypothetical examples of the association between response variable and expression levels when the effect of the fingerprint feature (FF) upon the response is significant. Each point represents a compound. Black and white points represent the presence/absence of a fingerprint feature, respectively. Upper row: scatterplots for the response versus the gene expression. Lower row: scatterplots for the residuals after adjusting for fingerprint effects.

16.5 Modeling Approach

16.5.1 The Joint Model

Let X be the gene expression matrix where X_{ij} is the jth gene expression of the ith compound, $i = 1, \ldots, n$ and $j = 1, \ldots, m$. Let Y_i denote the measurement for the bioassay data. Both gene expression and bioassay read-outs are assumed to be normally distributed. Let $\mathbf{Z}$ be the binary chemical structure or fingerprint feature matrix in which the ki^{th} element takes a value of one, $z_{ki} = 1$, or zero, $z_{ki} = 0$, if the kth fingerprint feature is respectively present/absent in the ith compound.

For a given fingerprint feature, the gene-specific joint model that allows testing for which gene is also differentially expressed and which gene is predictive of the response irrespective of the effect of the fingerprint feature is given by

$$\begin{pmatrix} X_{ij} \\ Y_i \end{pmatrix} \sim N \left[\begin{pmatrix} \mu_X + \alpha_j Z_i \\ \mu_Y + \beta Z_i \end{pmatrix}, \Sigma_j \right], \tag{16.1}$$

where the error terms have a joint zero-mean normal distribution with gene-specific covariance matrix, Σ_j:

$$\Sigma_j = \begin{pmatrix} \sigma_{jj} & \sigma_{jY} \\ \sigma_{jY} & \sigma_{YY} \end{pmatrix}. \tag{16.2}$$

The parameters α_j and β represent the fingerprint feature effects for the jth gene and the response, respectively, and μ_j and μ_Y are gene-specific and the response-related intercepts, respectively. Note that this model is identical to the joint model for a single-trial setting discussed in Chapter 3. Thus, the gene-specific association with the response can be obtained using the adjusted association (Buyse and Molenberghs, 1998), a coefficient that is derived from the covariance matrix, Σ_j, of gene-specific joint model (16.2):

$$\rho_j = \frac{\sigma_{jY}}{\sqrt{\sigma_{jj}\sigma_{YY}}}. \tag{16.3}$$

Indeed, $\rho_j = 1$ indicates a deterministic relationship between the gene expression and the response after accounting for the effect of a fingerprint feature.

16.5.2 Inference

As mentioned in Section 16.5.1, the model allows testing for differentially expressed genes, hence for each gene, we test the hypotheses:

$$\begin{aligned} H_{0_j} &: \alpha_j = 0, \\ H_{1_j} &: \alpha_j \neq 0. \end{aligned} \tag{16.4}$$

For a microarray with m genes, there are m null hypotheses to be tested, which implies that an adjustment for multiple testing should be applied. Throughout this chapter, we apply the false discovery rate (FDR) approach proposed by Benjamini and Hochberg (1995).

Moreover, in order to make inference about ρ_j, there is a need to test whether the expression level of a gene and the bioassay read-out are correlated, specifically, whether the expression level of a gene can predict the bioassay read-out. Thus, in addition to the hypotheses in (16.4), one needs to test the hypotheses:

$$\begin{aligned} H_{0_j} &: \rho_j = 0, \\ H_{1_j} &: \rho_j \neq 0, \end{aligned} \tag{16.5}$$

or equivalently

$$H_{0_j}: \sigma_{jY} = 0, \quad H_{1_j}: \sigma_{jY} \neq 0. \tag{16.6}$$

Under the null hypothesis, the joint model in (16.1) is reduced to

$$\begin{pmatrix} X_{ij} \\ Y_i \end{pmatrix} \sim N \left[\begin{pmatrix} \mu_j + \alpha_j Z_i \\ \mu_Y + \beta Z_i \end{pmatrix}, \Sigma_j = \begin{pmatrix} \sigma_{jj} & 0 \\ 0 & \sigma_{YY} \end{pmatrix} \right]. \tag{16.7}$$

Consequently, the inference for the adjusted association can be based on a likelihood ratio test by comparing models in (16.1) and (16.7). Asymptotically, the likelihood ratio statistic follows a χ^2-distribution with one degree-of-freedom. The Benjamini and Hochberg (1995) procedure is used to adjust for false discovery rate when testing for the null hypotheses of $H_{0_j}: \rho_j = 0$ for all the genes simultaneously per fingerprint feature.

16.5.3 Graphical Interpretation (II): Adjusted Association and Conditional Independence

As shown in Table 16.1, genes can be classified into subgroups according to the results obtained from the hypothesis testing in (16.4) and (16.5). For the first group of genes (a), the association between the gene expression and pIC50 exists regardless of the effect of a chemical substructure of the compound while the association from the second group of genes (b) is driven by the fingerprint feature. This association can also further expand our knowledge about the biological mechanisms of compounds to guide decision-making in lead selection. Ideally, results from the joint modeling of every fingerprint feature, gene, and activity data are generated. In this chapter, we only present the results of applying the joint model using a fingerprint feature that is mostly associated with the variation in compound activity.

16.6 Analysis of the EGFR and the ROS1 Projects

16.6.1 Application to the EGFR Project

This oncology project focuses on the inhibition of the epidermal growth factor receptor (EGFR), which has been identified in many human epithelial cancers, colorectal, breast, pancreatic, non-small-cell lung, and brain cancer (Shaib et al., 2013).

For this project, of the 55 fingerprint features that demonstrated differential effects on the primary bioassay, FF-442307337 came out first based on a

TABLE 16.1

Subclasses of genes using a hypothetical example. If both α and β are significantly different from zero, the correlation between the gene expression and bioactivity is present but in contrast with scenario (a), the gene expression in scenario (b) is correlated with the bioactivity variable only due to the effect of the fingerprint feature, hence its adjusted association is zero, $\rho_j = 0$. From the point of view of the structural optimization in the early drug development, the association observed in (b) is desirable while the one observed in (a) is an ideal genetic biomarker for bioactivity.

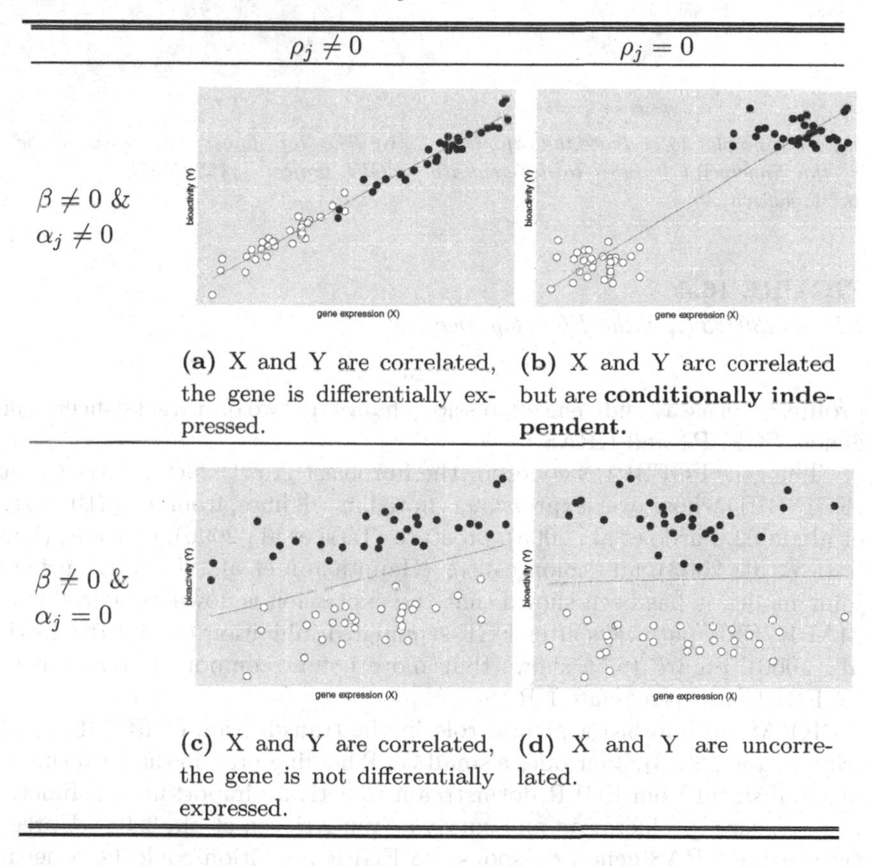

(a) X and Y are correlated, the gene is differentially expressed.

(b) X and Y are correlated but are **conditionally independent.**

(c) X and Y are correlated, the gene is not differentially expressed.

(d) X and Y are uncorrelated.

feature-by-feature two-sample t-test of bioactivity data (Figure 16.4a). This substructure is prominent in less potent compounds, i.e., those with pIC50 values less than 6.5 (Figure 16.4b).

Several genes correlate with the inhibitory activity against the target. Figure 16.5 highlights the linear association between pIC50 from the anti-

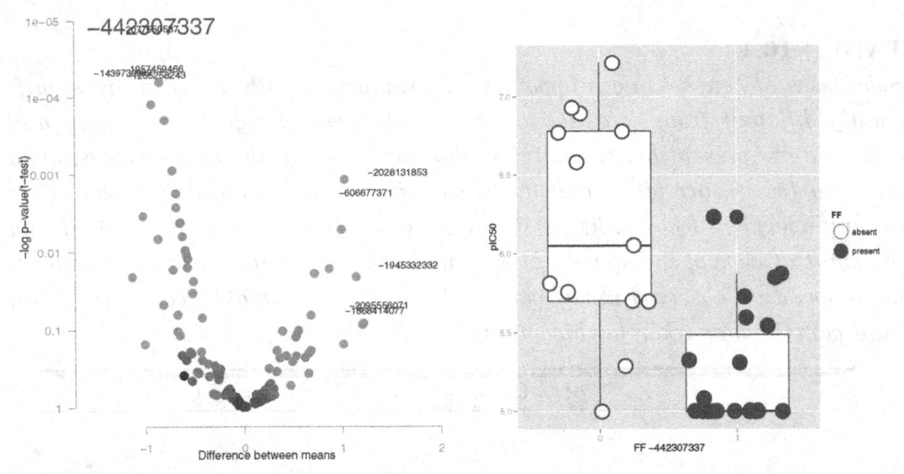

(a) *Volcano plot to evaluate the capacity of the fingerprint features to differentiate the bioactivity.*

(b) *The top fingerprint features for the EGFR project: -442307337.*

FIGURE 16.4
FF -442307337 for the EGFR project.

proliferation assay and gene expression changes of two on-target cancer-related genes: FGFBP1 and KRAS.

The gene FGFBP1 encodes for the fibroblast growth factor carrier protein (FGF-BP1) whose over-expression is noted in cell lines, from lung (Brattström et al., 2002; Pardo et al., 2003), prostate (Tassi et al., 2006), pancreas (Kuwahara et al., 2003), and colon cancer (Hauptmann et al., 2003). By using the joint model, it has been shown that the expression is down-regulated via the MAPK/ERK pathways after EGF-stimulated inhibition of EGFR (Harris et al., 2000). Figure 16.5a shows that more potent compounds down-regulate FGFBP1 but up-regulate KRAS.

KRAS protein has a pivotal role in the transduction of EGFR signaling (Shaib et al., 2013), it encodes a small GTP binding protein that transmits the original signal from EGFR downstream to activate important cell functions, in particular, proliferation and survival (van Krieken et al., 2008). Upregulation of the KRAS gene in response to EGFR inhibition could be a negative feedback mechanism of the cell to trigger cell survival. Several authors have indicated KRAS as part of a potential mechanism of resistance to EGFR inhibition, which makes KRAS a key target oncogene (Zimmerman et al., 2013; Collins and di Magliano, 2014). This gene participates in a large number of signaling pathways including MAPK, ErbB, VEGF, and a number of biological processes.

On the structure-activity side, the chemical feature, FF-442307337, is also

TABLE 16.2
Results for FF -442307337 (EGFR) at 5% FDR.

		ρ	
		$\neq 0$	0
α	$\neq 0$	396	61
	0	1099	2039

linked with differential expression of numerous genes. In addition, some of the correlations observed between the pIC50 and gene expression can be attributed to this substructure as the correlation changes after adjusting for this chemical feature (Figure 16.6).

Next, genes are classified into subgroups based on whether their expression changes are linked with the structure and/or the association remains linear after adjustments for the chemical structure. The number of genes for each subgroup are presented in Table 16.2.

KRAS and FGFBP1 seem to belong to different gene classes. Figure 16.7 shows the 5 most differentially expressed genes with the adjusted association remaining high after adjusting for the chemical structure including the gene FGFBP1, while the estimates for the top 10 genes are given in Table 16.3. The association observed between the gene FGFBP1 and pIC50 is still evident after adjusting for chemical structure (Figure 16.5b). Most of these genes are known to participate in biological processes involving cell proliferation (positive and negative), survival, and differentiation. Another set of differentially expressed genes following a similar pattern to gene KRAS is presented in Table 16.4 with the visualization of the top 5 genes in Figure 16.8. For this group, the joint model resulted in very low adjusted correlation (p-adj(ρ)>0.05) between the genes and the activity. Unlike FGFBP1, the adjustment has a considerable effect in the observed association (from unadjusted correlation, r=0.62 to adjusted correlation, ρ =0.34, see Figure 16.5b).

The substructure FF-442307337 is present in the majority of compounds that inhibit cell growth to a lesser extent than FGFBP1. Figure 16.9a shows the chemical structure of FF-442307337, an oxygen in ortho position of the aniline (highlighted substructure). The next compound is very similar to the less potent compound but without FF-442307337 and it is one of the highly potent compounds in this experiment (Figure 16.9b) along with the two reference compounds gefitinib and erlotinib (Figure 16.9c-d). However, other less potent compounds do not have this feature; this substructure is probably not the sole reason for compounds' lower activity.

TABLE 16.3
List of top 10 differentially expressed genes with high adjusted association (p-adj(ρ) < 0.05) after adjusting for FF -442307337 (EGFR).

Genes	Effect	p-adj(Effect)	r	ρ	p-adj(ρ)
FOSL1	1.19	0.01	−0.84	−0.76	0.00
FGFBP1	0.79	0.01	−0.84	−0.78	0.00
SEPP1	−0.64	0.01	0.81	0.73	0.00
SCGB2A1	−0.61	0.01	0.83	0.76	0.00
SH2B3	0.61	0.01	−0.79	−0.69	0.00
SLCO4A1	0.60	0.01	−0.79	−0.70	0.00
PHLDA1	0.58	0.01	−0.85	−0.77	0.00
RRM2	0.56	0.02	−0.77	−0.70	0.00
TXNIP	−0.53	0.00	0.75	0.58	0.00
CDC6	0.52	0.01	−0.80	−0.73	0.00

16.6.2 Application to the ROS1 Project

This project sought to develop compounds that inhibit ROS1 (reactive oxygen species), known to be over-expressed in several cancer types. Excessive quantities of ROS1 causes oxidative stress that is generally detrimental to cells (Gorrini, Harris, and Mak, 2013). A cellular assay for target inhibition showed several compounds with high inhibitory activity. FF -2086493472 came out to be the top fingerprint feature that can well separate the bioactivity of the compounds (Figure 16.10b). Here, the feature can be linked with lower potency since all compounds having the fingerprint feature have lower pIC50 values than those compounds not having the feature.

The joint modeling resulted in identification of genes that are associated with the pIC50. A number of genes showed positive correlation, like FNIP1, while TXNRD1 along with other genes showed negative correlation (Figure 16.11a).

Interestingly, TXNRD1, a key player in oxidative stress control, is also evaluated as a cancer drug target associated with aggressive tumor growth (Powis and Kirkpatrick, 2007; Eriksson et al., 2009). Elevated levels of this gene in many human cancers contribute to increased proliferation, resistance to cell death, and increased angiogenesis. Dai et al. (2013) show that simultaneous inhibition of TXNRD1 and AKT pathways (activated by ROS1) induced robust ROS1 production. Discovering potential inhibitors of this gene could contribute to cancer therapy (Urig and Becker, 2006). In this experiment, compounds with high ROS1 inhibitory activity also show inhibition of TXNRD1.

The joint model furthermore revealed that potent compounds with lower gene expression effects on TXNRD1 lack FF-2086493472. Moreover, the association between the pIC50 and the expression of gene TXRND1 can be fully

TABLE 16.4

List of top 10 differentially expressed genes with low adjusted association (p-adj(ρ) > 0.05) after adjusting for FF -442307337 (EGFR).

Genes	Effect	p-adj(Effect)	r	ρ	p-adj(ρ)
KRAS	−0.30	0.00	0.62	0.34	0.07
MAP9	−0.13	0.00	0.62	0.29	0.13
SMG1	−0.10	0.00	0.62	0.35	0.06
PTER	−0.10	0.00	0.61	0.35	0.06
ODZ3	−0.14	0.01	0.59	0.35	0.06
SCAF11	−0.16	0.00	0.59	0.30	0.12
PCYOX1	−0.23	0.00	0.58	0.30	0.12
PHACTR2	−0.13	0.01	0.58	0.35	0.06
USP3	−0.07	0.01	0.57	0.35	0.06
FBXO21	−0.12	0.00	0.57	0.27	0.16

explained by the absence/presence of this feature (Figure 16.11b). Table 16.5 shows a set of differentially expressed genes with the same type of association observed between TXNRD1 and pIC50 that disappears after adjusting for FF-2086493472 (Figure 16.13). Figure 16.12 shows how the correlation between the pIC50 and all genes changes after accounting for FF-2086493472.

Little is known about the biology of the FNIP1 gene, particularly relating to cancer. Hasumi et al. (2008) indicated that FNIP1 mRNA was significantly higher in renal cell carcinoma compared to normal kidney. Unlike TXNRD1, the correlation between the bioassay and the gene remains moderately strong after adjusting for the fingerprint feature. This implies that FNIP1 remains to be linearly associated with the efficacy data independent of this structural feature. Table 16.6 presents 9 other genes showing the same type of association with pIC50 as FNIP1 (Figure 16.14). The number of genes in each subclass is given in Table 16.7.

TABLE 16.5
List of top 10 differentially expressed genes with low adjusted association (p-adj(ρ) > 0.05) after adjusting for FF -2086493472 (ROS1).

Genes	Effect	p-adj(Effect)	r	ρ	p-adj(ρ)
TXNRD1	0.39	0.00	−0.65	−0.08	0.54
PFKFB3	0.57	0.00	−0.61	0.00	0.97
SNORD52	0.23	0.00	−0.65	−0.12	0.33
GDF15	−1.09	0.00	0.67	0.21	0.07
ZNF292	−0.30	0.00	0.59	0.01	0.95
CTPS	0.30	0.00	−0.63	−0.16	0.19
KIRREL	0.34	0.00	−0.64	−0.19	0.11
HMGCS1	0.77	0.00	−0.58	−0.04	0.77
TFPI	−0.46	0.00	0.60	0.11	0.37
HIST1H1A	0.49	0.00	−0.52	0.09	0.49

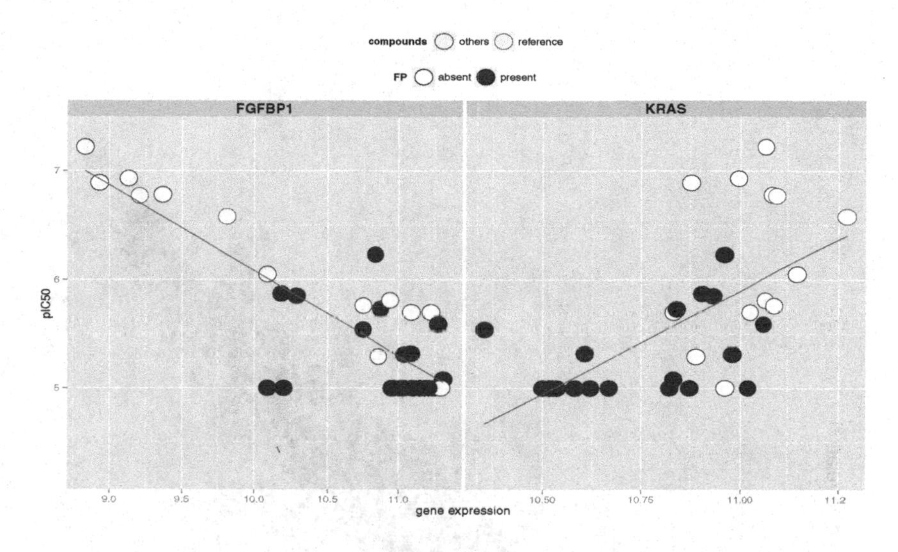

(a) Gene expression versus pIC50.

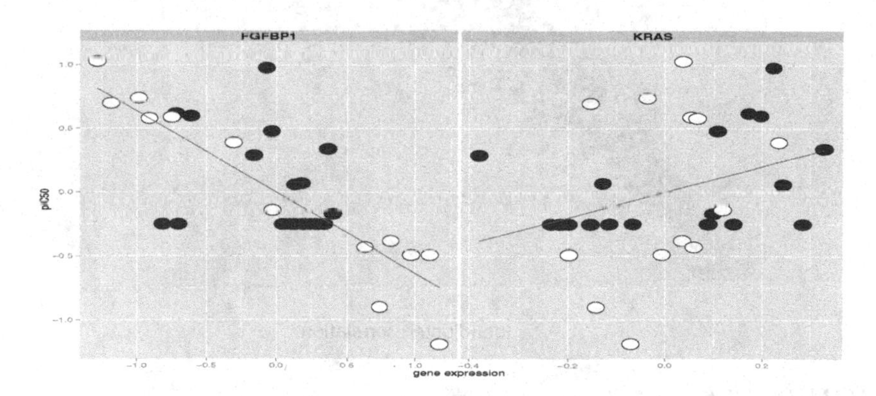

(b) Gene expression versus pIC50 after adjustment.

FIGURE 16.5
Two on-target genes that correlate with EGFR inhibition: FGFBP1 and KRAS. Each point is a compound with the two reference compounds as highlighted circles. The solid blue points indicate the presence of FF -442307337.

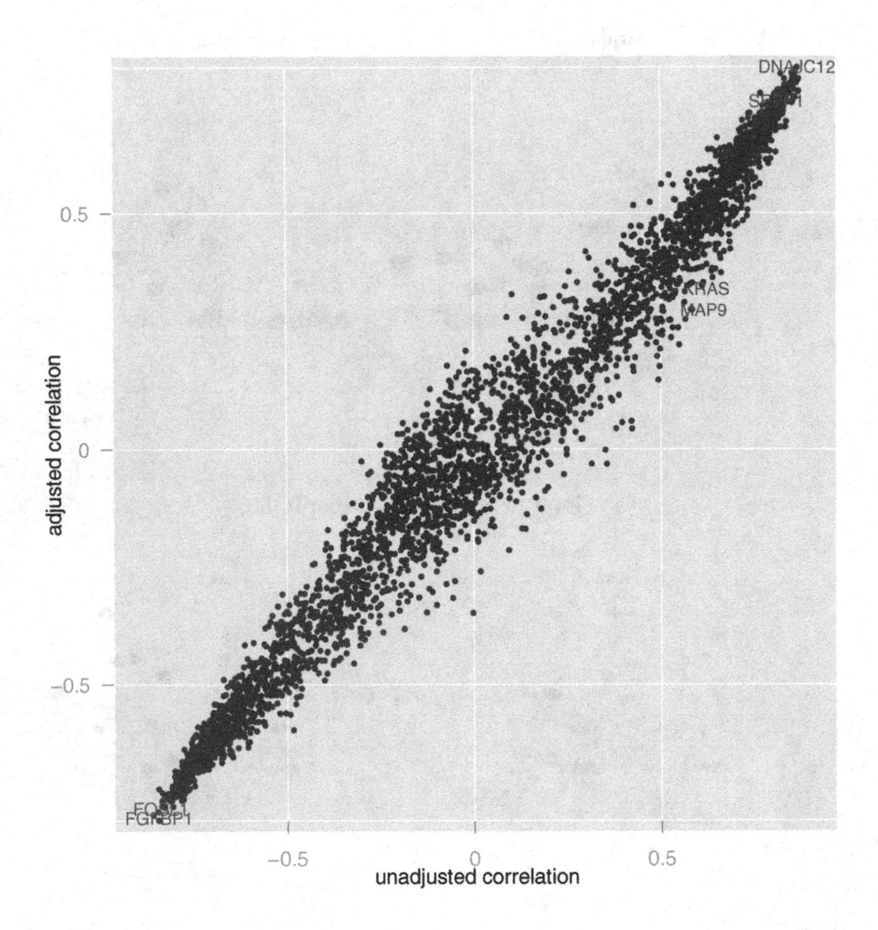

FIGURE 16.6

Unadjusted versus adjusted correlations. Each point is a gene. Genes that have high correlation but very low adjusted correlation indicates that the fingerprint feature is creating the association.

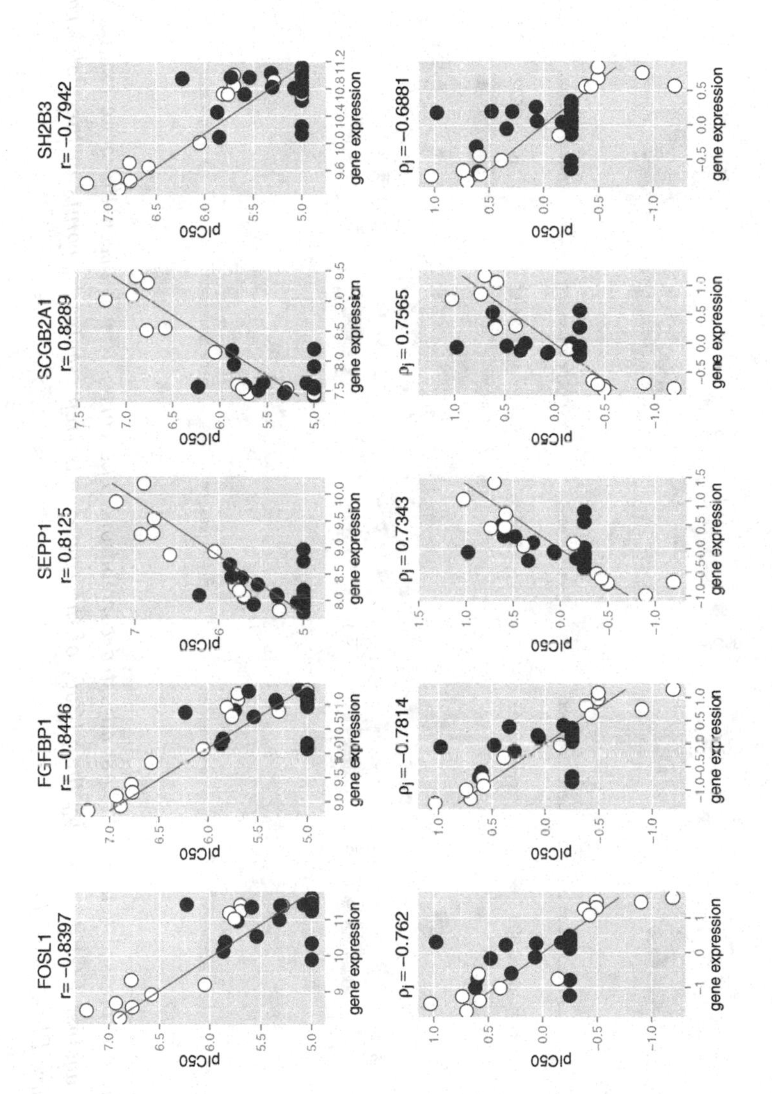

FIGURE 16.7
Top 5 differentially expressed genes with high adjusted correlation. The correlation between the gene expression and the inhibitory activity against EGFR, given by the pIC50, of the compounds (represented by points in the plots) can be explained by the substructure FF-44207337.

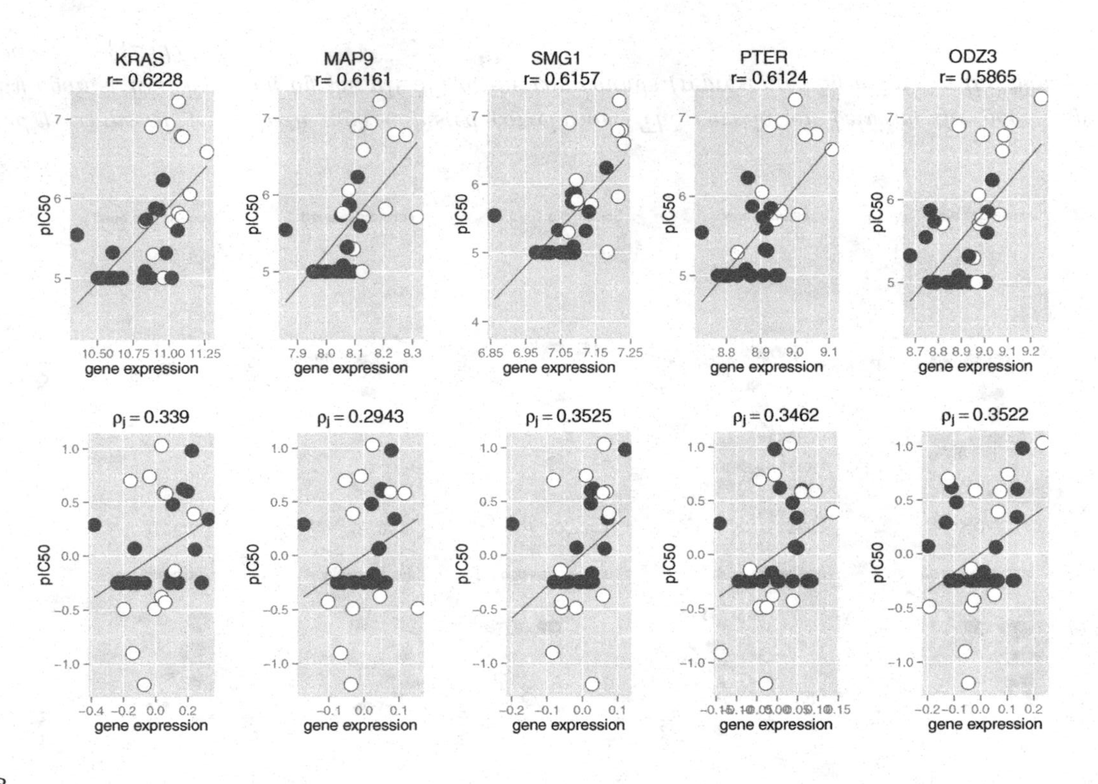

FIGURE 16.8

Top 5 differentially expressed genes with low adjusted correlation. The correlation between the gene expression and the inhibitory activity against EGFR, given by the pIC50, of the compounds (represented by points in the plots) can be explained by the substructure FF -442307337.

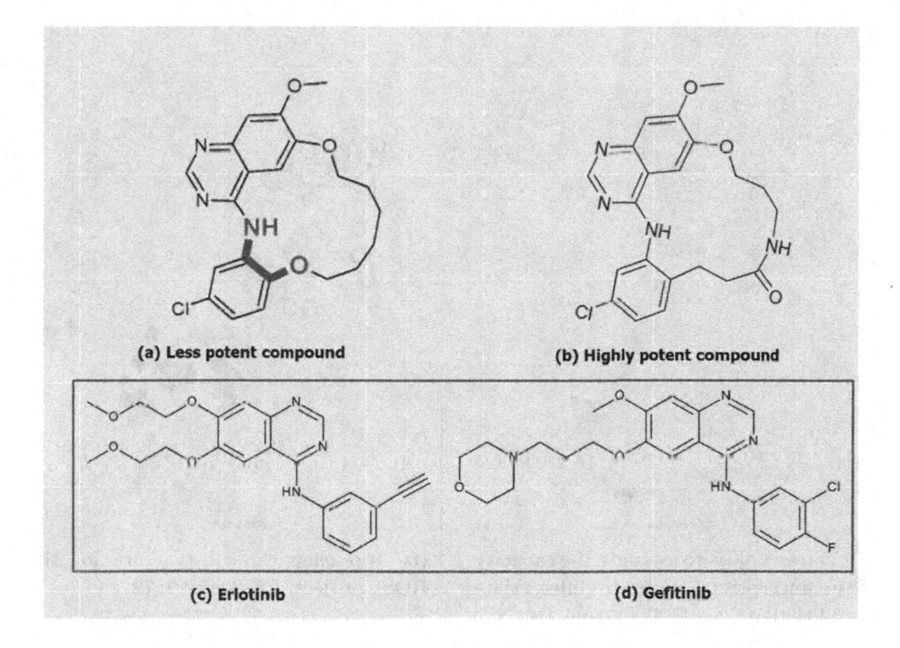

FIGURE 16.9
Chemical structures of (a) identified less potent compound; (b) highly potent compound in the EGFR project; and the two reference compounds in this experiment, (c) erlotinib and (d) gefitinib.

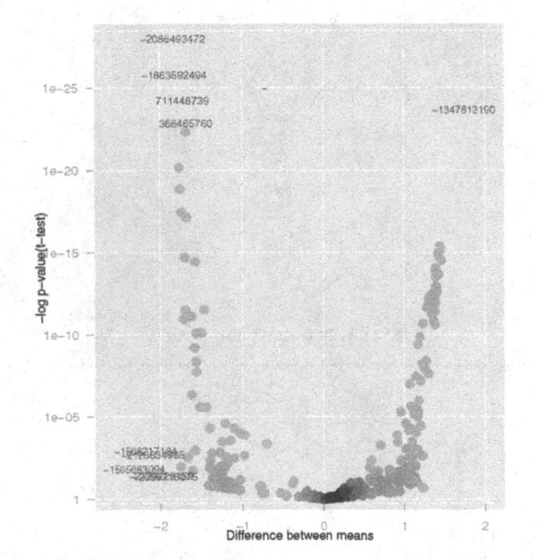

(a) Volcano plots to evaluate the capacity of the fingerprint features to differentiate the bioactivity.

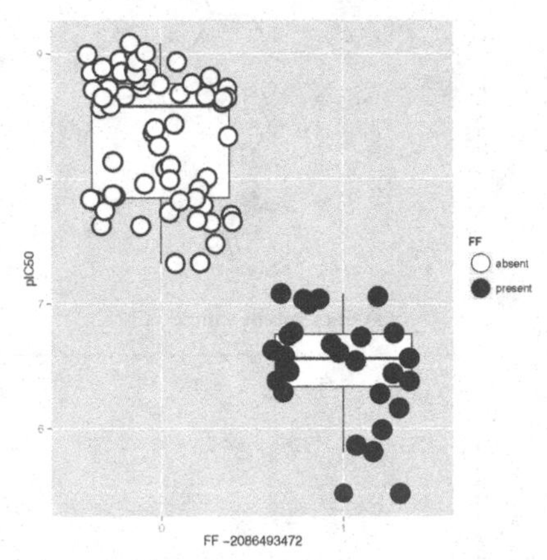

(b) Top chemical substructure for the ROS1 project: FF-2086493472.

FIGURE 16.10

Plots highlighting the most relevant fingerprint features for the ROS1 project.

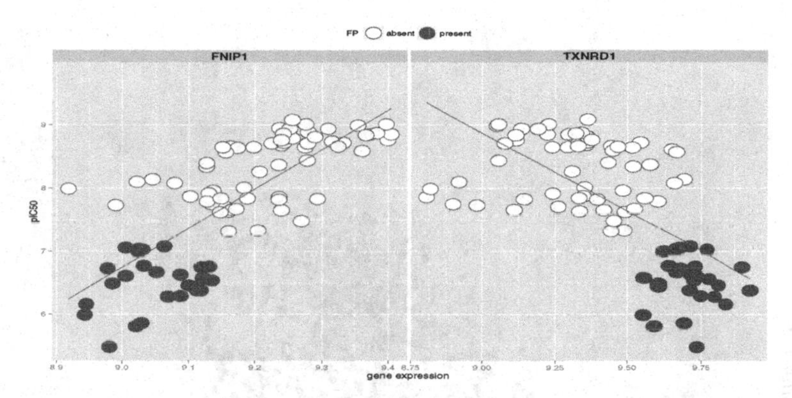

(a) Gene expression versus pIC50.

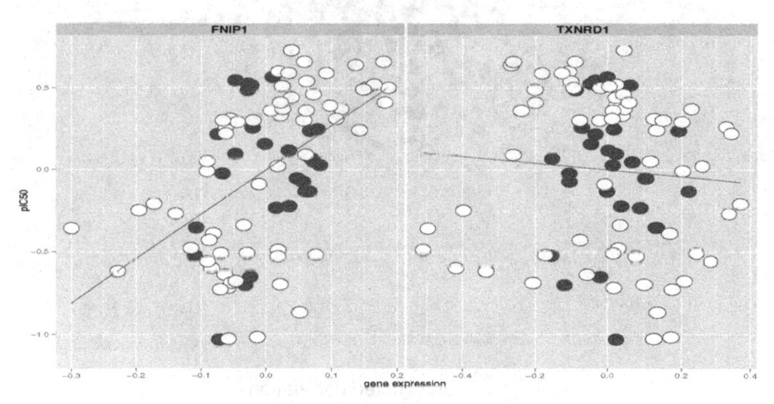

(b) Gene expression versus pIC50 after adjustment.

FIGURE 16.11
Two cancer-related genes that correlate with ROS1-inhibition: FNIP1 and TXNRD1. The solid points indicate the presence of FF -2086493472.

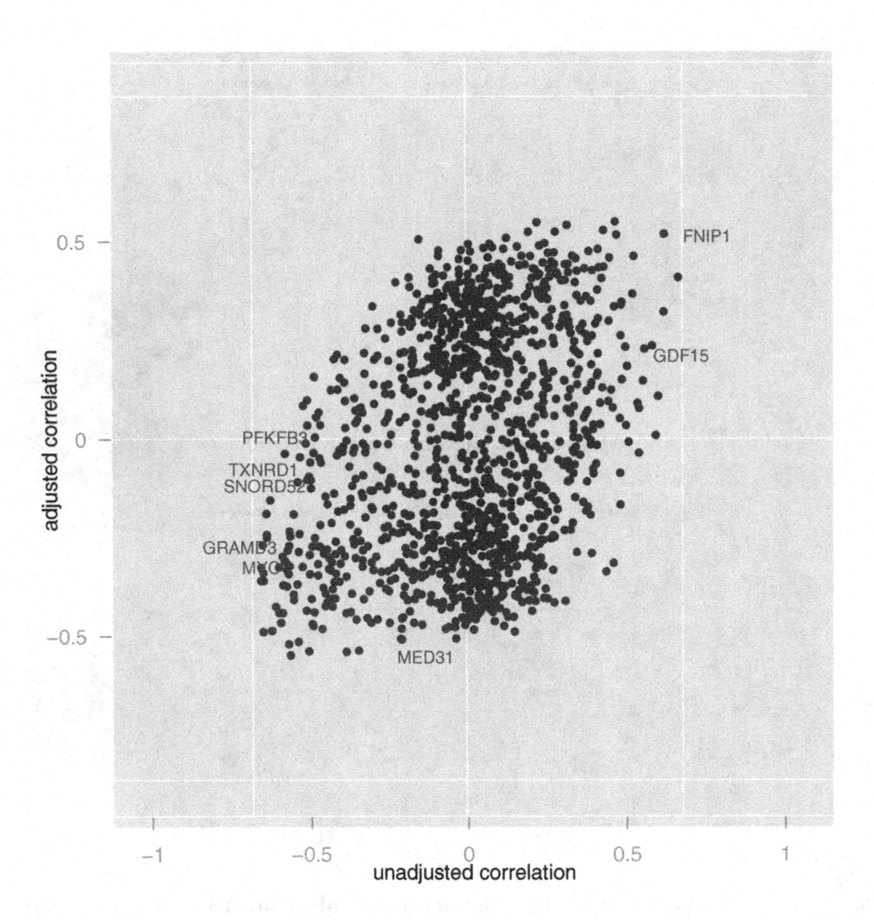

FIGURE 16.12
Unadjusted versus adjusted correlations. Each point is a gene. Genes that have high correlation but very low adjusted correlation indicates that the fingerprint feature is creating the association.

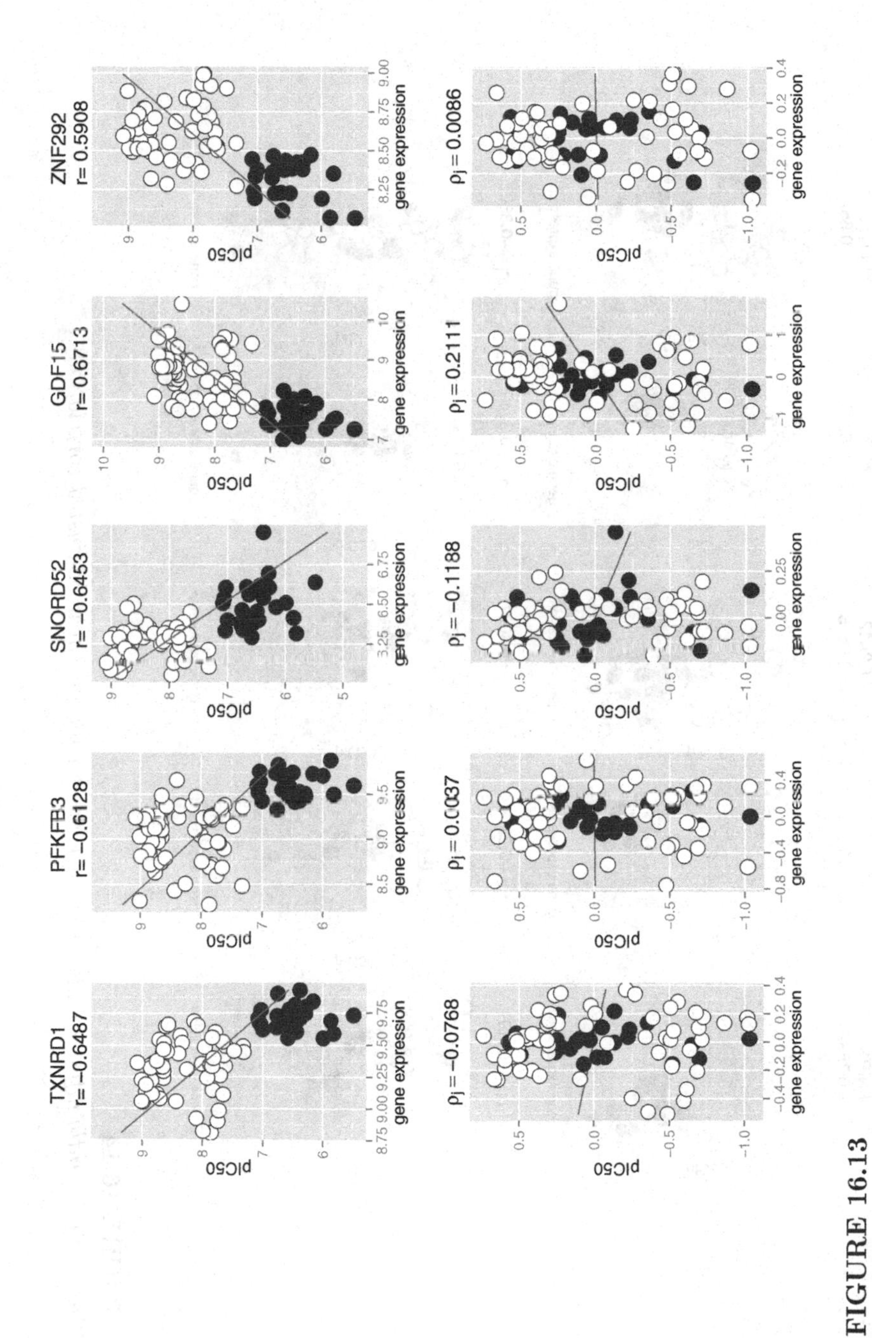

FIGURE 16.13
Top 5 differentially expressed genes with low adjusted correlation.

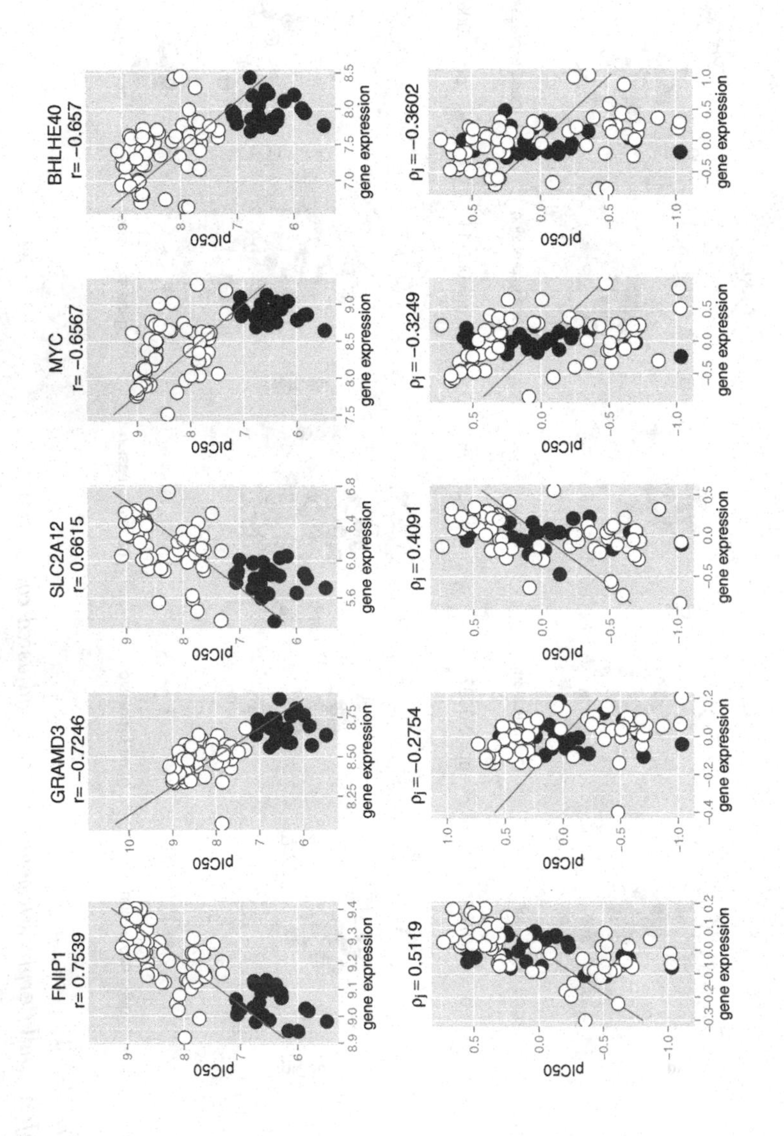

FIGURE 16.14
Top 5 significantly differentially expressed genes with significant adjusted correlation.

TABLE 16.6
List of top 10 differentially expressed genes with high adjusted association (p-adj(ρ) < 0.05) after adjusting for FF -2086493472 (ROS1).

Genes	Effect	p-adj(Effect)	r	ρ	p-adj(ρ)
FNIP1	−0.16	0.00	0.75	0.51	0.00
GRAMD3	0.20	0.00	−0.72	−0.27	0.02
SLC2A12	−0.37	0.00	0.66	0.41	0.00
MYC	0.52	0.00	−0.66	−0.33	0.00
BHLHE40	0.55	0.00	−0.66	−0.36	0.00
TGFB2	0.57	0.00	−0.66	−0.33	0.00
TMEM177	0.13	0.00	−0.65	−0.27	0.02
SNORD4B	0.25	0.00	−0.65	−0.49	0.00
TNFRSF12A	0.82	0.00	−0.65	−0.34	0.00
SNORD44	0.19	0.00	−0.65	−0.36	0.00

TABLE 16.7
Results for FF -2086493472 (ROS) at 5% FDR.

		ρ	
		$\neq 0$	0
α	$\neq 0$	139	239
	0	382	529

16.7 The R Package IntegratedJM

16.7.1 Identification of Biomarkers

In this section we describe the R package `IntegratedJM`, which can be used in order to conduct the analysis presented in this chapter. We use the EGFR project for illustration. The expression matrix X is stored in the R object `dat`. As mentioned in Section 16.3, the EGFR project consists of information on 3595 genes measured for 35 compounds.

```
> dim(dat)
Features  Samples
    3595       35
```

The vectors `responseVector` and `covariate` are the bioactivity (Y) and the fingerprint feature (Z) variables, respectively:

```
> length(responseVector)
```

```
[1] 35
> length(covariate)
[1] 35
```

The main function in the package, `fitJM()`, can be used to fit the joint model specified in (16.1):

```
> jmRes <- fitJM(dat=dat, responseVector=responseVector,
            covariate=covariate, methodMultTest = 'fdr')
```

Note that the argument `methodMultTest='fdr'` implies that the BH-FDR approach (Amaratunga, Cabrera, and Shkedy, 2014) is used for multiplicity adjustment. The list of the top genes is obtained using the function `topkGenes`. The argument `Effect` implies that a subset of differentially expressed genes will be selected. The ranking argument specifies how to rank the genes within the selected subset. For the EGFR project, the gene `KRAS` has the highest absolute value for unadjusted association (see also Table 16.4):

```
> topkGenes(jointModelResult=jmRes, subset_type ="Effect",ranking = "Pearson"
, k=10, sigLevel = 0.05)
     Genes   FP-Effect p-adj(Effect) Unadj.Asso. Adj.Asso. p-adj(Adj.Asso.)
1     KRAS -0.29738661  0.0008707120   0.6228461 0.3390398       0.07048685
2     MAP9 -0.13059460  0.0002435665   0.6160688 0.2942768       0.12538775
3     SMG1 -0.09732380  0.0019501488   0.6157263 0.3524950       0.05841850
4     PTER -0.10177997  0.0019501488   0.6123932 0.3462307       0.06378699
5     ODZ3 -0.13710657  0.0055083660   0.5864808 0.3521713       0.05866836
6   SCAF11 -0.16406685  0.0017160848   0.5852470 0.2951218       0.12404584
7   PCYOX1 -0.22745115  0.0019501488   0.5823441 0.2950562       0.12410166
8  PHACTR2 -0.12632673  0.0061587590   0.5793338 0.3488484       0.06155341
9     USP3 -0.06771665  0.0070062886   0.5735814 0.3453967       0.06445048
10  FBXO21 -0.12135041  0.0022172747   0.5670778 0.2748839       0.15757229
```

The gene `FOSL1` is the top ranked gene in the subset of differentially expressed and correlated genes, when ranked based on the absolute value of the fingerprint effect on the gene expression (see Table 16.3):

```
> topkGenes(jointModelResult=jmRes, subset_type ="Effect and Correlation",
          ranking = "CovEffect1", k=10, sigLevel = 0.05)

      Genes  FP-Effect p-adj(Effect) Unadj.Asso.  Adj.Asso. p-adj(Adj.Asso.)
1     FOSL1  1.1942768   0.005728185  -0.8396638 -0.7619553     4.590942e-06
2    FGFBP1  0.7872531   0.008023226  -0.8446045 -0.7813558     2.422426e-06
3     SEPP1 -0.6360825   0.008776129   0.8124630  0.7342640     7.168442e-06
4  SCGB2A1 -0.6139309   0.008017638   0.8288709  0.7565218     4.633984e-06
5     SH2B3  0.6106726   0.005601205  -0.7942338 -0.6880690     2.586543e-05
6   SLCO4A1  0.5988076   0.009534114  -0.7903577 -0.7028792     1.633291e-05
7    PHLDA1  0.5752853   0.005132267  -0.8465864 -0.7683447     3.543378e-06
8      RRM2  0.5645259   0.016186359  -0.7703687 -0.6957629     2.011019e-05
9     TXNIP -0.5267830   0.002845200   0.7453539  0.5827579     5.588912e-04
10     CDC6  0.5210562   0.011427699  -0.8022046 -0.7280215     8.268421e-06
```

Figure 16.15 shows the expression levels versus the bioactivity for `FGFBP1` and the corresponding plot for the residuals and was produced using the function `plot1gene()`.

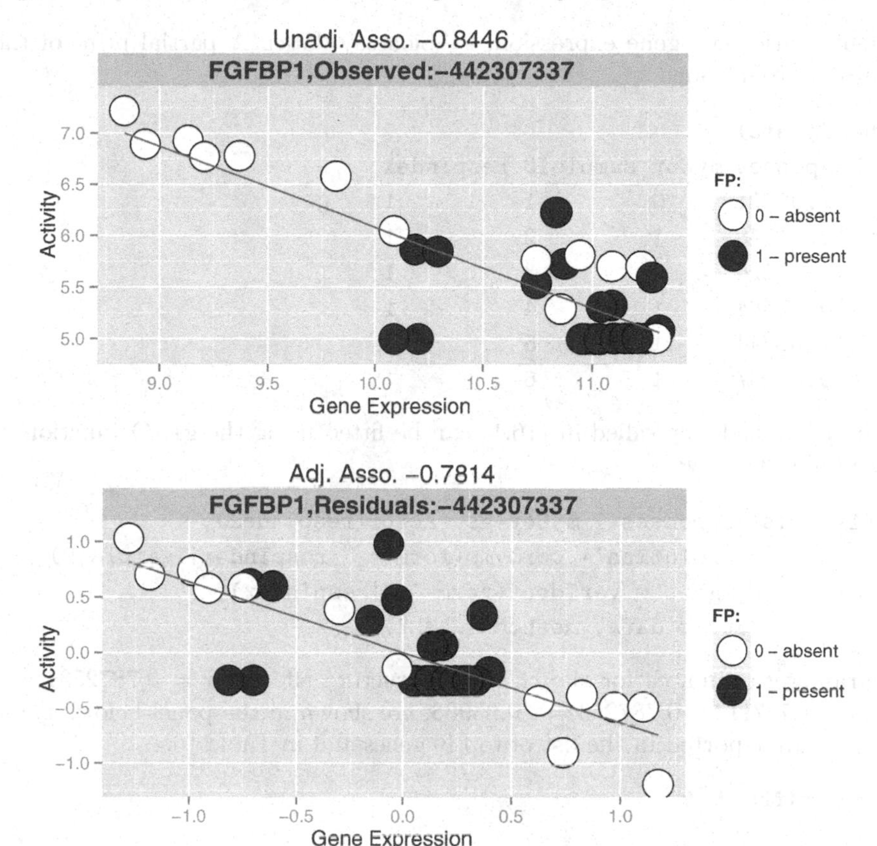

FIGURE 16.15
Expression levels versus bioactivity gene FGFBP1: raw data (upper panel) and corresponding residuals (lower panel).

```
>plot1gene(geneName="FGFBP1",fp=covariate,fpName = "-442307337"
,responseVector=responseVector,dat=dat,resPlot=TRUE,
colP = "blue",colA = "white")
```

16.7.2 Analysis of One Gene Using the gls Function

The main function in the package, `fitJM()`, fits a joint model for the gene expression and the bioactivity data. In this section we discuss the implementation in R for an analysis of a particular gene using the `gls()` function. For illustration we use the data for the gene `FGFBP1` in the EGFR dataset. The object `data` contains the variables `Responses` (gene expression and bioassay data), `myCov` (the fingerprint feature) `sampleID` and `respIndex` (endpoint identification: 1—gene expression, 2—bioassay data). A partial print of the data is given below.

```
>head(data)
  Responses myCov sampleID respIndex
1  11.08821     0        1         1
2  10.18648     1        2         1
3  11.22024     0        3         1
4  10.74484     1        4         1
5  11.08644     1        5         1
6  10.87207     1        6         1
```

The joint model specified in (16.1) can be fitted using the **gls()** function in the following way:

```
>f1<- gls(Responses ~ myCov*as.factor(respIndex),
         correlation = corSymm(form = ~ respIndex| sampleID),
         weights = varIdent(form=~ 1|respIndex),
         data = data, method = "ML")
```

Parameter estimates for the chemical structure effects, $\hat{\alpha} = 0.7872531$ and $\hat{\beta} = -1.727113 + 0.787253 = -0.93986$, are shown in the panel below. These values are reported in the list of top K genes and in Table 16.4.

```
summary(f1)

Coefficients:
                                Value Std.Error   t-value p-value
(Intercept)                 10.116852 0.1776370  56.95240   0e+00
myCov                        0.787253 0.2240557   3.51365   8e-04
as.factor(respIndex)2       -3.926083 0.3043475 -12.90000   0e+00
myCov:as.factor(respIndex)2 -1.727113 0.3838773  -4.49913   0e+00
```

The adjusted association, $\hat{\rho} = -0.781$, can be found in the correlation structure panel:

```
Correlation Structure: General
 Formula: ~respIndex | sampleID
 Parameter estimate(s):
 Correlation:
   1
2 -0.781
```

To test the null hypothesis $H_0 : \rho = 0$, we fit a reduced model in which the covariance between gene expression and the bioactivity data is zero in the following way:

```
>f2 <- gls(Responses ~ myCov*as.factor(respIndex),
          weights = varIdent(form=~ 1|respIndex),
          data = data, method="ML")
```

The likelihood ratio test is used to test the null hypothesis. For the gene FGFBP1, the null hypothesis is rejected:

```
>anova(f1,f2)

   Model df       AIC      BIC    logLik   Test  L.Ratio p-value
f1     1  7  98.77017 114.5096 -42.38508
f2     2  6 129.77289 143.2639 -58.88644 1 vs 2 33.00272  <.0001
```

16.8 The IntegratedJM Shiny App

The joint model formulated in (16.1) is implemented in the `IntegratedJM` Shiny App, which is an online graphical user interface (GUI) that can be downloaded from `http://ibiostat.be/online-resources`. More details about Shiny Apps are provided in Chapter 14.

We use the EGFR data for illustration. Three different data sources, gene expression matrix, the bioactivity, and the fingerprint features are required for the analysis and can be uploaded using the screen shown in Figure 16.16.

Note that genes, bioactivity data, and fingerprint features are the rows of the three matrices while the compounds are in the columns. Hence, as seen in Figure 16.16, the three datasets have an equal number of columns (n). The model is fitted using the tab *Joint Modeling*. Note that we can choose to perform the analysis for one specific gene (for example, *PLOT 1 GENE*) or on all the genes (*JM*). It is possible to upload the bioactivity and fingerprint matrices as row vectors (i.e., the analysis is done for one bioactivity variable and one fingerprint).

Once the data is uploaded and the *JM* tab is selected, we need to choose

- the bioactivity variable and one fingerprint feature in the left panel of Figure 16.17,
- the overall significance level for inference (for example, `alpha=0.05`),
- the multiple testing correction procedure (`"fdr","holm", "hochberg", "hommel", "bonferroni", "BY","none"`).

The right panel in Figure 16.17 shows the output for the analysis. Note that the table contains a selected subset of genes is identical to Table 16.3.

Several graphical displays can be produced. For example, Figure 16.12

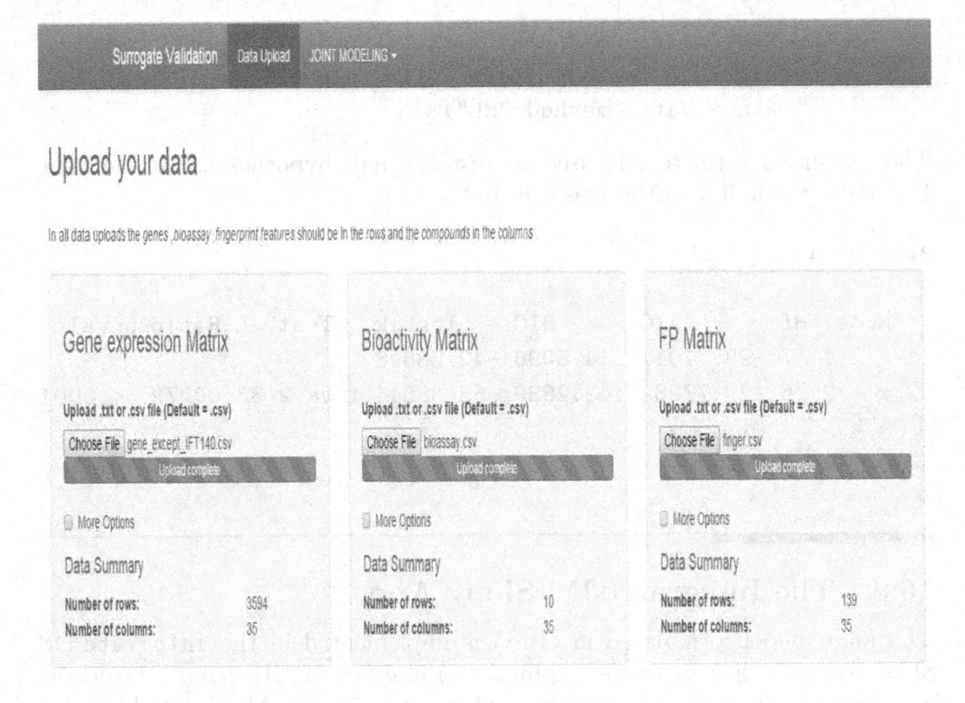

FIGURE 16.16
The IntegratedJM Shiny App: loading the three data sources.

and classification of genes (presented in Table 16.2) can be produced using the specification presented in Figure 16.18.

Once a gene of interest is identified, the tab PLOT 1 GENE allows us to perform the analysis on a single gene (see for example Figure 16.19, which is identical to Figure 16.15).

16.9 Concluding Remarks

The joint modeling framework facilitates an integration of multi-source data in the early drug development phase, particularly the associations between chemical structures, biological activity, and gene expressions, in order to identify potential leads in the early phase of drug discovery alongside the development of genomic biomarkers for efficacy of compounds. Selecting and evaluating biomarkers in early drug discovery can substantially shorten development time or the time to reach a critical decision point, such as candidate selection, in drug development.

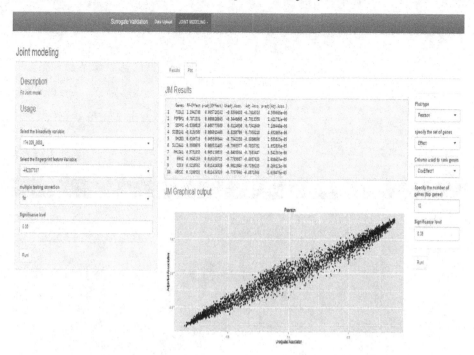

FIGURE 16.17

The IntegratedJM Shiny App. Left Panel: Specification of the variables for the analysis. Right Panel: Top K genes and adjusted/unadjusted association.

The joint modeling approach, although implemented using only one feature at a time for every data source, facilitates the extraction of valuable insights into the associations between chemical structures and mechanism of actions. Although we focused in this chapter on one fingerprint feature and on-target assay per project, this method can easily be run in loops. In a pharmaceutical pipeline implementation, this model can be applied to all or a defined set of interesting chemical substructures, genes, and biological assays (efficacy or toxicity related). The large amount of output can then be collated and filtered for vital information that can help the research team, especially, the medicinal chemist and biologist in taking the next step.

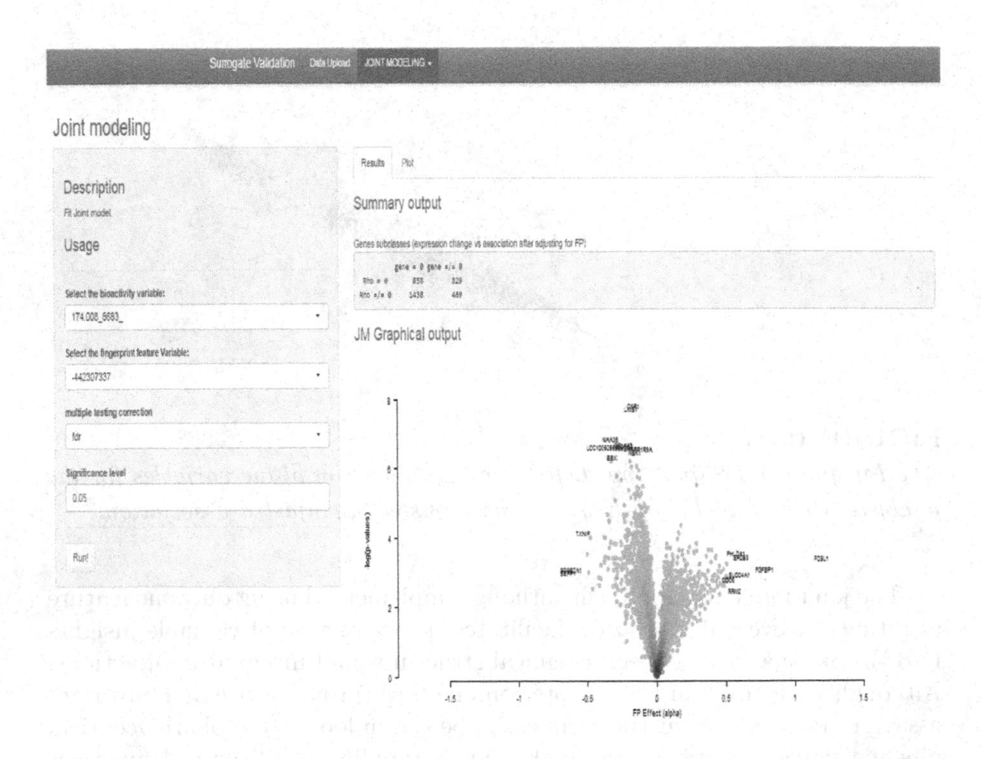

FIGURE 16.18
The Integrated Shiny App: Classification of genes and volcano plot.

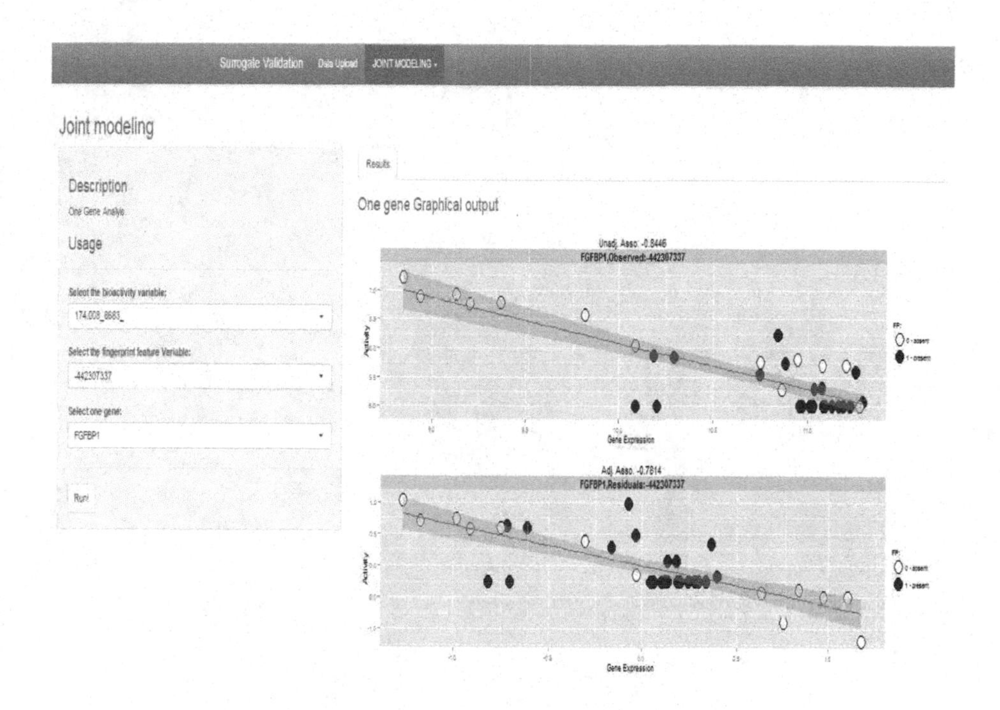

FIGURE 16.19
The IntegratedJM Shiny App: Gene-specific analysis.

17

Evaluation of Magnetic Resonance Imaging as a Biomarker in Alzheimer's Disease

Leacky Muchene, Ziv Shkedy

Hasselt University, Belgium

Luc Bijnens, Nikolay Manyakov, Tom Van De Casteele, Tom Jacobs

Janssen Pharmaceutica, Belgium

Marleen Verhoye, Jelle Praet, Annemie Van der Linden

University of Antwerp, Belgium

Astrid Bottelbergs, Mark Schmidt

Janssen Pharmaceutica, Belgium

Darrel Pemberton

Janssen Pharmaceutica, Belgium

CONTENTS

17.1 Introduction

17.1.1 Alzheimer's Disease

Alzheimer's disease (AD), the most common cause of dementia, is an irreversible age-related condition resulting in an increase in dependency on care providers for basic functioning. Clinical symptoms of sporadic AD manifest mostly in the elderly population (at least 65 years) and include progressive deterioration of specific cognitive functions such as memory, speech, motor skills and perception (McKhann et al., 1984). A proper diagnosis of AD suffers from the lack of diagnostic tools that can accurately distinguish AD from other causes of cognitive impairment especially at an early stage of the disease (Blennow, 2004; Chetelat and Baron, 2003; Galvin and Sadowsky, 2012). Moreover, AD results in multiple pathological changes in the brain, which do not manifest the same way in all patients. The most common AD-related pathological changes in the brain include amyloid-beta protein plague deposition (Masters et al., 1985; Hardy and Selkoe, 2002), neurofibrillary tangle (hyperphosphorylated tau) formation, and neuro-degeneration (Hol et al., 2003; Serrano-Pozo et al., 2011). How these changes influence the progression of AD is unfortunately not clearly understood since the onset of clinical symptoms of AD occurs much later than the onset of the pathological changes associated with the disease (Agronin, M.E., 2007). Considering the fact that there is no known cure for AD, an early diagnosis of the disease would therefore be preferable in order to allow for the introduction of treatments that may delay the progression of the disease such as a lifestyle intervention or novel therapeutic management of the patients.

From a practical point of view, although the pathological markers of AD are indicative of the disease progression, they can only be measured cross-sectionally (once per patient). This is due to the fact that pathological histology staining involves post-mortem examination, whose acquisition comes too late from a diagnostic point of view (Perl, 2010). Thus, potential biomakers which can be easily acquired in clinical follow-up of patients would be of interest in early diagnosis of the disease (Hampel et al., 2009). One of the challenges in current AD research is the availability of a suitable animal model, fully representative for the disease pathology. On the other hand, the advantage of using an animal model exhibiting only one pathological indication of AD is that it enables us to study the influence of one aspect of the disease, without the interaction of other pathological indications. The existing animal models mainly target one or a few aspects of the disease (Duff and Suleman, 2004). An animal model with over-expressed Amyloid Precursor Protein (APP) gene and Presenilin (PS) results in variants of mouse models such as the APP/PS1 mouse model that was used in this experiment (Götz and Götz, 2009).

17.1.2 Magnetic Resonance Imaging and Histology Parameters

Non-invasive neuro-imaging-based technologies such as Positron Emission Tomography (PET) scan and Magnetic Resonance Imaging (MRI), if adequately validated, hold the most promise for adoption in both diagnosis and clinical follow-up of disease progression in AD (Dickerson and Sperling, 2005). Using neuro-imaging, differences in brain anatomy, chemistry, and physiology can be detected via the measured MRI parameters. Additionally, longitudinal MRI studies enable the assessment of neuro-anatomical changes as the animal ages. MRI technology is highly advanced with different scanning technologies resulting in different measures. Diffusion Tensor Imaging (DTI) has been shown to characterize AD progression in white matter (Alexander et al., 2007; Klohs et al., 2013), and DTI quantifies the diffusivity of water molecules in the brain microstructure, which is hypothesized to follow a Gaussian distribution. Diffusion Kurtosis Imaging (DKI) aims at simultaneously quantifying both the Gaussian (diffusion tensor) and non-Gaussian (diffusion kurtosis) behavior of water. Several studies have reported the superiority of DKI over DTI in detecting AD pathology in both white and gray matter (Hui et al., 2008; Cheung et al., 2009; Veraart et al., 2011).

The degree of neuronal myelination was determined by immunohistochemical visualization of myelin basic protein (MBP), the major protein component of myelin sheaths. In addition, Glial Fibrillary Acidic Protein (GFAP) and Ionizing Calcium-Binding Adaptor molecule 1 (IBA-1) were used as markers for astrocytes and microglia, respectively. Finally, 4G8 labeling was performed to detect amyloid-beta in the brains of APP/PS1 transgenic mice.

In this chapter, we apply the methodology presented in Chapter 4 to evaluate the potential of MRI parameters as biomarkers for histology features in different regions of the brain. Although, the experimental setting we discuss in this chapter is not the same as the clinical trial setting discussed in previous

TABLE 17.1
Summary of the data: Number of animals per age and genotype.

Age	2	4	6	8	10
Transgenic	10	10	9	9	3
Wildtype	2	2	2	2	2

chapters, we propose to use the surrogacy framework for the evaluation of MRI parameters as biomarkers for specific histology features, using a similar approach within the normal-normal surrogacy setting. After a description of the case study in Section 17.2, we present an elaborate discussion of the similarity to the surrogacy setting in Section 17.3. A two-stage modeling approach is presented in Section 17.4. Sections 17.5 and 17.6 are devoted to the application of the proposed methodology in the case study, while software issues are discussed in Sections 17.7 and 17.8.

17.2 The AD Mouse Model for MRI and Histology Data

Data from an APP/PS1 transgenic mouse model experiment is used to evaluate if MRI parameters can be used as biomarkers for histology. Up to five cohorts of mice aged 2, 4, 6, 8, and 10 months were scanned (sample sizes are given in Table 17.1). The experiment comprised two mouse genotypes: (1) transgenic APP/PS1 mice, which over-expressed the KM670/671NL APP mutation and the L166P PS1 mutation and (2) wildtype mice, which represents a healthy control group.

Diffusion weighted data were acquired on a 7T Bruker Pharmascan system: 28 slices with resolution $(0.2136 \times 0.214 \times 0.2)\,\text{mm}^3$; 3 x (20 diffusion gradient directions), $\delta = 5\,\text{ms}$, $\Delta = 12\,\text{ms}$, 7 b-values $(400 - 800 - 1200 - 1600 - 2000 - 2400 - 2800)\,\text{s/mm}^2$. Seven diffusion parameter maps were estimated (Veraart et al., 2013), including Axial Kurtosis (MRI-AK), Radial Kurtosis (MRI-RK), Mean Kurtosis (MRI-MK), Axial Diffusivity (MRI-AD), Radial Diffusivity (MRI-RD), Mean Diffusivity (MRI-MD), and Fractional Anisotropy (MRI-FA). In addition, four pathological histology stains were applied: GFAP and IBA-1 staining for neuroinflammation, MBP staining for myelination, and 4G8 staining for amyloid-beta. For all four histology stains, the histology feature used in the analyses presented in this chapter was percentage of area stained.

In total, data was available from 23 brain Regions of Interest (ROI) covering both the white and gray matter. For each region, the averages of each of the seven MRI parameters and four histology stains (each quantified by

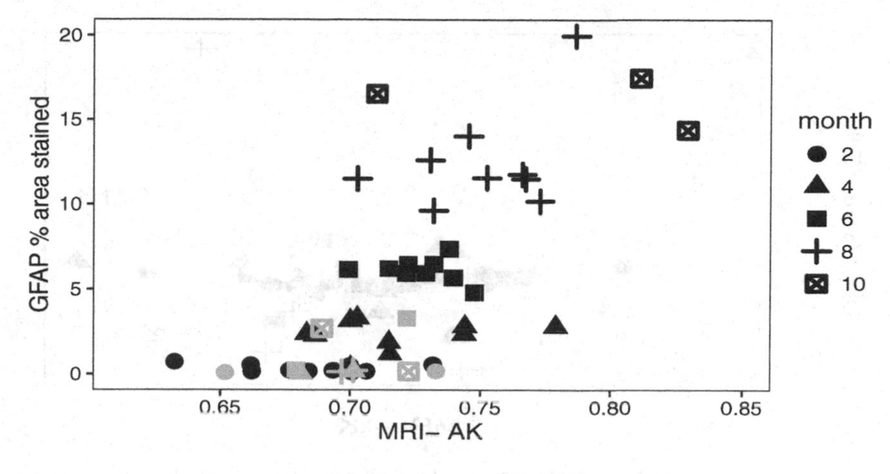

(a) *Histology versus MRI.*

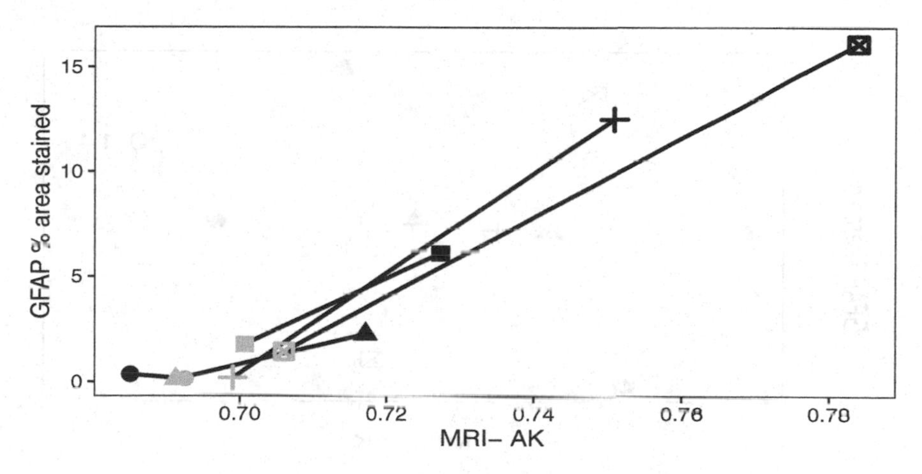

(b) *Age-dependent AD progression effect.*

FIGURE 17.1

The motor cortex region. Panel a: the observed data. Panel b: the means per age group. The solid line connects the means of the transgenic group with the means of age-matched wildtype group. Gray symbols: wildtype mice. Black symbols: transgenic mice.

the percentage of area stained) are available for each animal. Figures 17.1 and 17.2 show examples of an MRI parameter (MRI-AK) versus GFAP percentage of area stained measured in the motor cortex region.

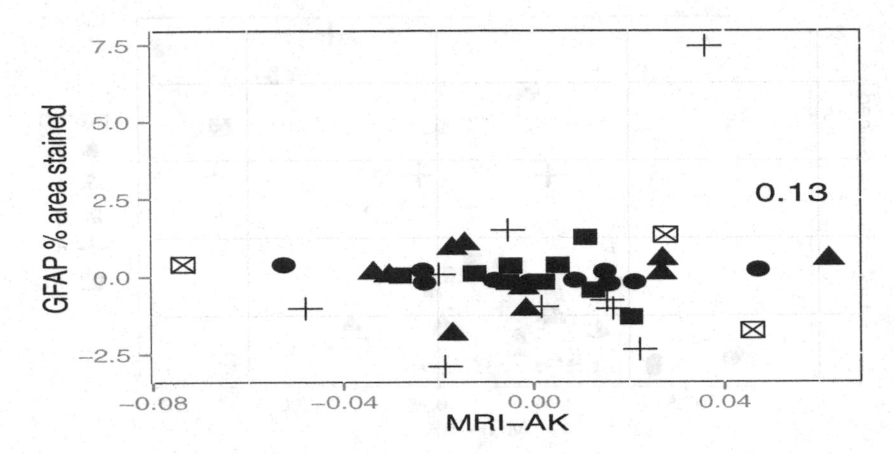

(a) Transgenic: Residuals after subtracting the age-matched means.

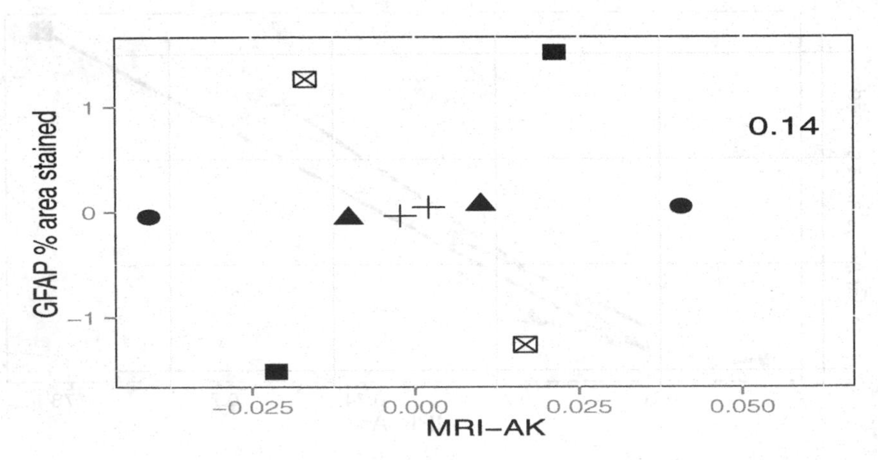

(b) Wildtype: Residuals after subtracting the age-matched means.

FIGURE 17.2
The motor cortex region. Panels a and b: the residuals after the group means for each age group were subtracted.

17.3 Two Levels of Surrogacy

Panels a and b in Figure 17.3 show an illustrative example in which a histology feature is plotted against a specific MRI parameter at 2 and 8 months, respectively. The effect of the disease progression is translated to a shift in

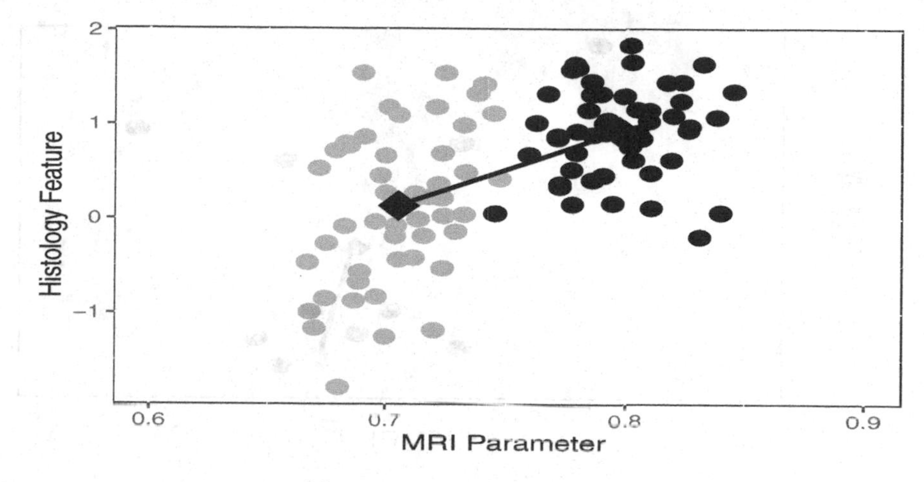

(a) *Simulated data at 2 months.*

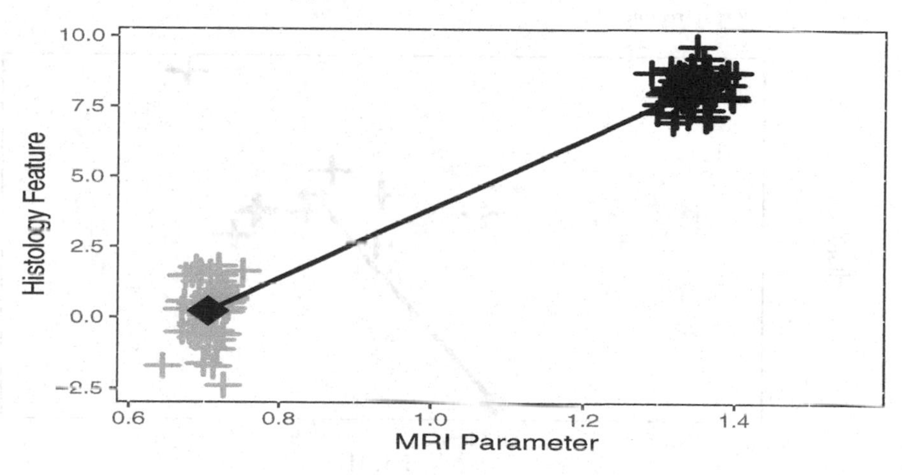

(b) *Simulated data at 8 months.*

FIGURE 17.3

Illustrative example: The effect of AD progression on an MRI parameter and a specific histology feature at two time points for simulated data. The solid line connects the means of the two genotypes. Gray symbols: wildtype mice. Black symbols: transgenic mice.

both the MRI parameter and histology feature in the transgenic group. Panels a and b of Figure 17.4 show the data at 2 and 8 months respectively, which will be analyzed in this chapter. Note that the slope of the lines connecting the means of the two clouds in panel b of Figures 17.3 and 17.4 corresponds to the relative effect (RE), discussed in Chapter 3.

Figures 17.5 and 17.6 illustrate two aspects of the association between an

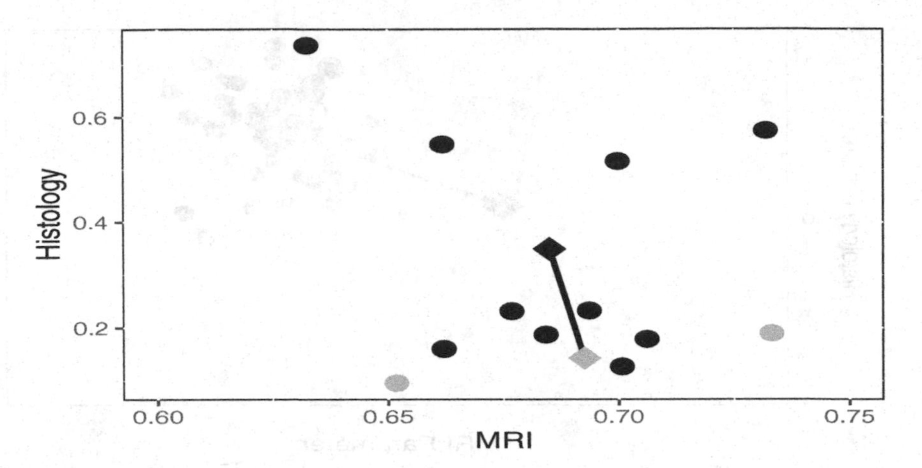

(a) *MRI-AK parameter versus GFAP percentage of area stained. Observed data at 2 months in the motor cortex region.*

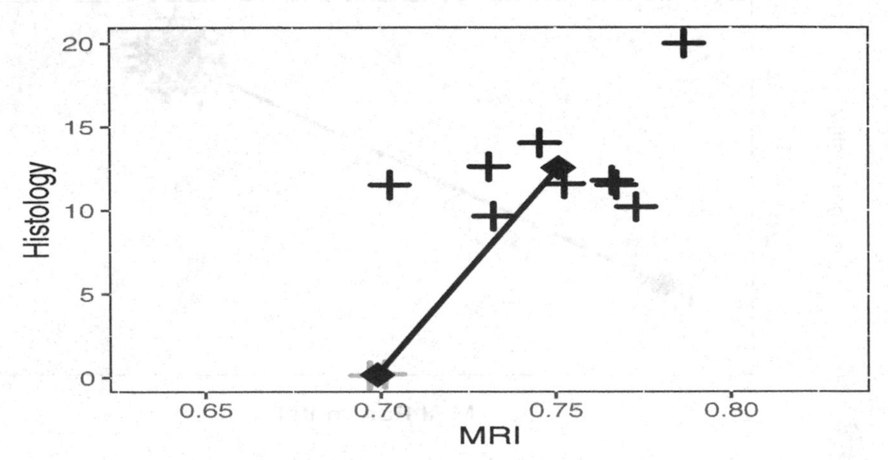

(b) *MRI-AK parameter versus GFAP percentage of area stained. Observed data at 8 months in the motor cortex region.*

FIGURE 17.4
Illustrative example: The effect of AD progression on an MRI parameter and a specific histology feature at two time points for real data. The solid line connects means of the two genotypes. Gray symbols: wildtype mice. Black symbols: transgenic mice.

MRI parameter and a given histology feature: the effect of AD progression (characterized by continual amyloid-beta deposition) and the correlation between the two variables. Panels a and b show the data and the residuals after subtracting the means, respectively. From Figure 17.5, the AD progression effect can be seen clearly in panel a, while panel b indicates that, conditional on AD progression effect, the two variables are not correlated. Using surrogacy terminology, Figure 17.5b indicates that, on an individual level, MRI is a poor biomarker for histology. A second illustrative example is shown in Figures 17.6a and b. For this example, the AD progression effect (shown in Figure 17.6a) has the same magnitude of the effects as in the first example. Note that the relative effects in the two examples are similar. Figure 17.6b reveals a substantial difference between the two examples on an individual level. For the second example, after adjusting for the AD progression effects, MRI and histology are correlated (Figure 17.6b). Hence, at an individual level, MRI is a good biomarker for histology. Note that we can use the adjusted association, discussed in Chapter 3, to evaluate MRI as a biomarker for histology at an individual level.

In the next example, presented in Figures 17.7 and 17.8, we "translate" the two aspects of the association between MRI and histology into two surrogacy measures: individual-level surrogacy and disease-level surrogacy. The latter corresponds to the trial-level surrogacy, discussed in Chapter 4. The examples presented in Figures 17.5 and 17.6 correspond to a single-trial setting and allow us to evaluate the quality of MRI as a biomarker for histology only at the individual level. On the other hand, the animal model for AD allows us to estimate surrogacy measures in both levels since MRI parameters and histology features are measured at 5 time points. Figure 17.7 shows a scenario in which an MRI parameter and a histology feature are not correlated, given the progression effect of AD but the disease effects (on both MRI and histology), shown in panel (c), are correlated. This suggests a scenario for which the disease-level surrogacy is high while individual-level surrogacy is low. In other words, the effect of AD progression on histology features can be predicted using the AD progression effects observed on MRI parameters, while at individual level, MRI values are not predictive for histology features. A scenario in which MRI parameters and histology features are associated at both disease and individual levels is shown in Figure 17.8.

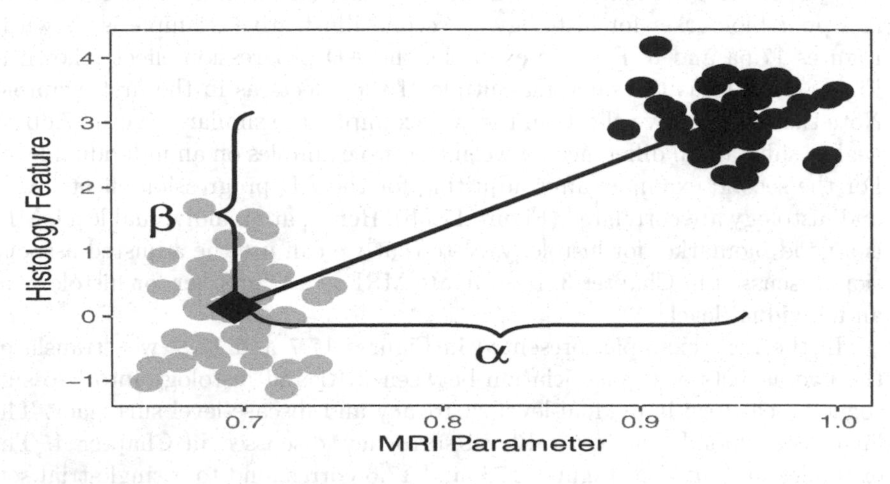

(a) *Histology versus MRI.*

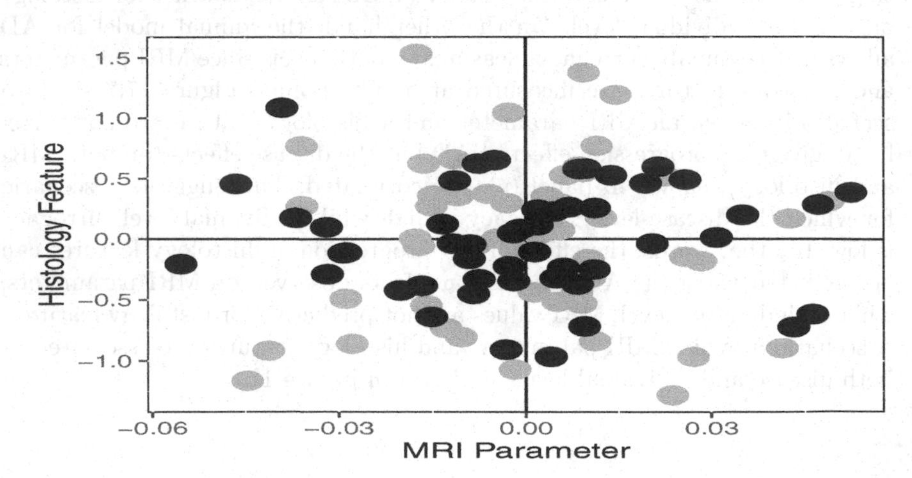

(b) *Residuals after subtracting the group means.*

FIGURE 17.5

Illustrative examples demonstrating the effect of AD progression on an MRI parameter and a histology feature at two time points, without correlation between MRI and histology parameters. Larger symbols denote the group means. Gray symbols: wildtype mice. Black symbols: transgenic mice.

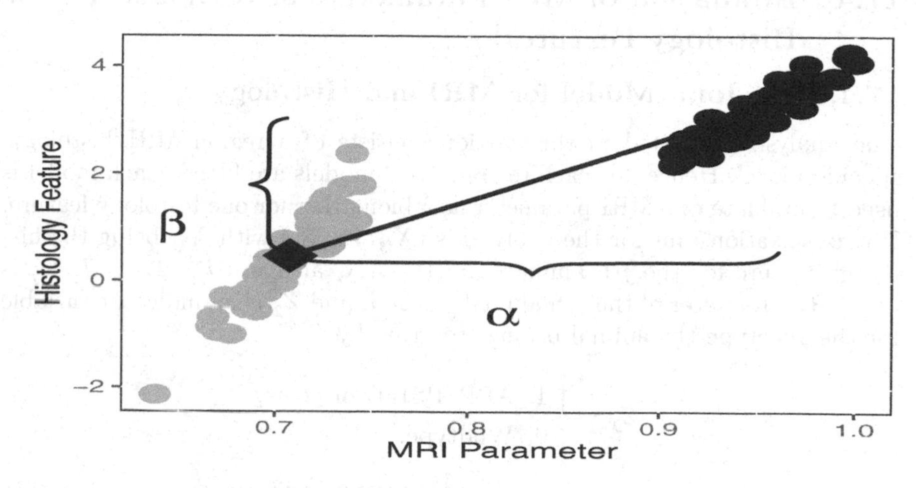

(a) *Histology versus MRI.*

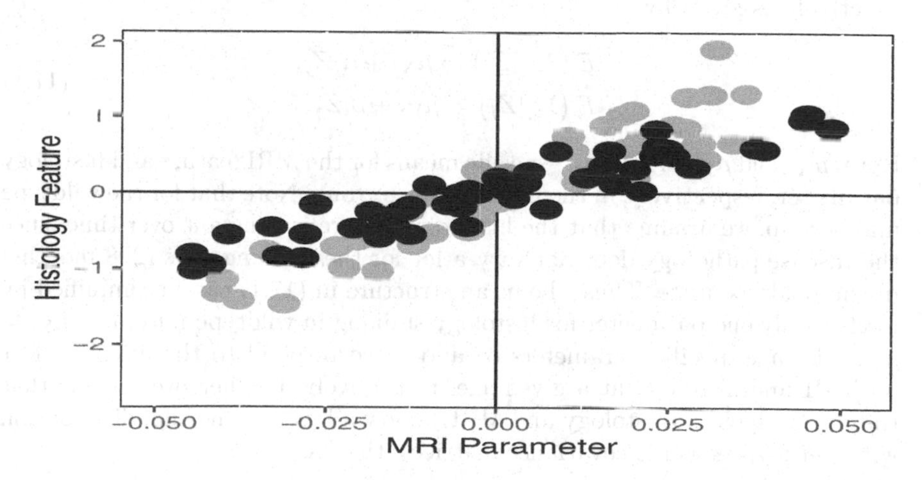

(b) *Residuals after subtracting the group means.*

FIGURE 17.6

Illustrative examples demonstrating the effect of AD progression on an MRI parameter and a histology feature at two time points, with correlation between MRI and histology parameters. Larger symbols denote the group means. Gray symbols: wildtype mice. Black symbols: transgenic mice.

17.4 Evaluation of MRI Parameters as a Biomarker for Histology Features

17.4.1 A Joint Model for MRI and Histology

The analysis presented in this section consists of a region/MRI/histology-specific model. Hence, for each region, 4×7 models are fitted. Each model is used to evaluate one MRI parameter as a biomarker for one histology feature. The observation unit for the analysis is (X_{ij}, Y_{ij}, Z_i) with X_{ij} being the histology feature for the jth animal, $j = 1, \ldots, N_i$ at age i, $i = 1, \ldots, I$; Y_{ij} is the MRI parameter of the jth animal at age i; and Z_j is an indicator variable for the genotype the animal belongs to given by

$$Z_j = \begin{cases} 1, & \text{APP/PS1 Transgenic,} \\ 0, & \text{Wildtype.} \end{cases}$$

We assume that the mean structure for MRI and histology parameters, respectively, is given by

$$\begin{aligned} E\left(X_{ij}|Z_j\right) &= \mu_{Xi} + \alpha_i Z_j, \\ E\left(Y_{ij}|Z_j\right) &= \mu_{Yi} + \beta_i Z_j. \end{aligned} \tag{17.1}$$

Here, μ_{Xi} and μ_{Yi} are the age-specific means for the MRI feature and histology parameter, respectively, in the wildtype mice group. Note that for the wildtype mice group, we assume that the histology feature is constant over time since the disease pathology does not vary a lot for these young ages (2–8 months) in the wildtype mice. Thus, the mean structure in (17.1) can be simplified by having only one parameter for histology staining in wildtype mice, i.e., $\mu_{Yi} = \mu_Y$. The age-specific parameters α_i and β_i correspond to the disease effect on MRI and histology at a given age, respectively. Further, we assume that the two endpoints (histology and MRI) follow a bivariate normal distribution with genotype-specific covariance matrices, that is,

$$\begin{pmatrix} X_{ij} \\ Y_{ij} \end{pmatrix} \sim N\left(\begin{bmatrix} \mu_{Xi} + \alpha_i Z_j \\ \mu_{Yi} + \beta_i Z_j \end{bmatrix}, \Sigma\right). \tag{17.2}$$

Here, Σ is a 2×2 genotype-specific covariance matrix given for transgenic and wildtype mice, respectively, by

$$\Sigma_{\mathrm{T}} = \begin{pmatrix} \sigma^2_{\mathrm{A_m}} & \sigma_{\mathrm{A_{hm}}} \\ \sigma_{\mathrm{A}_{hm}} & \sigma^2_{\mathrm{A}_h} \end{pmatrix} \text{ and } \Sigma_{\mathrm{W}} = \begin{pmatrix} \sigma^2_{\mathrm{W}_m} & \sigma_{\mathrm{W_{hm}}} \\ \sigma_{\mathrm{W_{hm}}} & \sigma^2_{\mathrm{W_h}} \end{pmatrix}. \tag{17.3}$$

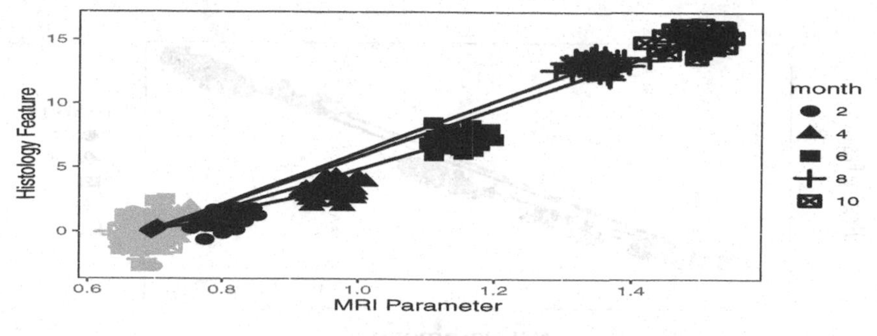

(a) *Histology versus MRI.*

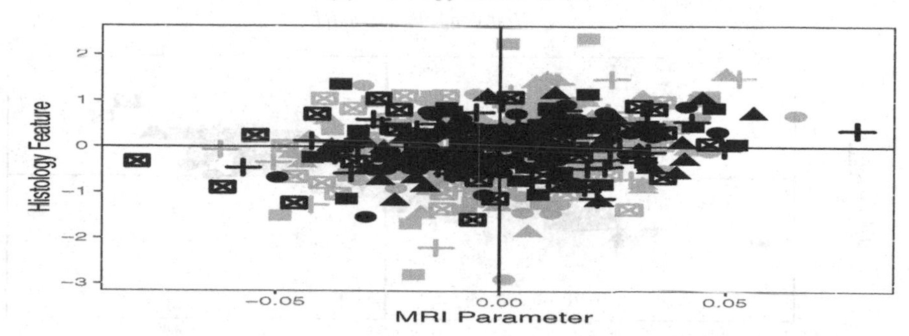

(b) *Residuals after subtracting the means.*

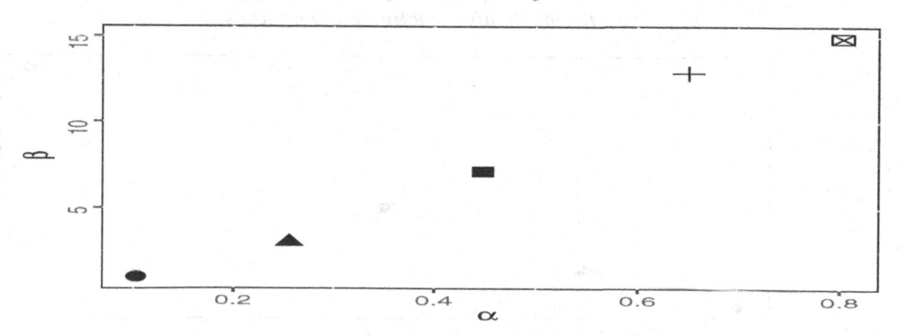

(c) *Age-dependent AD progression effect.*

FIGURE 17.7
Illustration of simulated individual- and disease-level surrogacy using the AD animal model for a scenario with low individual-level surrogacy. The solid lines in panel a connect the means of the transgenic and wildtype groups at each age. The slope of these lines is equal to the RE (at each age). Panel b shows the association between a histology feature and the MRI parameter. Panel c presents the disease effects β on a histology feature versus the disease effects α on an MRI parameter. Gray symbols: wildtype mice. Black symbols: transgenic mice.

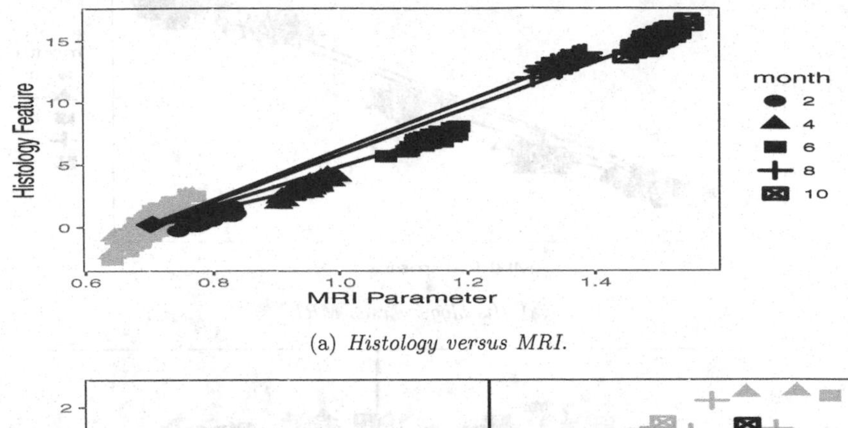

(a) *Histology versus MRI.*

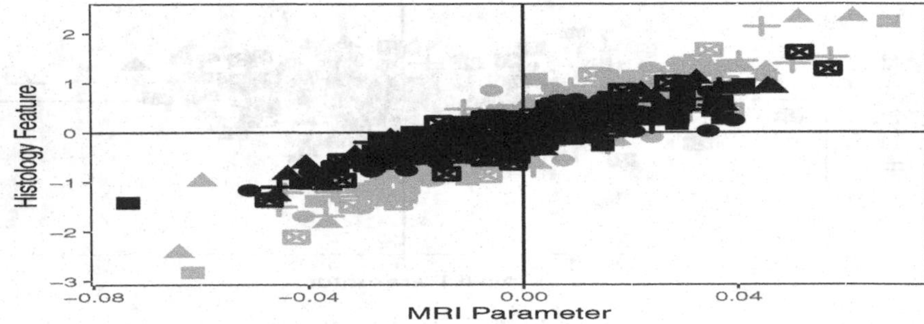

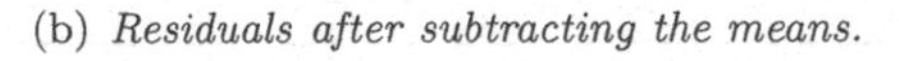

(b) *Residuals after subtracting the means.*

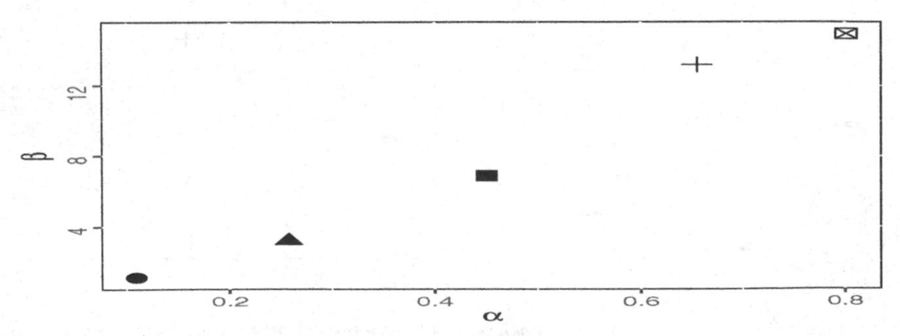

(c) *Age dependent AD progression effect.*

FIGURE 17.8
Illustration of simulated individual and disease-level surrogacy using the AD animal model for a scenario with high individual-level surrogacy. The solid lines in panel a connect the means of the transgenic and wildtype groups at each age. The slope of these lines is equal to the RE (at each age). Panel c presents the disease effects β on a histology feature versus the disease effects α on an MRI parameter. Gray symbols: wildtype. Black symbols: transgenic.

The joint model specified in (17.1) allows us to model two sources (or aspects) of the association between a specific histology feature and an MRI parameter: (1) the association between the disease evolution effects (with respect to age) of the two endpoints and (2) the association between the two endpoints adjusted for the time evolution of the disease. In what follows, we show that the two sources of association can be interpreted as individual- and disease-level surrogacy. The latter is similar to the trial-level surrogacy discussed in Chapter 4.

17.4.2 Genotype-Specific Individual-Level Surrogacy

Based on the covariance matrices specified in (17.3), we can derive the adjusted correlation between an MRI parameter and a specific histology feature for each genotype given by

$$\rho_{\mathrm{T}} = \frac{\sigma_{A_{hm}}}{\sqrt{\sigma^2_{A_h} \times \sigma^2_{A_m}}}, \text{ and } \rho_{\mathrm{W}} = \frac{\sigma_{W_{hm}}}{\sqrt{\sigma^2_{W_h} \times \sigma^2_{W_m}}}. \tag{17.4}$$

The genotype-specific adjusted correlations ρ_W and ρ_T measure the association between the two endpoints adjusted for the time evolution of the disease and can be interpreted in the same way as the adjusted association in the surrogacy model presented in Chapter 3. A large absolute values of the adjusted correlation implies a better surrogacy at an individual level. Note that, in contrast with the models discussed in Chapter 4, we do not assume that the association between MRI and histology is equal in the two groups.

17.4.3 Disease-Level Surrogacy

The joint model specified in (17.1) allows us to estimate the age and genotype-specific parameters $(\alpha_1, \alpha_2, \alpha_3, \alpha_4, \alpha_5)$ and $(\beta_1, \beta_2, \beta_3, \beta_4, \beta_5)$. Our aim is to establish a relationship between α_i and β_i, and in particular, to assess whether AD evolution observed for the MRI parameter is predictive for the AD evolution observed for a particular histology feature. In other words, we wish to evaluate whether an MRI parameter can be used as a biomarker for a given histology feature in an AD mouse model at a disease level. Disease-level surrogacy can be measured using R^2 obtained from the regression model in a similar way as done in Chapter 4 for trial-level surrogacy. From (17.5), η and γ are regression coefficients, while ε_i denotes the measurement error for the regression model:

$$\widehat{\beta}_i = \eta + \gamma\widehat{\alpha}_i + \varepsilon_i, \quad i = 1, \ldots, I. \tag{17.5}$$

TABLE 17.2
The motor cortex region: Parameter estimate (standard error) of AD progression effects. β: the disease effect on GFAP percentage of area stained. α: the disease effects on MRI-AK.

Age	$\widehat{\beta}$ (s.e.)	$\widehat{\alpha}$ (s.e.)
2	−0.35 (0.51)	−0.01 (0.02)
4	1.58 (0.51)	0.03 (0.02)
6	5.43 (0.53)	0.03 (0.02)
8	11.83 (0.53)	0.05 (0.02)
10	15.43 (0.92)	0.08 (0.03)

17.5 the MRI Project Data: Examples of Region-Specific Models

The joint model specified in (17.1) was applied for each combination of the seven MRI parameters and the four histology stains in each of the 23 ROIs (shown in Figure 17.15). In this section, we discuss the results in the motor cortex (Section 17.5.1) and the caudate-putamen (Section 17.5.2) regions. Note that, as explained in Section 17.4, the joint model (17.1) is formulated with a constant effect of histology in the wildtype mice ($\mu_{Yi} = \mu_Y$).

17.5.1 The Motor Cortex: GFAP Staining and MRI-AK

The observed data for GFAP percentage of area stained and MRI-AK are shown in Figure 17.9a where an age-dependent shift of MRI and histology measurements for older transgenic mice is observed. Parameter estimates obtained for the joint model are presented in Table 17.2. The estimated regression model, shown in Figure 17.9b is given by $\widehat{\beta}_i = 0.064 + 192.675\widehat{\alpha}_i$. The surrogacy measure at disease level $\widehat{R}^2_D = 0.91$ indicates that MRI-AK is a good predictive biomarker for GFAP staining. At an individual level, after adjusting for the disease effect, there is low correlation between the residuals ($\widehat{\rho_A} = \widehat{\rho_W} = 0.13$) indicating a low individual-level surrogacy (Figure 17.10a and b).

Figure 17.11a presents the disease-level surrogacy measures for all seven MRI parameters and four histology stains in the motor cortex region. Note that the MRI-AK parameter is found to be predictive for 4G8 staining ($R^2_D = 0.94$) and GFAP staining ($R^2_D = 0.91$), while it has relatively low predictive value for the IBA-1 ($R^2_D = 0.60$) and MBP ($R^2_D = 0.47$) staining. MRI-MD was found to be predictive at the disease-level for 4G8 ($R^2_D = 0.87$), GFAP ($R^2_D = 0.90$), and IBA-1 ($R^2_D = 0.76$) stainings, respectively. In addition,

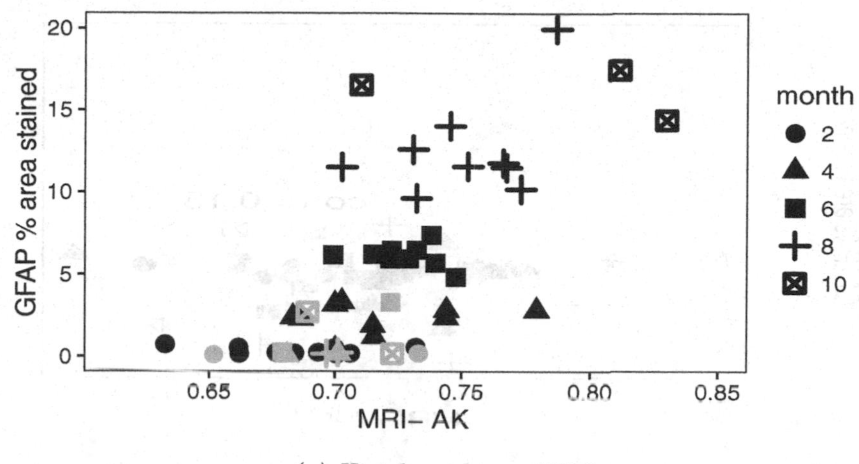

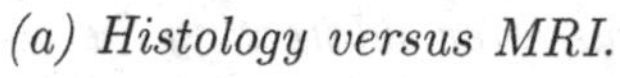
(a) Histology versus MRI.

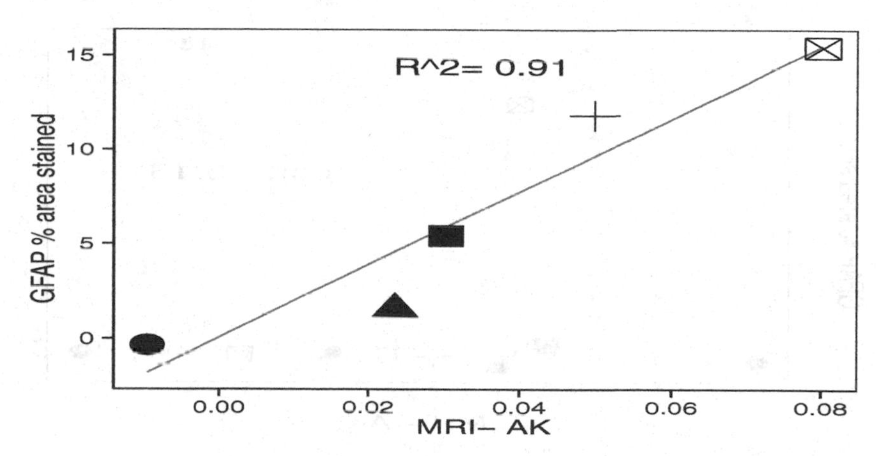

(b) Age-dependent AD progression effect.

FIGURE 17.9
The motor cortex region: Evaluation of surrogacy for MRI-AK and GFAP percentage of area stained. Gray symbols: wildtype mice. Black symbols: transgenic mice.

MRI-RD was predictive for MBP staining with $R^2_D = 0.83$. The results for individual-level surrogacy are shown in Figure 17.11, which reveals that MRI parameters were not predictive for histology at an individual-level in both transgenic (Figure 17.11b) and wildtype mice (Figure 17.11c).

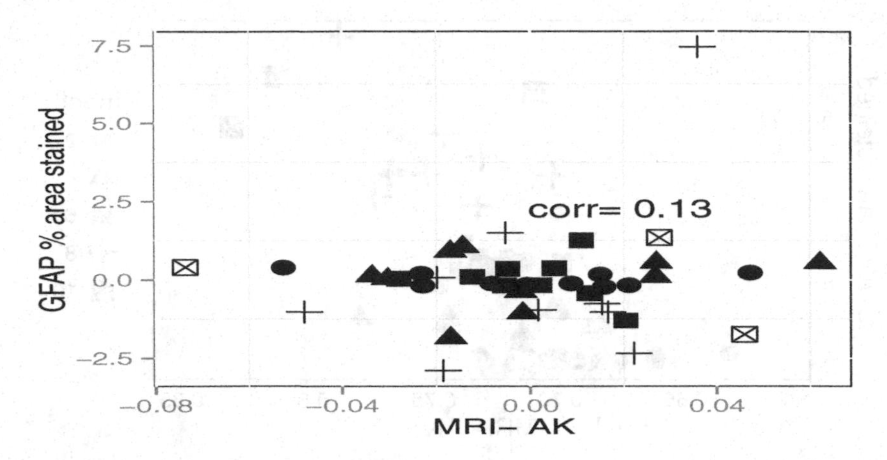

(a) Transgenic: Residuals after subtracting the age-matched group means.

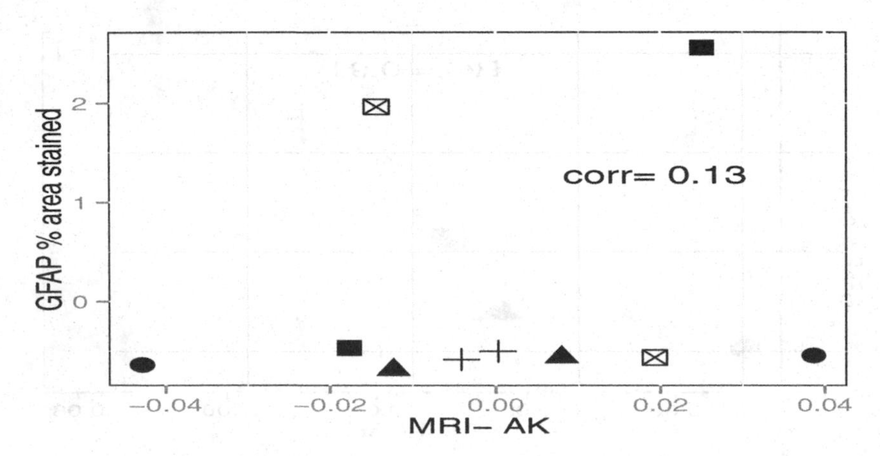

(b) Wildtype: Residuals after subtracting the age-matched group means.

FIGURE 17.10
The motor cortex region: Evaluation of surrogacy for MRI-AK and GFAP percentage of area stained. Residuals.

17.5.2 The Caudate-Putamen: GFAP Staining and MRI-AK

A similar analysis was conducted for the caudate-putamen region. The observed data for GFAP percentage of area stained and MRI-AK shown in Figure 17.12a indicates an age-dependent shift in histology values for transgenic mice and a relatively small shift in MRI-AK values. The estimated disease-level surrogacy is relatively low at $R_D^2 = 0.596$ (see Figure 17.12b). Moreover,

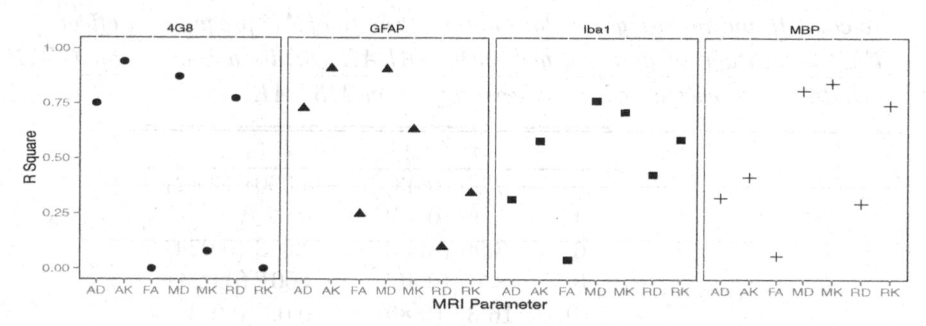

(a) Disease-level surrogacy for all MRI parameters and histology staining.

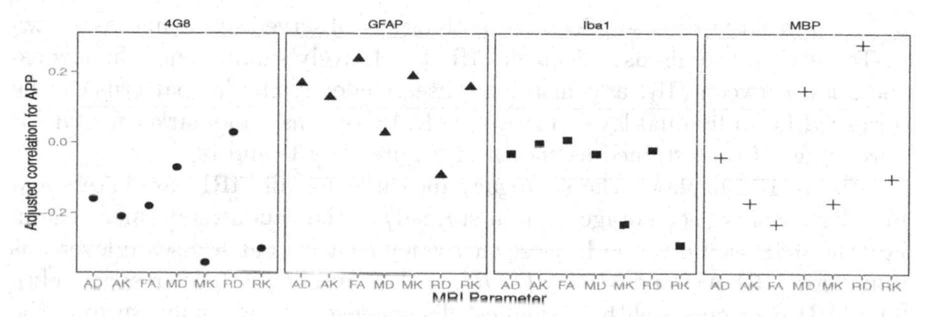

(b) Transgenic mice: Individual-level surrogacy for all MRI parameters and histology staining.

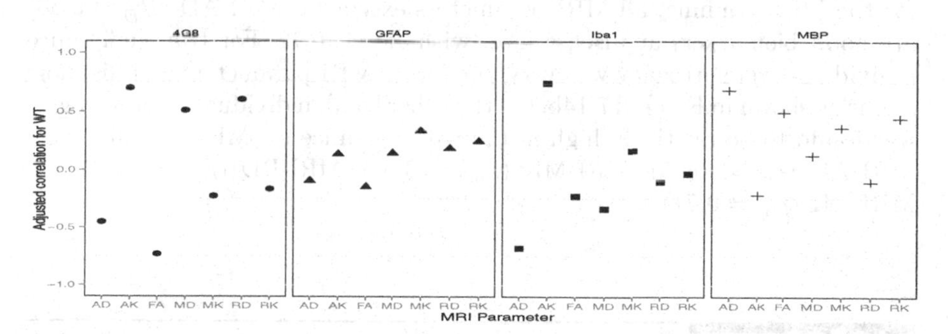

(c) Wildtype mice: Individual-level surrogacy for all MRI parameters and histology staining.

FIGURE 17.11

The motor cortex region: Individual and disease-level surrogacy for all MRI parameters and histology stains (percentage of area stained).

TABLE 17.3

The caudate-putamen region: Parameter estimate of AD progression effects for GFAP percentage of area stained with MRI-AK. β: disease effect on GFAP percentage of area stained. α: disease effect on MRI-AK.

Age	$\widehat{\beta}$ (s.e.)	$\widehat{\alpha}$ (s.e.)
2	0.35 (0.43)	−0.0001 (0.02)
4	1.05 (0.43)	0.02 (0.02)
6	3.99 (0.46)	−0.013 (0.024)
8	8.75 (0.46)	0.0001 (0.024)
10	16.37 (0.80)	0.09 (0.03)

although a large disease effect on histology is observed over time as shown in Table 17.3, the disease effect on MRI is relatively small, hence the low association between MRI and histology disease effects. Similar patterns can be observed for individual-level surrogacy of MRI-AK as a biomarker for GFAP percentage of area stained as shown in Figures 17.13a and b.

Figure 17.14a shows the surrogacy measures for all MRI parameters and histology stains (percentage of area stained) in the caudate-putamen region. For the 4G8 staining, the highest surrogacy measures at a disease level was found for MRI-AD and MRI-MD ($R^2_D = 0.62$ and $R^2_D = 0.61$, respectively). The MRI parameters with the highest disease-level surrogacy measures in the caudate-putamen region were MRI-MD, MRI-MK, and MRI-RD for the GFAP staining with $R^2_D = 0.83$, $R^2_D = 0.87$, and $R^2_D = 0.86$, respectively. Note that for the MBP staining, all MRI parameters except for MRI-AD ($R^2_D = 0.35$), are good biomarkers at disease level with $R^2_D \geq 0.72$. For transgenic mice, individual-level surrogacy was very low for all MRI parameters and histology stains as shown in Figure 17.14b. On the other hand, individual-level surrogacy was found to be relatively high in the wildtype mice for MBP staining using MRI-AK ($\widehat{\rho}_W = 0.95$), MRI-MK ($\widehat{\rho}_W = 0.94$), MRI-RD ($\widehat{\rho}_W = 0.94$), and MRI-RK ($\widehat{\rho}_W = 0.71$).

17.6 The Surrogacy Map of the Brain

The joint model allows us to evaluate the surrogacy pattern in the brain for all combinations of MRI parameters and histology stains. Figure 17.15 shows a heatmap of the disease-level surrogacy in the 23 ROI. Clearly, surrogacy is highly dependent on the region, MRI parameter and histology stain. For regions such as the amygdala and olfactory bulb, none of the MRI parameters is useful as a biomarker for any of the histology stains. GFAP percentage

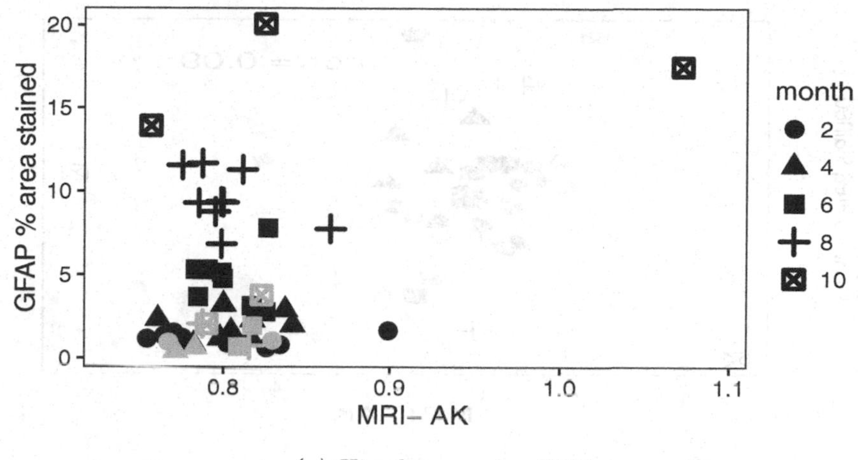

(a) Histology versus MRI.

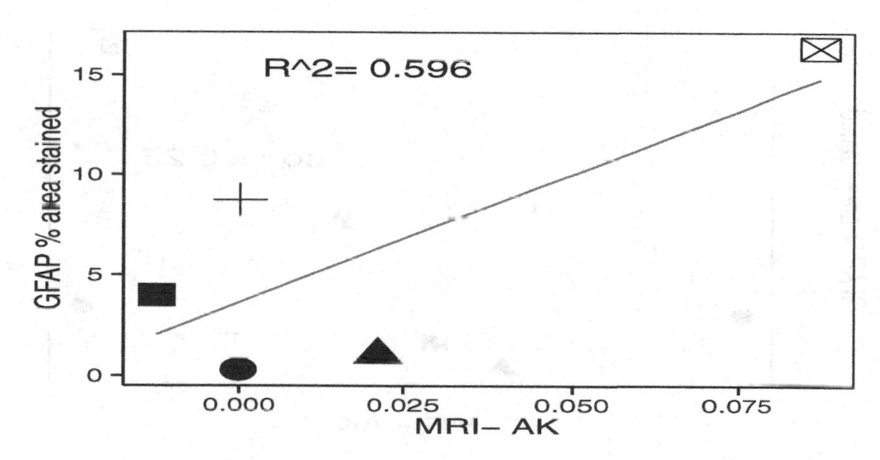

(b) Age-dependent AD progression effect.

FIGURE 17.12

The caudate-putamen region: Evaluation of surrogacy with MRI-AK and GFAP percentage of area stained. Gray symbols: wildtype mice. Black symbols: transgenic mice.

of area stained can be predicted by several MRI parameters in the caudate-putamen, cerebellum, and several cortex regions. For IBA-1 staining, good disease-level surrogacy was observed in the septal nucleus region using all MRI parameters (apart from MRI-AD and MRI-AK). The relatively high level of surrogacy of MRI parameters with 4G8 staining was observed in the cortex regions. Thus, since these four histology stains evaluate different aspects of the

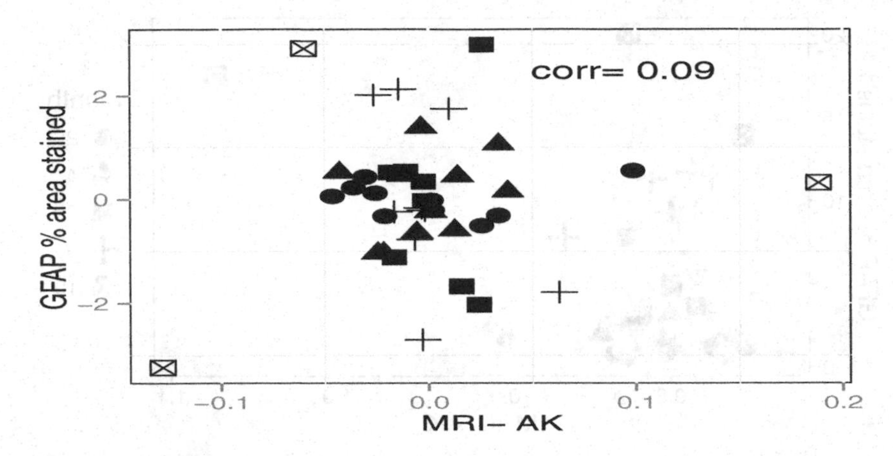

(a) Transgenic: Residuals after subtracting the mean.

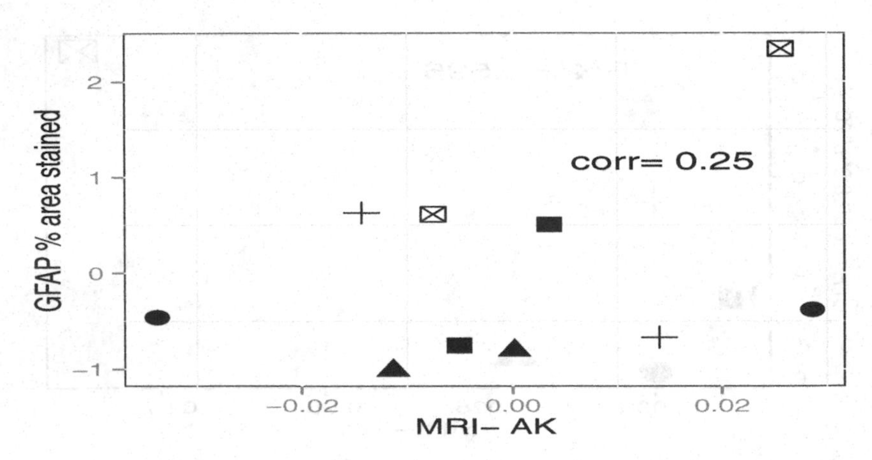

(b) Wildtype: Residuals after subtracting the mean.

FIGURE 17.13

The caudate-putamen region: Evaluation of surrogacy with MRI-AK and GFAP percentage of area stained. Residuals.

disease morphology, there is need to evaluate surrogacy at the different brain regions using MRI parameters with high surrogacy level for the particular histology stains. A surrogacy map for individual-level surrogacy in transgenic mice is presented in Figure 17.16a. Overall, a low individual-level surrogacy is observed, an indication that prediction of histology at an individual level is not practical using MRI parameters. For the wildtype mice, however, individual-

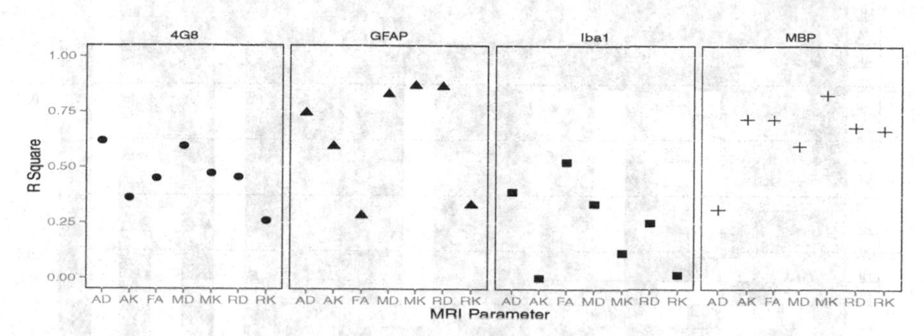

(a) Disease-level surrogacy.

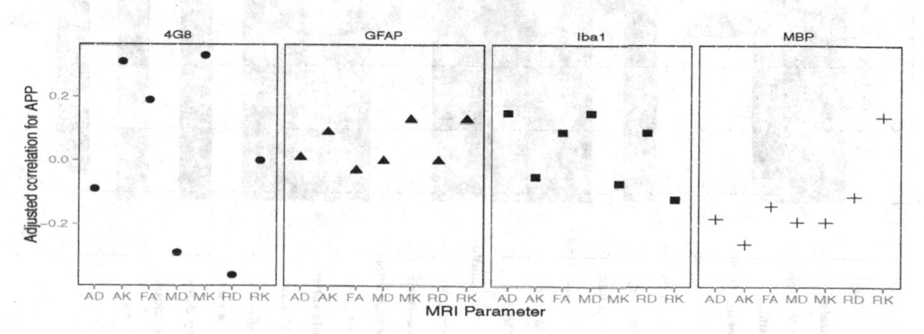

(b) Individual-level surrogacy in transgenic mice.

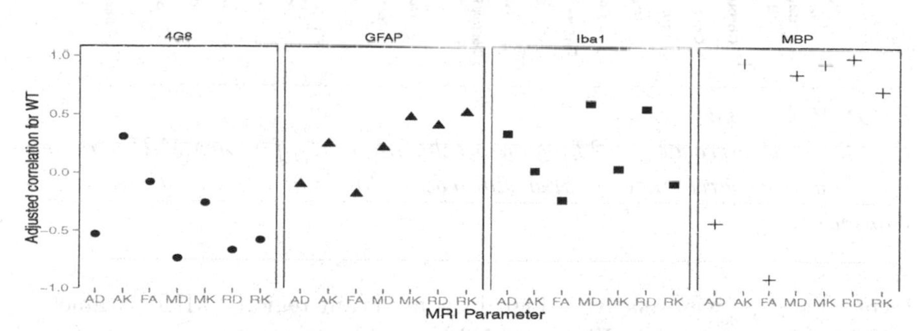

(c) Individual-level surrogacy in wildtype mice.

FIGURE 17.14
The caudate-putamen region: Individual and disease-level surrogacy map for all MRI parameters, and histology stains (percentage of area stained).

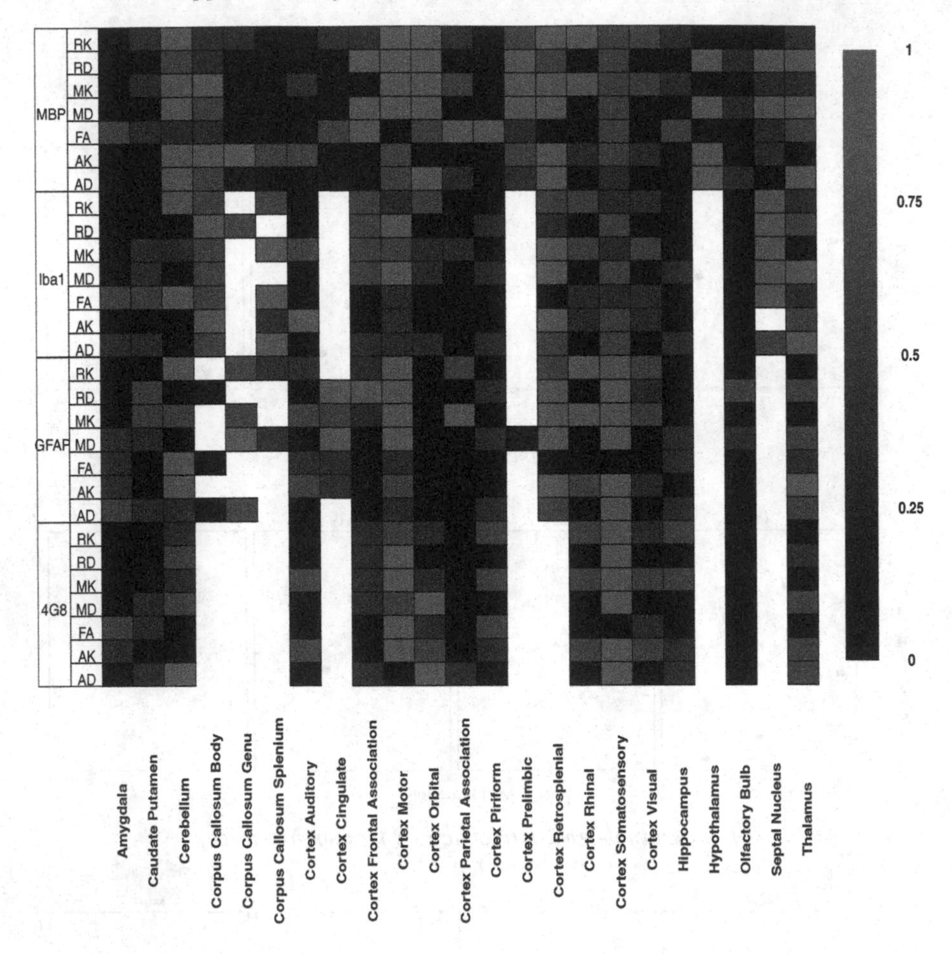

FIGURE 17.15

Disease-level surrogacy in 23 regions of the brain (R^2_D for each MRI parameter and histology percentage of area stained). White fill: surrogacy measure not computed.

level surrogacy was relatively high in some brain regions, MRI parameters, and histology stains (see Figure 17.16b).

17.7 Implementation in SAS

In this section, we discuss the implementation of the joint model discussed in Section 17.4 in SAS using data from the motor cortex with a pair of MRI-AK

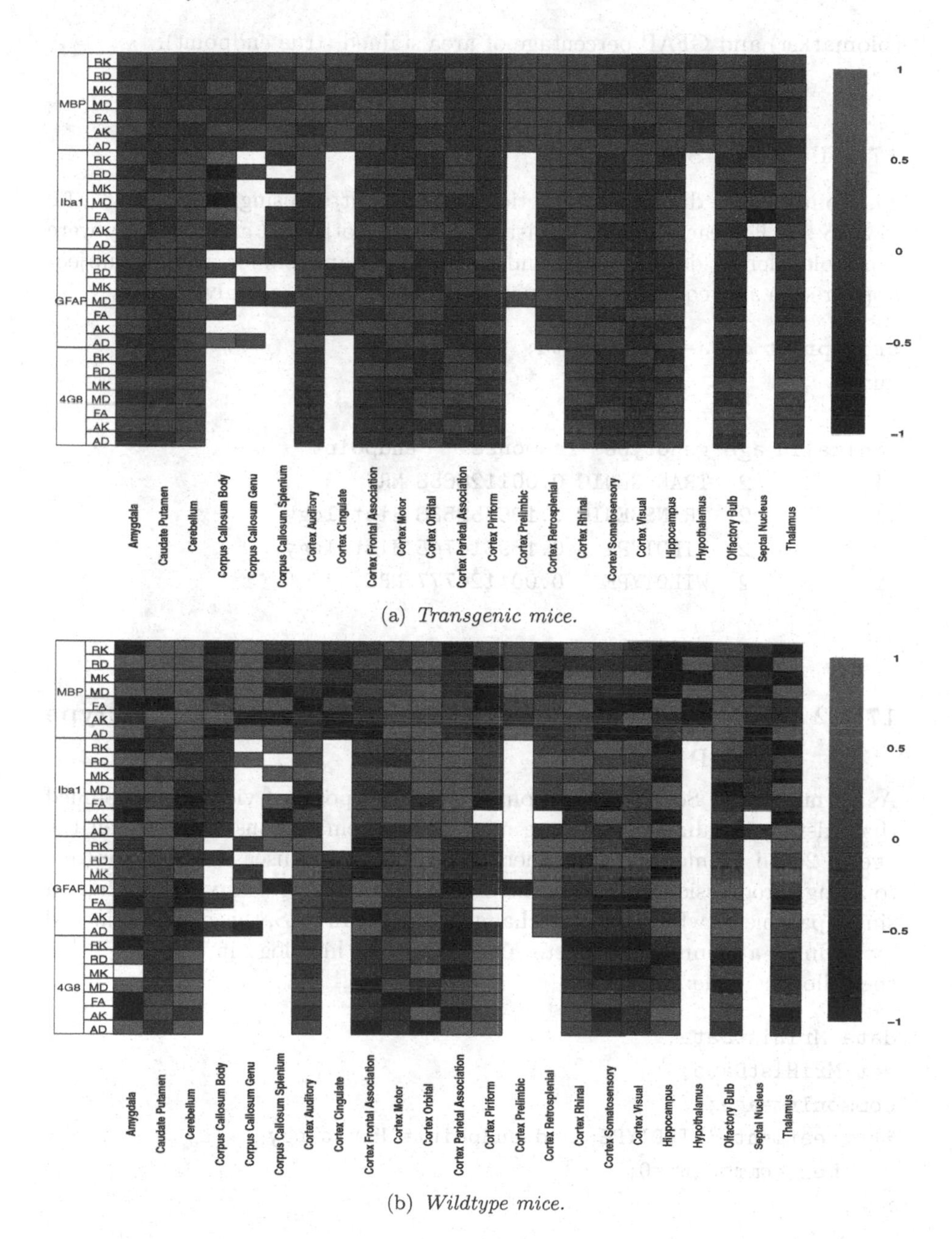

(a) *Transgenic mice.*

(b) *Wildtype mice.*

FIGURE 17.16

Individual-level surrogacy in 23 regions of the brain ($\widehat{\rho}_T$ and $\widehat{\rho}_W$, respectively, for each MRI parameter and histology percentage of area stained). White fill: surrogacy measure not computed.

(biomarker) and GFAP percentage of area stained (true endpoint).

17.7.1 Data Structure

The joint model, discussed in Section 17.4, was fitted using procedure `MIXED` in SAS 9.4. For each subject, measurements for both MRI and histology were available. Hence, data for MRI and histology parameters for a single subject appeared in subsequent rows. A partial print of the data is given below:

```
proc print data=MriHistData;
run

 animalid age genotype  response    endpoint
 1          2  TRANSGENIC 0.001128658 MRI
 1          2  TRANSGENIC 0.126652588 Histology
 2          2  WILDTYPE   0.189814745 Histology
 2          2  WILDTYPE   0.001124777 MRI
```

17.7.2 Common Parameter for Histology in the Wildtype Group

As mentioned in Section 17.4, from a biological point of view, it is assumed that histology values of wildtype mice should remain constant between the age of 2 and 10 months, since there is no significant disease pathology (due to aging) progression. Hence, in the model for histology, wildtype mice have a single parameter which does not change with age. In SAS, this can be achieved by defining a common parameter `CommonInt` for histology in wildtype using the following code:

```
data MriHistData;
set MriHistData;
commonInt=age;
if treatment='WILDTYPE' and endpoint='Histology'
   then commonInt=0;
run;
```

The association between MRI and histology is modeled using the `REPEATED` statement. The option `GROUP=genotype` allows for genotype-specific covariance matrices (17.3). The estimated disease effects on both MRI and histology are output by passing the `solution` option and stored in a dataset named fixedeffects using the SOLUTIONF option in the ODS OUTPUT command. The complete SAS code used to fit the joint model is:

```
proc mixed data=surrogate;
class genotype animalid endpoint commonint(ref='0');
model response=commonint*endpoint commonint*endpoint*genotype
    / solution noint;
repeated endpoint / sujbect=animalid*commonint
                    type=un group=genotype R=1,4 rcorr=1,4;
ods output solutionf=fixedeffects;
run;
```

Parameter estimates for the disease progression effects (in both endpoints) are shown in Figure 17.17. The individual-level surrogacy for wildtype and transgenic mice is computed using the estimated covariance matrices (Figure 17.18). To compute disease-level surrogacy, a linear regression model is fitted using PROC GLM in SAS.

```
proc glm data=fixedeffectsProcessed;
model effectstrue=effectssurrogate;
run;
```

In the above code, effectstrue corresponds to the estimated disease effects on the true endpoint $\widehat{\beta}$, while effectssurrogate corresponds to the estimated disease effects on the surrogate endpoint $\widehat{\alpha}$. The reported measure for disease-level surrogacy corresponds to R^2 obtained from the linear regression model (Figure 17.19).

17.7.3 Age-Specific Parameters for Histology in the Wildtype Model

Rather than assume a common histology parameter in wildtype mice, an age-specific parameter can be specified by substituting commonint with age. In order to obtain age and genotype-specific estimates for the disease effect on both MRI and histology, we include in the model an interaction term age*endpoint*genotype.

```
proc mixed data=MriHistData;
class genotype animalid endpoint age;
model response=age*endpoint age*endpoint*genotype
                / solution noint;
repeated endpoint / subject=animalid*age type=un
                    group=genotype R=1,4 rcorr=1,4;
ods output solutionf=fixedeffects;
```

Solution for Fixed Effects								
Effect	**treatment**	**endpoint**	**int**	**Estimate**	**Standard Error**	**DF**	**t Value**	**Pr > |t|**
int			2	0.6946	0.02220	4	31.29	<.0001
int			4	0.6935	0.02220	4	31.24	<.0001
int			6	0.6969	0.02220	4	31.39	<.0001
int			8	0.7010	0.02220	4	31.57	<.0001
int			10	0.7036	0.02220	4	31.69	<.0001
int			0	0.7304	0.3799	4	1.92	0.1269
treatme*endpoint*int	TRANSGENIC	surrogate	2	-0.00964	0.02404	31	-0.40	0.6910
treatme*endpoint*int	TRANSGENIC	surrogate	4	0.02359	0.02404	31	0.98	0.3341
treatme*endpoint*int	TRANSGENIC	surrogate	6	0.03035	0.02424	31	1.25	0.2198
treatme*endpoint*int	TRANSGENIC	surrogate	8	0.04985	0.02424	31	2.06	0.0482
treatme*endpoint*int	TRANSGENIC	surrogate	10	0.08022	0.02787	31	2.88	0.0072
treatme*endpoint*int	TRANSGENIC	true	2	-0.3455	0.5051	31	-0.68	0.4990
treatme*endpoint*int	TRANSGENIC	true	4	1.5811	0.5051	31	3.13	0.0038
treatme*endpoint*int	TRANSGENIC	true	6	5.4260	0.5324	31	10.19	<.0001
treatme*endpoint*int	TRANSGENIC	true	8	11.8291	0.5324	31	22.22	<.0001
treatme*endpoint*int	TRANSGENIC	true	10	15.4263	0.9215	31	16.74	<.0001
treatme*endpoint*int	WILDTYPE	surrogate	2	0	.	.	.	.
treatme*endpoint*int	WILDTYPE	surrogate	4	0	.	.	.	.
treatme*endpoint*int	WILDTYPE	surrogate	6	0	.	.	.	.
treatme*endpoint*int	WILDTYPE	surrogate	8	0	.	.	.	.
treatme*endpoint*int	WILDTYPE	surrogate	10	0	.	.	.	.
treatme*endpoint*int	WILDTYPE	true	0	0	.	.	.	.

FIGURE 17.17
SAS fixed-effects parameter estimates.

```
run;
```

17.8 Implementation in R

The proposed model can easily be implemented in R using the `gls` function from the `nlme` package.

Estimated R Matrix for animalid 1		
Row	Col1	Col2
1	0.000851	0.006179
2	0.006179	2.5462

Estimated R Matrix for animalid 4		
Row	Col1	Col2
1	1.4433	0.005111
2	0.005111	0.001000

Estimated R Correlation Matrix for animalid 1		
Row	Col1	Col2
1	1.0000	0.1327
2	0.1327	1.0000

Estimated R Correlation Matrix for animalid 4		
Row	Col1	Col2
1	1.0000	0.1345
2	0.1345	1.0000

FIGURE 17.18
SAS covariance matrix estimates for individual-level surrogacy.

17.8.1 Common Parameter for Histology in the Wildtype Group

We adopt a dummy coding for the variables of interest as shown in the partial print of the `MriHistData.dummy` data object (Figure 17.20). The model can be fitted using the following R code:

```
library(nlme)
fit <- gls(response~-1+endpoint+mu_SURRO_wt4+mu_SURRO_wt6+
    mu_SURRO_wt8+mu_SURRO_wt10 +beta_TRANS_TRUE_2
    +alpha_TRANS_TRUE_4+alpha_TRANS_TRUE_6+alpha_TRANS_TRUE_8
    +alpha_TRANS_TRUE_10+beta_TRANS_SURRO_2
```

R-Square	Coeff Var	Root MSE	true Mean
0.910071	34.23266	2.322145	6.783421

FIGURE 17.19
Disease-level surrogacy: GLM regression model output.

```
+beta_TRANS_SURRO_4 +beta_TRANS_SURRO_6
+beta_TRANS_SURRO_8 +beta_TRANS_SURRO_10,
        data=MriHistData.dummy,
        correlation=corSymm(form = ~ 1| animalid ),
        weight=varIdent(form=~1|endpoint*genotype))
```

By specifying `endpoint` in the right-hand side of the `formula`, we allow for a common parameter estimate for histology (true endpoint) in wildtype as well as a parameter for MRI (surrogate endpoint) at 2 months for wildtype mice. The variables `alpha_TRANS_TRUE_2`- `alpha_TRANS_TRUE_10` correspond to β_1–β_5 while `beta_TRANS_SURRO_2`- `beta_TRANS_SURRO_10` correspond to α_1–α_5 in (17.1).

The argument `correlation=...` allows for the specification of correlated outcomes within a subject. Further, we specify an unstructured correlation using the `corSym` construct. In order to define heterogeneous variances, that is, endpoint and genotype-specific variance covariance matrices as defined in (17.3), the argument `weight=varIdent(...)` is used. The output for the disease progression parameters is shown in Figure 17.21.

The estimated correlation estimates for disease-level surrogacy (17.4) are shown in the panel below.

```
Transgenic.covmat <- getVarCov(fit, individual=1)
cov2cor(Transgenic.covmat )
Marginal variance covariance matrix
        [,1]     [,2]
[1,] 1.00000 0.13295
[2,] 0.13295 1.00000
Wildtype.covmat <- getVarCov(fit, individual=4)
cov2cor(Wildtype.covmat)
```

```
> head(MriHistData.dummy, 10)
   animalid age   genotype  endpoint   response commonint mu_TRUE_wt mu_SURRO_wt2 mu_SURRO_wt4 mu_SURRO_wt6 mu_SURRO_wt8 mu_SURRO_wt10 alpha_TRANS_TRUE_2 alpha_TRANS_TRUE_4
1        37   2 TRANSGENIC      true 0.57389482         2          0            1            0            0            0             0                  1                  0
52       37   2 TRANSGENIC surrogate 0.73209081         2          0            1            0            0            0             0                  0                  0
42       39   2   WILDTYPE      true 0.18981475         0          1            0            0            0            0             0                  0                  0
93       39   2   WILDTYPE surrogate 0.73324633         2          0            1            0            0            0             0                  0                  0
44        6   4   WILDTYPE      true 0.04817485         0          1            0            0            0            0             0                  0                  0
95        6   4   WILDTYPE surrogate 0.68116338         4          0            0            1            0            0             0                  0                  0
18       49   4 TRANSGENIC      true 2.39414174         4          0            0            1            0            0             0                  0                  1
69       49   4 TRANSGENIC surrogate 0.68341699         4          0            0            1            0            0             0                  0                  0
46       15   6   WILDTYPE      true 3.28905565         0          1            0            0            0            0             0                  0                  0
97       15   6   WILDTYPE surrogate 0.72204392         6          0            0            0            1            0             0                  0                  0
   alpha_TRANS_TRUE_6 alpha_TRANS_TRUE_8 alpha_TRANS_TRUE_10 beta_TRANS_SURRO_2 beta_TRANS_SURRO_4 beta_TRANS_SURRO_6 beta_TRANS_SURRO_8 beta_TRANS_SURRO_10
1                   0                  0                   0                  0                  0                  0                  0                   0
52                  0                  0                   0                  1                  0                  0                  0                   0
42                  0                  0                   0                  0                  0                  0                  0                   0
93                  0                  0                   0                  0                  0                  0                  0                   0
44                  0                  0                   0                  0                  0                  0                  0                   0
95                  0                  0                   0                  0                  0                  0                  0                   0
18                  0                  0                   0                  0                  0                  0                  0                   0
69                  0                  0                   0                  0                  1                  0                  0                   0
46                  0                  0                   0                  0                  0                  0                  0                   0
97                  0                  0                   0                  0                  0                  0                  0                   0
```

FIGURE 17.20

Partial print of the `MriHistData.dummy` *data object.*

```
> round(summary(fit)$tTable,3)
                      Value Std.Error t-value p-value
endpointtrue          0.730     0.380   1.923   0.058
endpointsurrogate     0.695     0.022  31.281   0.000
mu_SURRO_wt4         -0.001     0.031  -0.036   0.971
mu_SURRO_wt6          0.002     0.031   0.076   0.939
mu_SURRO_wt8          0.006     0.031   0.202   0.840
mu_SURRO_wt10         0.009     0.031   0.286   0.775
alpha_TRANS_TRUE_2   -0.381     0.632  -0.604   0.548
alpha_TRANS_TRUE_4    1.545     0.632   2.444   0.017
alpha_TRANS_TRUE_6    5.390     0.654   8.237   0.000
alpha_TRANS_TRUE_8   11.793     0.654  18.022   0.000
alpha_TRANS_TRUE_10  15.390     0.997  15.436   0.000
beta_TRANS_SURRO_2   -0.010     0.024  -0.400   0.690
beta_TRANS_SURRO_4    0.024     0.024   0.982   0.329
beta_TRANS_SURRO_6    0.030     0.024   1.250   0.215
beta_TRANS_SURRO_8    0.050     0.024   2.057   0.043
beta_TRANS_SURRO_10   0.080     0.028   2.877   0.005
```

FIGURE 17.21
R gls output for the surrogacy model.

```
Marginal variance covariance matrix
        [,1]    [,2]
[1,] 1.00000 0.13355
[2,] 0.13355 1.00000
```

To obtain the disease-level surrogacy, a linear regression is fitted to the disease progression effects and the model R^2 obtained.

```
summary(lm(alpha~beta, data=fixedEffectsProcessed))$r.squared
[1] 0.9101327
```

17.8.2 Age-Specific Parameters for Histology in the Wild-type Group

A partial print of the dataset for the model with age-specific parameters for histology in the wildtype group is shown below.

```
> head(MriHistData)
   animalid age   genotype  endpoint   response
30        1  10 TRANSGENIC      true 17.4715576
81        1  10 TRANSGENIC surrogate  0.8114934
31        2  10 TRANSGENIC      true 16.5277908
82        2  10 TRANSGENIC surrogate  0.7101217
32        3  10 TRANSGENIC      true 14.3902328
83        3  10 TRANSGENIC surrogate  0.8296881
```

The model is fitted using `age` and `endpoint` as factor variables. The interaction term `endpoint:age` denotes the age-specific average readout for MRI and histology in wildtype mice, while the three-way interaction term `endpoint:genotype:age` denotes the age-specific disease effect (transgenic compared to wildtype mice).

```
fit2 <- gls(response~endpoint:age+endpoint:genotype:age -1,
       data=MriHistData,
       correlation=corSymm( form = ~ 1| animalid ),
       weight=varIdent(form=~1|endpoint*genotype))
```

Parameter estimates are shown in Figure 17.22. Note that in this case, the coefficients for histology in wildtype mice are more imprecise (since at each age, only two observations are available). The estimation of disease-level surrogacy follows as in the previous case of the model with a common histology parameter in wildtype mice.

```
> round(summary(fit)$tTable,3)
                                          Value Std.Error t-value p-value
endpointtrue:month2                       0.143     0.882   0.162   0.872
endpointsurrogate:month2                  0.693     0.022  30.955   0.000
endpointtrue:month4                       0.111     0.882   0.126   0.900
endpointsurrogate:month4                  0.691     0.022  30.900   0.000
endpointtrue:month6                       1.776     0.882   2.015   0.047
endpointsurrogate:month6                  0.701     0.022  31.318   0.000
endpointtrue:month8                       0.190     0.882   0.216   0.829
endpointsurrogate:month8                  0.699     0.022  31.246   0.000
endpointtrue:month10                      1.432     0.882   1.624   0.108
endpointsurrogate:month10                 0.706     0.022  31.558   0.000
endpointtrue:month2:genotypeTRANSGENIC    0.206     1.016   0.203   0.840
endpointsurrogate:month2:genotypeTRANSGENIC -0.008  0.024  -0.313   0.755
endpointtrue:month4:genotypeTRANSGENIC    2.164     1.016   2.130   0.036
endpointsurrogate:month4:genotypeTRANSGENIC 0.026   0.024   1.065   0.290
endpointtrue:month6:genotypeTRANSGENIC    4.347     1.030   4.222   0.000
endpointsurrogate:month6:genotypeTRANSGENIC 0.027   0.024   1.092   0.278
endpointtrue:month8:genotypeTRANSGENIC   12.340     1.030  11.984   0.000
endpointsurrogate:month8:genotypeTRANSGENIC 0.052   0.024   2.122   0.037
endpointtrue:month10:genotypeTRANSGENIC  14.698     1.275  11.527   0.000
endpointsurrogate:month10:genotypeTRANSGENIC 0.078  0.028   2.776   0.007
```

FIGURE 17.22
R gls output for the age-specific surrogacy model.

17.9 Concluding Remarks

The joint model specified in Section 17.4 was developed in order to model the association between MRI and histology, taking into account the disease progression effects on both endpoints. The observation unit that we have used in this chapter is the triplet (Genotype$_j$, MRI$_{ij}$, Histology$_{ij}$). Figure 17.23 illustrates the two sources of association presented in this chapter. For a given age, the effect of the disease on MRI α_i and the effect of the disease on histology β_i is represented by the shift in the distribution of both MRI and histology parameters as illustrated in panel b. Panel a illustrates the genotype-specific association in the residuals after adjusting for the disease effects α_i and β_i.

We have shown that, using a two-stage approach, we can estimate a genotype-specific adjusted association $\widehat{\rho}_W$ and $\widehat{\rho}_A$ using the joint model (17.1) in the first stage, while the prediction of the disease progression effects on histology can be done in the second stage using a linear regression model for $\widehat{\beta}_i$ and $\widehat{\alpha}_i$. Although, the experimental setting discussed in this chapter is completely different from the one discussed in Chapter 4, the same association structure (as illustrated in Figure 17.23a) implies that the same modeling

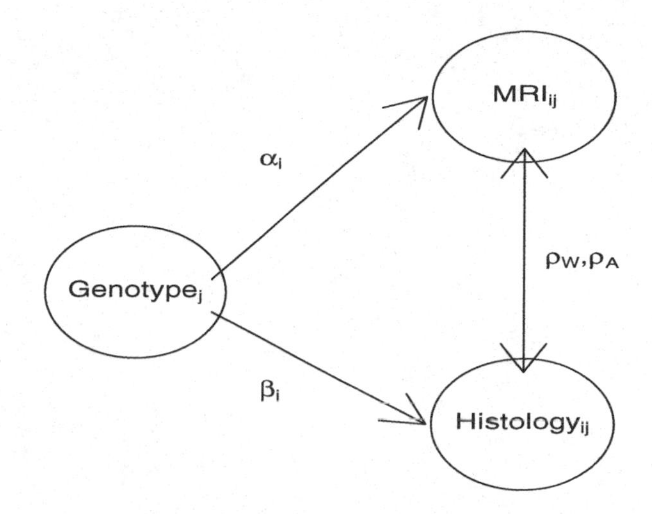

(a) *Association between age and endpoints.*

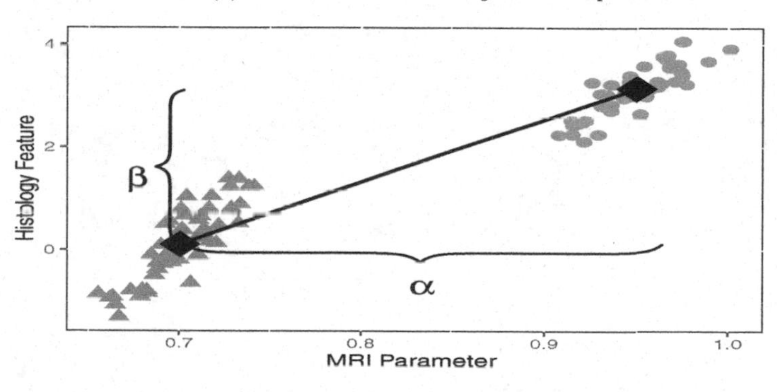

(b) *Histology versus MRI at age j.*

FIGURE 17.23
Illustration of the joint modeling framework: The association between MRI and histology after adjusting for the disease effects.

approach can be used in order to evaluate the quality of MRI as a biomarker for histology. We have shown that the use of MRI as a biomarker for histology depends on the brain region, MRI parameters, and histology staining.

The case studies presented in this chapter posed two challenges with regard to sample size: (1) there were only five age groups, which implies that estimation of the linear regression line in the second stage is based on only five observations and (2) there were only two control mice at each age group. Therefore, the genotype-specific coefficients μ_{Yi} in (17.2) are based on two observations, hence they may have higher variability.

Bibliography

Acquaviva, J., Wong, R., and Charest, A. (2009). The multifaceted roles of the receptor tyrosine kinase ros in development and cancer. *Biochimica et Biophysica Acta*, **1795**, 37–52.

Agresti, A. (2014). *Categorical Data Analysis.* John Wiley & Sons.

Agronin, M.E. (2007). *Alzheimer Disease and Other Dementias: A Practical Guide.* Philadelphia: Lippincott Williams & Wilkins.

Alexander, A.L., Lee, J.-E., Lazar, M., and Field, A.-S. (2007). Diffusion tensor imaging of the brain. *Neurotherapeutics*, **4**, 316–329.

Allison, P.D. (2008). Convergence failures in logistic regression. In: *SAS Global Forum 2008*, pp. 1–11. Cary, NC: SAS Press.

Alonso, A., Geys, H., Molenberghs, G., and Kenward, M.G. (2003). Validation of surrogate markers in multiple randomized clinical trials with repeated measures. *Biometrical Journal*, **45**, 931–945.

Alonso, A., Geys, H., Molenberghs, G., and Kenward, M.G. (2004a). Validation of surrogate markers in multiple randomized clinical trials with repeated measurements: Canonical correlation approach. *Biometrics*, **60**, 845–853.

Alonso, A., and Molenberghs, G. (2007). Surrogate marker evaluation from an information theoretic perspective. *Biometrics*, **63**, 180–186.

Alonso A. and Molenberghs G. (2008). Evaluating time to cancer recurrence as a surrogate marker for survival from an information theory perspective. *Statistical Methods in Medical Research* **17**, 497–504.

Alonso, A., Molenberghs, G., Burzykowski, T., Renard, D., Geys, H., Shkedy, Z., Tibaldi, F., Abrahantes, J., and Buyse, M. (2004b). Prentice's approach and the meta-analytic paradigm: A reflection on the role of statistics in the evaluation of surrogate endpoints. *Biometrics* **60**, 724–728.

Alonso, A., Molenberghs, G., Geys, H., and Buyse, M. (2006). A unifying approach for surrogate marker validation based on Prentice's criteria. *Statistics in Medicine*, **25**, 205–211.

Alonso, A.A., Molenberghs, G., and van Breukelen, G. (2014). Statistical validation of surrogate markers in clinical trials. In: *Developments in Statistical Evaluation of Clinical Trials.* K. van Montfort, J. Oud, and W. Ghidey (eds.). Berlin-Heidelberg: Springer.

Alonso, A., Van der Elst, W., Molenberghs, G., Buyse, M., and Burzykowski, T. (2015). On the relationship between the causal-inference and meta-analytic paradigms for the validation of surrogate endpoints. *Biometrics*, **71**, 15-24.

Alonso, A., Van der Elst, W., Molenberghs, G., Buyse, M., and Burzykowski, T. (2016). An information-theoretic approach for the evaluation of surrogate endpoints based on causal inference. *Biometrics*, doi: 10.1111/biom.12483.

Amaratunga, D., Cabrera, J., and Shkedy, Z. (2014). *Exploration and Analysis of DNA Microarray and Other High-Dimensional Data.* New York: John Wiley & Sons.

American Psychiatric Association (2000). *Diagnostic and Statistical Manual of Mental Diseases.* Washington, DC: American Psychiatric Association.

Anderson, J.R., Cain, K.C., and Gelber, R.D. (1983). Analysis of survival by tumour response. *Journal of Clinical Oncology*, **1**, 710-719.

Armstrong, A.J., Garrett–Mayer, E., Yang, Y.C.O., Carducci, M.A., Tannock, I., de Wit, R., and Eisenberger, M. (2007). Prostate-specific antigen and pain surrogacy analysis in metastatic hormone-refractory prostate cancer. *Journal of Clinical Oncology*, **25**, 3965–3970.

Assam, P., Tilahun A., Alonso, A., Molenberghs G. (2011). Information theoretic approach to surrogate markers evaluation with failure time endpoints. *Journal of Lifetime Data Analysis*, **17**, 195–204.

Benjamini, Y. and Hochberg, Y. (1995). Controlling the false discovery rate: A practical and powerful approach to multiple testing. *Journal of the Royal Statistical Society, Series B*, **57**, 289–300.

Biomarkers Definition Working Group. (2001). Biomarkers and surrogate endpoints: Preferred definitions and conceptual framework. *Clinical Pharmacology and Therapeutics*, **69**, 89–95.

Blennow, K. (2004). Cerebrospinal fluid protein biomarkers for Alzheimer's disease. *Journal of the American Society for Experimental NeuroTherapeutics*, **1**, 213–225.

Bonini, S., Eichler H.G., Wathion, N., and Rasi, G. (2014). Transparency and the European Medicines Agency sharing of clinical trial data. *New England Journal of Medicine*, **271**, 2452–2455.

Brattström, D., Bergqvist, M., Hesselius, P., Larsson, A., Lamberg, K., Wernlund, J., Brodin, O., and Wagenius, G. (2002). Elevated preoperative serum levels of angiogenic cytokines correlate to larger primary tumours and poorer survival in non-small cell lung cancer patients. *Lung Cancer*, **7**, 57–63.

Brillinger, R.D. (2004). Some data analyses using mutual information. *Brazilian Journal of Probability and Statistics*, **18**, 163–182.

Bruce, E.D., Autenrieth, R.L., Burghardt, R.C., Donnelly, K.C., and McDonald, T.J. (2008). Using quantitative structure-activity relationships (QSAR) to predict toxic endpoints for polycyclic aromatic hydrocarbons (PAH). *Journal of Toxicology and Environmental Health. Part A*, **71**, 1073–1084.

Burzykowski, T. and Buyse, M. (2006). Surrogate threshold effect: An alternative measure for meta-analytic surrogate endpoint validation. *Pharmaceutical Statistics* **5**, 173–186.

Burzykowski, T., Buyse, M., Piccart-Gebhart, M.J., Sledge, G., Carmichael, J., Lck, H.J., Mackey, J.R., Nabholtz, J.M., Paridaens, R., Biganzoli, L., Jassem, J., Bontenbal, M., Bonneterre, J., Chan, S., Atalay Basaran, G., and Therasse, P. (2008). Evaluation of tumor response, disease control, progression-free survival, and time to progression as potential surrogate endpoints in metastatic breast cancer. *Journal of Clinical Oncology*, **26**, 1987–1992.

Burzykowski, T. and Cortiñas Abrahantes, J. (2005). Validation in the case of two failure-time endpoints. In: *The Evaluation of Surrogate Endpoints*. T. Burzykowski, G. Molenberghs, and M. Buyse (eds.). New York: Springer.

Burzykowski, T., Molenberghs, G., and Buyse, M. (2004). The validation of surrogate endpoints using data from randomized clinical trials: A case-study in advanced colorectal cancer. *Journal of the Royal Statistical Society, Series A*, **167**, 103–124.

Burzykowski, T., Molenberghs, G., and Buyse, M. (2005). *The Evaluation of Surrogate Endpoints*. New York: Springer.

Burzykowski, T., Molenberghs, G., Buyse, M., Geys, H., and Renard, D. (2001). Validation of surrogate endpoints in multiple randomized clinical trials with failure-time endpoints. *Applied Statistics*, **50**, 405–422.

Buyse M. (2009). Use of meta-analysis for the validation of surrogate endpoints and biomarkers in cancer trials. *Cancer Journal*, **15**, 421–425.

Buyse, M., Burzykowski, T., Carroll, K., Michiels, S., Sargent, D.J., Elfring, G.L., Pignon, J.P., and Piedbois, P. (2007). Progression-free survival is a surrogate for survival in advanced colorectal cancer. *Journal of Clinical Oncology*, **25**, 5218–5224.

Buyse, M., Burzykowski, T., and Saad, E.D. (2016). Neoadjuvant as future for drug development in breast cancer (Letter). *Clinical Cancer Research*, **22**,268.

Buyse, M., Michiels, S., Squifflet, P., Lucchesi, K.J., Hellstrand, K., Brune, M.L., Castaigne, S., and Rowe, J.M. (2011). Leukemia-free survival as a surrogate endpoint for overall survival in the evaluation of maintenance therapy for patients with acute myeloid leukemia in complete remission. *Haematologica*, **96**, 1106–1112.

Buyse, M., and Molenberghs, G. (1998). The validation of surrogate endpoints in randomized experiments. *Biometrics*, **54**, 1014–1029.

Buyse, M., Molenberghs, G., Burzykowski, T., Renard, D., and Geys, H. (2000). The validation of surrogate endpoints in meta-analyses of randomized experiments. *Biostatistics*, **1**, 49–67.

Buyse, M., Molenberghs, G., Paoletti, X., Oba, K., Alonso, A., Van der Elst, W., and Burzykowski, T. (2016). Statistical evaluation of surrogate endpoints with examples from cancer trials. *Biometrical Journal*, **58**, 104–132.

Buyse, M., Thirion, P., Carlson, R.W., Burzykowski, T., Molenberghs, G., and Piedbois, P. (2000). Tumour response to first line chemotherapy improves the survival of patients with advanced colorectal cancer. *Lancet*, **356**, 373–378.

Buyse, M., Vangeneugden, T., Bijnens, L., Renard, D., Burzykowski, T., Geys, H., and Molenberghs, G. (2003). Validation of biomarkers as surrogates for clinical endpoints. In: *Biomarkers in Clinical Drug Development*, J.C. Bloom, R.A. Dean, (eds.), pp. 149–168. New York: Marcel Dekker.

Cardiac Arrhythmia Suppression Trial (CAST) Investigators. (1989). Preliminary Report: Effect of encainide and flecainide on mortality in a randomized trial of arrhythmia suppression after myocardial infraction. *New England Journal of Medicine*, **321**, 406–412.

Charest, A. Wilker, E.W., McLaughlin, M.E., Lane, K., Gowda, R., Coven, S., McMahon, K., Kovach, S., Feng, Y., Yaffe, M.B., Jacks, T., and Housman, D. (2006). ROS fusion tyrosine kinase activates a SH2 domain-containing phosphatase-2/phosphatidylinositol 3-kinase/mammalian target of rapamycin signaling axis to form glioblastoma in mice. *Cancer Research*, **66**, 7473–7481.

Chetelat, G. and Baron, J.C. (2003). Early diagnosis of Alzheimer's disease: Contribution of structural neuroimaging. *NeuroImage*, **18**, 525–541.

Cheung, M.M., Hui, E.S., Chan, K.C., Helpern, J.A., Qi, L., and Wu, E.X. (2009). Does diffusion kurtosis imaging lead to better neural tissue characterization? A rodent brain maturation study. *NeuroImage*, **45**, 386–392.

Choi, S., Lagakos, S., Schooley, R.T., and Volberding, P.A. (1993). CD4+ lymphocytes are an incomplete surrogate marker for clinical progression in persons with asymptomatic HIV infection taking zidovudine. *Annals of Internal Medicine*, **118**, 674–680.

Ciani, O., Buyse, M., Garside, R., Pavey, T., Stein, K., Sterne, J.A.C., Taylor, R.S. (2013). Comparison of treatment effect sizes associated with surrogate and final patient relevant outcomes in randomised controlled trials: Meta-epidemiological study. *British Medical Journal*, **346**, f457.

Ciani, O., Davis, S., Tappenden, P., Cantrell, A., Garside, R., Stein, K., Saad, E., Buyse, M., and Taylor, R.S. (2014). Validation of surrogate endpoints in advanced solid tumors: Systematic review of statistical methods, results, and implications for policy makers. *International Journal of Technology Assessment in HealthCare*, **30**, 1–13.

Clayton, D.G. (1978). A model for association in bivariate life tables and its application in epidemiological studies of familial tendency in chronic disease incidence. *Biometrika*, **65**, 141–151.

Ciani, O., Buyse, M., Garside, R., Peters, J., Saad, E.D., Stein, K., and Taylor, R.S. (2015). Validation of surrogate outcomes for overall survival in advanced colorectal cancer: A systematic review and meta-analysis of randomised controlled trials. *Journal of Clinical Epidemiology*, **68**, 833–842.

Collette, L., Burzykowski, T., Carroll, K.J., Newling, D., Morris, T., and-Schroeder, F.H. (2005). Is prostate-specific antigen a valid surrogate end point for survival in hormonally treated patients with metastatic prostate cancer? *Journal of Clinical Oncology*, **23**, 6139–6148.

Collette, L., Burzykowski, T., and Buyse, M. (2007). Are prostate-specific antigen changes valid surrogates for survival in hormone-refractory cancer? A meta-analysis is needed! (Letter to the Editor). *Journal of Clinical Oncology*, **25**, 5673–5674.

Collins, M.A. and di Magliano, M.P. (2014). KRAS as a key oncogene and therapeutic target in pancreatic cancer. *Frontiers in Physiology*, **4**, 407.

Cortazar, P., Zhang, L., Untch, M., Mehta, K., Costantino, J.P., Wolmark, N., Bonnefoi, H., Cameron, D., Gianni, L., Valagussa, P., Swain, S.M., Prowell, T. Loibl, S. Wickerham, D.L., Bogaerts, J., Baselga, J., Perou, C., Blumenthal, G., Blohmer, J., Mamounas, E.P., Bergh, J., Semiglazov, V., Justice, R., Eidtmann, H., Paik, S., Piccart, M., Sridhara, R., Fasching, P.A., Slaets, L., Tang, S., Gerber, B., Geyer, C.E., Pazdur, R., Ditsch, N., Rastogi, P., Eiermann, W., and von Minckwitz, G. (2014). Pathological complete response and long-term clinical benefit in breast cancer: The CT-NeoBC pooled analysis. *Lancet*, **384**, 164–172.

Cortiñas Abrahantes, J., Molenberghs, G., Burzykowski, T., Shkedy, Z., and Renard, D. (2004). Choice of units of analysis and modeling strategies in multilevel hierarchical models. *Computational Statistics and Data Analysis*, **47**, 537–563.

Cortiñas Abrahantes, J., Shkedy, Z., and Molenberghs, G. (2008). Alternative methods to evaluate trial level surrogacy. *Clinical Trials*, **5**, 194–208.

Cover, T. and Tomas, J. (1991). *Elements of Information Theory.* New York: John Wiley & Sons.

Cox, D.R. (1972). Regression models and life-tables. *Journal of the Royal Statistical Society, Series B*, **34**, 187–202.

Cox, D.R. and Oakes, D. (1984). *Analysis of Survival Data.* London: Chapman & Hall/CRC.

Dai, B., Yoo, S.Y., Bartholomeusz, G., Graham, R.A., Majidi, M., Yan, S., Meng, J., Ji, L., Coombes, K., Minna, J.D., Fang, B., and Roth, J.A. (2013). KEAP1-dependent synthetic lethality induced by AKT and TXNRD1 inhibitors in lung cancer. *Cancer Research*, **73**, 5542–5543.

Dale, J.R. (1986). Global cross ratio models for bivariate, discrete, ordered responses. *Biometrics*, **42**, 909–917.

D'Amico, A.V., Chen, M.H., de Castro, M., Loffredo, M., Lamb, D.S., Steigler, A., Kantoff, P.W., and Denham, J.W. (2012). Surrogate endpoints for prostate cancer-specific mortality after radiotherapy and androgen suppression therapy in men with localized or locally advanced prostate cancer: An analysis of 2 randomized trials. *Lancet Oncology*, **13**, 189–195.

Daniels, M. J., and Hughes, M. D. (1997). Meta-analysis for the evaluation of potential surrogate markers. *Statistics in Medicine*, **16**, 1515–1527.

Dearden, J.C. (2003). In silico prediction of drug toxicity. *Journal of Computer-Aided Molecular Design*, **17**, 119–127.

DeGruttola, V., Fleming, T.R., Lin, D.Y., and Coombs, R. (1997). Validating surrogate markers - Are we being naive? *Journal of Infectious Diseases*, **175**, 237–246.

DeGruttola, V. and Tu, X.M. (1994). Modelling progression of CD-4 lymphocyte count and its relationship to survival time. *Biometrics*, **50**, 1003–1014.

DeMichele, A., Yee, D., Berry, D.A., Albain, K.S., Benz, C.C., Boughey, J., Buxton, M., Chia, S.K., Chien, A.J., and Chui, S.Y. (2015). The neoadjuvant model is still the future for drug development in breast cancer. *Clinical Cancer Research*, **21**, 2911–2915.

DeMichele, A., Yee, D., Paoloni, M., Berry, D.A., Esserman, L.J. (2016). Neoadjuvant as future for drug development in breast cancer (Letter). *Clinical Cancer Research*, **22**, 269.

Dempster, A.P., Laird, N.M., and Rubin, D.B. (1977). Maximum likelihood from incomplete data via the EM algorithm (with discussion). *Journal of the Royal Statistical Society, Series B*, **39**, 1–38.

Denham, J.W., Steigler, A., Wilcox, C., Lamb, D.S.,Joseph, D.,Atkinson, C., Matthews, J.,Tai, K.H.,Spry, N.A.,Christie, D.,Gleeson, P.S.,Greer, P.B., D'Este, C., and Trans-Tasman Radiation Oncology Group 96.01 Trialists. (2008). Time to biochemical failure and prostate-specific antigen doubling time as surrogates for prostate cancer-specific mortality: Evidence from the TROG 96.01 randomised controlled trial. *Lancet Oncology*, **9**, 1058–1068.

Dickerson, B.C. and Sperling, R.A. (2005). Neuroimaging biomarkers for clinical trials of disease-modifying therapies in Alzheimer's disease. *NeuroRx*, **2**, 348–360.

Duff, K. and Suleman, F. (2004). Transgenic mouse models of Alzheimer's disease: How useful have they been for therapeutic development? *Briefings in Functional Genomics & Proteomics*, **3**, 47–59.

Eriksson, S., Prast-Nielsen, E., Flaberg, E., Szekely, L., and Arner, E.S. (2009). High levels of thioredoxin reductase 1 modulate drug-specific cytotoxic efficacy. *Free Radical Biology & Medicine*, **47**, 1661–1671.

Ferentz, A.E. (2002). Integrating pharmacogenomics into drug development. *Pharmacogenomics*, **3**, 453–467.

Firth, D. (1993). Bias reduction of maximum likelihood estimates. *Biometrika*, **80**, 27–38.

Fleming, T.R. (1994). Surrogate markers in AIDS and cancer trials. *Statistics in Medicine* **13**, 1423–1435.

Fleming, T.R. and DeMets, D.L. (1996). Surrogate end points in clinical trials: Are we being misled? *Annals of Internal Medicine* **125**, 605–613.

Foster, N.R., Renfro, L.A., Schild, S.E., Redman, M.W., Wang, X.F., Dahlberg, S.E., Diny, K., Bradbury, P.A., Ramalingam, S.S., Gandame, D.R., Shibata, T., Saijo, N., Vokes, E.E., Adjei, A.A., and Mandrekar, S.J. (2015). Multitrial evaluation of progression-free survival as a surrogate end point for overall survival in first-line extensive-stage small-cell lung cancer. *Journal of Thoracic Oncology*, **10**, 1099-1106.

Frangakis, C.E., and Rubin, D.B. (2002). Principal stratification in causal inference. *Biometrics*, **58**, 21–29.

Freedman, L.S. (2001). Confidence intervals and statistical power of the "validation" ratio for surrogate and intermediate endpoints. *Journal of Statistical Planning and Inference*, **96**, 143–153.

Freedman, L.S., Graubard, B.I., and Schatzkin, A. (1992). Statistical validation of intermediate endpoints for chronic diseases. *Statistics in Medicine*, **11**, 167–178.

Gail, M.H., Pfeiffer, R., van Houwelingen, J.C., and Carroll, R.J. (2000). On meta-analytic assessment of surrogate outcomes. *Biostatistics*, **1**, 231–246.

Galvin, J.E. and Sadowsky, C.H. (2012). Practical guidelines for the recognition and diagnosis of dementia. *Journal of the American Board of Family Medicine*, **25**, 367–382.

GASTRIC (Global Advanced/Adjuvant Stomach Tumor Research International Collaboration) Group. (2010). Benefit of adjuvant chemotherapy for resectable gastric cancer: A meta-analysis. *Journal of the American Medical Association*, **303**, 1729–1737.

GASTRIC (Global Advanced/Adjuvant Stomach Tumor Research International Collaboration) Group. (2013). Role of chemotherapy for advanced / recurrent gastric cancer: An individual-patient-data meta-analysis. *European Journal of Cancer*, **49**, 1565–1577.

Geys, H (2005). Validation using single-trial data: Mixed binary and continuous outcomes. In: *The Evaluation of Surrogate Endpoints*, T. Burzykowski, G. Molenberghs, and M. Buyse (eds.). pp. 83–93. New York: Springer.

Ghosh, D., Taylor, J.M.G., and Sargent, D.J. (2012). On meta-analytic assessment of meta-analysis for surrogacy: Accelerated failure time models and semicompeting risks modeling. *Biometrics*, **68**, 226–232.

Göhlmann, H. and Talloen, W. (2009). *Gene Expression Studies Using Affymetrix Microarrays*. Boca Raton: Chapman & Hall/CRC.

Gorrini, C., Harris, I.S., and Mak, T.W. (2013). Modulation of oxidative stress as an anticancer strategy. *Nature Reviews Drug Discovery*, **12**, 931–947.

Götz, J. and Götz, N.N. (2009). Animal models for Alzheimer's disease and frontotemporal dementia: A perspective. *ASN Neuro*, **1**, e00019.

Guy, W. (1976). Clinical Global Impression. In *ECDEU Assessment Manual for Psychopharmacology (revised)*. pp. 217–221. National Institute of Mental Health.

Halabi, S., Armstrong, A.J., Sartor, O., de Bono, J., Kaplan, E., Lin, C.Y., Solomon, N.C., and Small, E.J. (2013). Prostate-specific antigen changes as surrogate for overall survival in men with castration-resistant prostate cancer treated with second-line chemotherapy. *Journal of Clinical Oncology*, **31**, 3944–2950.

Hampel, H., Broich, K., Hoessler, Y., and Pantel, J. (2009). Biological markers for early detection and pharmacological treatment of Alzheimer's disease. *Dialogues in Clinical Neuroscience*, **11**, 141–157.

Hardy, J., and Selkoe, D.J. (2002). The amyloid hypothesis of Alzheimer's disease: Progress and problems on the road to therapeutics. *Science*, **297**, 353–356.

Harris, V.K., Coticchia, C.M., Kagan, B.L., Ahmad, S., Wellstein, A., and Riegel, A.T. (2000). Induction of the angiogenic modulator fibroblast growth factor-binding protein by epidermal growth factor is mediated through both MEK/ERK and P38 signal transduction pathways. *The Journal of Biological Chemistry*, **275**, 10802–10811.

Hasumi, H., Baba, M., Hong, S.B., Hasumi, Y., Huang, Y., Yao, M., Valera, V.A., Linehan, W.M., and Schmidt, L.S. (2008). Identification and characterization of a novel folliculin-interacting protein FNIP2. *Gene*, **415**, 60–67.

Hauptmann, S., Siegert, A., Berger, S., Denkert, C., Köbel, M., Ott, S., Siri, A., and Borsi, L. (2003). Regulation of cell growth and the expression of extracellular matrix proteins in colorectal adenocarcinoma: A fibroblast-tumor cell coculture model to study tumor-host interactions in vitro. *European Journal of Cell Biology*, **82**, 1–8.

Heinze, G. and Schemper, M. (2002). A solution to the problem of separation in logistic regression. *Statistics in Medicine*, **21**, 2409–2419.

Henderson, R., Diggle, P., and Dobson, A. (2000). Joint modelling of longitudinal measurements and event time data. *Biostatistics*, **1**, 465-480.

Hermans, L., Molenberghs, G., Kenward, M.G., Van der Elst, W., Nassiri, V., Aerts, M., and Verbeke, G. (2015). Clusters with random size: Maximum likelihood versus weighted estimation. In: *Proceedings of the 30th International Workshop on Statistical Modelling.* International Statistical Modeling Society.

Hol, E.M., Roelofs, R.F., Moraal, E., Sonnemans, M.A.F., Sluijs, J.A., Proper, E.A., de Graan, P.N.E., Fischer, D.F., and van Leeuwen, F.W. (2003). Neuronal expression of GFAP in patients with Alzheimer pathology and identification of novel GFAP splice forms. *Molecular Psychiatry*, **8**, 786–796.

Hougaard, P. (1986). Survival models for heterogeneous populations derived from stable distributions. *Biometrika*, **73**, 387–396.

Hsu P.L. (1941). On the limiting distribution of the canonical correlation. *Biometrika* **32**, 38–45.

Hui, E.S., Cheung, M.M., Qi, L., and Wu, E.X. (2008). Towards better MR characterization of neural tissues using directional diffusion kurtosis analysis. *NeuroImage*, **42**, 122–134.

ICECaP Working Group. (2015). The development of intermediate clinical endpoints in cancer of the prostate (ICECaP). *Journal of the National Cancer Institute,* **107**,12, doi:10.1093/jnci/djv261.

Institut für Qualität und Wirtschaftlichkeit im Gesundheitswesen. (2011). Validity of surrogate endpoints in oncology. (https://www.iqwig.de/download/A10–05_Executive_Summary_v1–1_Surrogate_endpoints_in_oncology.pdf), *IQWiG Reports, Commission,* No. A10–05.

International Conference on Harmonisation of technical requirements for registration of pharmaceuticals for human use. (1998). ICH Harmonised Tripartite Guideline. Statistical principles for clinical trials. (http://www.ich.org/pdfICH/e9.pdf), *Federal Register 63*, No. 179, 49583.

Joe, H. (1989). Relative entropy measures of multivariate dependence. *Journal of the American Statistical Association*, **84**, 157–164.

Joffe, M.M. and Greene, T. (2008). Related causal frameworks for surrogate outcomes. *Biometrics*, **64**, 1–10.

Johnson, M. and Maggiora, G. (1990). *Concepts and Applications of Molecular Similarity.* New York: John Wiley & Sons.

Johnson, R. A., and Wichern, D. W. (2007). *Applied Multivariate Statistical Analysis.* Upper Saddle River, NJ: Pearson Prentice-Hall.

Jones, T.C. (2001). Call for a new approach to the process of clinical trials and drug registration. *British Medical Journal*, **322**, 920–923.

Kalbfleisch J. and Prentice R.L. (1980). *The Statistical Analysis of Failure Time Data.* New York: John Wiley & Sons.

Kane, J., Honigfeld, G., Singer, J., and Meltzer, H. (1988). Clozapine for the treatment-resistant schizophrenic. A double-blind comparison with chlorpromazine. *Archives of General Psychiatry, 45*, 789–796.

Kendall, M.G. and Stuart, A. (1966). *The Advanced Theory of Statistics.* London: Griffin.

Kent, T., J. (1983). Information gain and a general measure of correlation. *Biometrika*, **70**, 163–173.

Klohs, J., Politano, I.W., Deistung, A., Grandjean, J., Drewek, A., Dominietto, M., Keist, R., Schweser, F., Reichenbach, J.R., Nitsch, R.M., Knuesel, I., and Rudin, M. (2013). Longitudinal assessment of amyloid pathology in transgenic ArcAβ mice using multi-parametric magnetic resonance imaging. *PLoS ONE*, **8**, e66097.

Korn, E.L., McShane, L.M., and Freidlin, B. (2013). Statistical challenges in the evaluation of treatments for small patient populations. *Science Translational Medicine*, **178**, 1–14.

Kullback, S. and Leibler, R. (1951). On information and sufficiency. *Annals of Mathematical Statistics*, **22**, 79–86.

Kuwahara, K., Sasaki, T., Kuwada, Y., Murakami, M., Yamasaki, S., and Chayama, K. (2003). Expressions of angiogenic factors in pancreatic ductal carcinoma: A correlative study with clinicopathologic parameters and patient survival. *Pancreas*, **26**, 344–349.

Lagakos, S.W. and Hoth, D.F. (1992). Surrogate markers in AIDS: Where are we? Where are we going? *Annals of Internal Medicine*, **116**, 599 601.

Laird, N.M. and Ware, J.H. (1982). Random effects models for longitudinal data. *Biometrics*, **38**, 963–974.

Laporte, S., Squifflet, P., Baroux, N., Quinaux, E., Fossella, F., Georgoulias, V., Pujol, J.L., Kudoh, S., Douillard, J.Y., Pignon, J.P., and Buyse, M. (2013). Prediction of survival benefits from progression-free survival benefits in advanced non small cell lung cancer: evidence from a pooled analysis of 2,334 patients randomized in 5 trials. *British Medical Journal Open*, **3**, 3.03.

Lassere, M.N. (2008). The Biomarker-Surrogacy Evaluation Schema: A review of the biomarker-surrogate literature and a proposal for a criterion-based, quantitative, multidimensional hierarchical levels of evidence schema for evaluating the status of biomarkers as surrogate endpoints. *Statistical Methods in Medical Research* **17**, 303–340.

Lassere, M.N., Johnson, K., Boers, M., Tugwell, P., Brooks, P., Simon, L., Strand, V., Conaghan, P., Ostergaard, M., Maksymowych, W.P., Landewe, R., Bresnihan, B., Tak, P.P., Wakefield, R., Mease, P., Bingham, C.O. III, Hughes, M., Altman, D., Buyse, M., Galbraith, S., and Wells, G. (2007). Definitions and validation criteria for biomarkers and surrogate endpoints: Development and testing of a quantitative hierarchical levels of evidence schema. *Journal of Rheumatology*, **34**, 607–615.

Lassere, M.N., Johnson, K.R., Schiff, M., and Rees, D. (2012). Is blood pressure reduction a valid surrogate endpoint for stroke prevention? An analysis incorporating a systematic review of randomised controlled trials, a by-trial weighted errors-in-variables regression, the surrogate threshold effect (STE) and the Biomarker-Surrogacy (BioSurrogate) Evaluation Schema (BSES). *BMC Medical Research Methodology*, **12**, 27.

le Cessie, S. and van Houwelingen, J.C. (1992). Ridge estimators in logistic regression. *Applied Statistics*, **41**, 191–201.

Lesaffre, E. (2008). Use and misuse of the *p*-value. *Bulletin of the NYU Hospital for Joint Diseases*, **66**, 146–149.

Lesko, L.J. and Atkinson, A.J. (2001). Use of biomarkers and surrogate endpoints in drug development and regulatory decision making: Criteria, validation, strategies. *Annual Review of Pharmacological Toxicology*, **41**, 347–366.

Leucht, S., Kane, J. M., Kissling, W., Hamann, J., Etschel, E., and Engel, R. (2005). Clinical implications of the Brief Psychiatric Rating Scale Scores. *British Journal of Psychiatry*, **187**, 366–371.

Li, Y., Taylor, J.M.G., and Elliott, M.R. (2010). A Bayesian approach to surrogacy assessment using principal stratification in clinical trials. *Biometrics*, **58**, 21–29.

Li, Y., Taylor, J.M.G., Elliott, M.R., and Sargent, D.R. (2011). Causal assessment of surrogacy in a meta-analysis of colorectal clinical trials. *Biostatistics*, **12**, 478–492.

Liang, K.Y., and Zeger, S.L. (1986) Longitudinal data analysis using generalized linear models, *Biometrika*, **73**, 13–22.

Lin, D.Y. (1994). Cox regression analysis of multivariate failure time data: The marginal approach. *Statistics in Medicine*, **13**, 2233–2247.

Lin, D.Y., Fischl, M.A., and Schoenfeld, D.A. (1993). Evaluating the role of CD4 lymphocyte counts as surrogate endpoints in human immunodeficiency virus clinical trials. *Statistics in Medicine*, **12**, 835-842.

Lin, D.Y., Fleming, T.R., and De Gruttola, V. (1997). Estimating the proportion of treatment effect explained by a surrogate marker. *Statistics in Medicine, 16,* 1515–1527.

Lin, D.Y., Shkedy, Z., Molenberghs, G., Talloen, W., Göhlmann, H., and Bijnens, L. (2010). Selection and evaluation of gene-specific biomarkers in pre-clinical and clinical microarray experiments. *Online Journal of Bioinformatics*, **11**, 106–127.

Lin, D.Y., and Wei, L.J. (1989). The robust inference for the Cox proportional hazards model. *Journal of the American Statistical Society*, **84**, 1074–1078.

Lindstrom, M. J., and Bates, D. M. (1988). Newton-Raphson and EM algorithms for linear mixed-effects models for repeated-measures data. *Journal of the American Statistical Association*, **83**, 1014–1022.

Linfoot, E.H. (1957). An informational measure of correlation. *Information and Control*, **1**, 85–89.

Lipsitz, S.R., Kim, K., and Zhao, L. (1994). Analysis of repeated categorical data using generalized estimating equations. *Statistics in Medicine*, **13**, 1149–1163.

Martin, Y.C., Kofron, J.L., and Traphagen, L.M. (2002). Do structurally similar molecules have similar biological activity? *Journal of Medicinal Chemistry*, **45**, 4350–4358.

Masters, C.L., Simms, G., Weinman, N.A., Multhaup, G., McDonald, B.L., and Beyreuther, K. (1985). Amyloid plaque core protein in Alzheimer disease and Down syndrome. *Proceedings of the National Academy of Sciences*, **82**, 4245–4249.

Matsui, S., Buyse, M., and Simon, R. (2015). *Design and Analysis of Clinical Trials for Predictive Medicine.* New York: Chapman & Hall/CRC.

Mauguen, A., Pignon, J.P., Burdett, S., Domerg, C., Fisher, D., Paulus, R., Mandrekar, S.J., Belani, C.P., Shepherd, F.A., Eisen, T. Pang, H., Collette, L., Sause, W.T., Dahlberg, S.E., Crawford, J., O'Brien, M., Schild, S.E., Parmar, M., Tierney, J.F., Le Pechoux, C., and Michiels, S. on behalf of the Surrogate Lung Project Collaborative Group. (2013). Surrogate endpoints for overall survival in chemotherapy and radiotherapy trials in operable and locally advanced lung cancer: A re-analysis of meta-analyses of individual patients' data. *Lancet Oncology*, **14**, 619–626.

McKhann, G., Drachman, D., Folstein, M., Katzman, R., Price, D., and Stadlan, E.M. (1984). Clinical diagnosis of Alzheimer's disease: Report of the NINCDS-ADRDA Work Group under the auspices of Department of Health and Human Services Task Force on Alzheimer's Disease. *Neurology*, **34**, 939.

Michiels, S., Le Maître, A., Buyse, M., Burzykowski, T., Maillard, E., Bogaerts, J., Vermorken, J.B., Budach, W., Pajak, T.F., Ang, K.K., Bourhis, J., and Pignon, J.P. on behalf of the MARCH and MACH-NC Collaborative Groups. (2009). Surrogate endpoints for overall survival in locally advanced head and neck cancer: Meta-analyses of individual patient data. *Lancet Oncology* **10**, 341–350.

Molenberghs, G., Alonso Abad, A., Van der Elst, W., Burzykowski, T., and Buyse, M. (2013). Surrogate endpoints: When should they be used? *Clinical Investigation*, **3**, 1147–1155.

Molenberghs, G., Burzykowski, T., Alonso Abad, A., Assam, P., Tilahun, A., and Buyse, M. (2010). A unified framework for the evaluation of surrogate endpoints in mental-health clinical trials. *Statistical Methods in Medical Research*, **19**, 205–236.

Molenberghs, G., Buyse, M., Geys, H., Renard, D., and Burzykowski, T. (2002). Statistical challenges in the evaluation of surrogate endpoints in randomized trials. *Controlled Clinical Trials* **23**, 607–625.

Molenberghs, G., and Kenward, M. G. (2007). *Missing Data in Clinical Studies.* New York: John Wiley & Sons.

Molenberghs, G., and Verbeke, G. (2005) *Models for Discrete Longitudinal Data*. New York: Springer.

Mortimer, A. M. (2007). Symptom rating scales and outcome in schizophrenia. *British Journal of Psychiatry, 191,* s7–s14.

Nantasenamat, C., Isarankura-Na-Ayudhya, C., Naenna, T., and Prachayasittikul, V. (2009). A practical overview of quantitative structure-activity relationship. *EXCLI Journal*, **8**, 74–78.

Nassiri, V., Molenberghs, G., and Verbeke, G. (2016). Finite information limit variance-covariance structures: Is the entire dataset needed for analysis? (2016). *Submitted for publication.*

Nelsen, R.B. (2006). *An Introduction to Copulas* (2nd ed.). New York: Springer.

Nisen, P. and Rockhold, F. (2013). Access to patient-level data from GlaxoSmithKline clinical trials. *New England Journal of Medicine*, **369**, 475–478.

Nyquist, H. (1924). Certain factors affecting telegraph speed. *Bell System Technical Journal*, **3**, 324–346.

Oba, K., Paoletti, X., Alberts, S., Bang, Y.J., Benedetti, J., Bleiberg, H., Catalano, P., Lordick, F., Michiels, S., Morita, S., Ohashi, Y., Pignon, J.P., Rougier, P., Sasako, M., Sakamoto, J., Sargent, D., Shitara, K., Van Cutsem, E., Buyse, M., and Burzykowski, T. on behalf of the GASTRIC group. (2013). Disease-free survival as a surrogate for overall survival in adjuvant trials of gastric cancer: A meta-analysis. *Journal of the National Cancer Institute*, **50**, 1600–1607.

O'Quigley J. and Flandre P. (2006). Quantification of the Prentice criteria for surrogate endpoints. *Biometrics*, **62**, 297–300.

Ovarian Cancer Meta-Analysis Project (1991). Cyclophosphamide plus cisplatin plus adriamycin versus cyclophosphamide, doxorubicin, and cisplatin chemotherapy of ovarian carcinoma: A meta-analysis. *Classic Papers and Current Comments*, **3**, 237–234.

Overall, J. and Gorham, D. (1962). The Brief Psychiatric Rating Scale. *Psychological Reports*, **10**, 799–812.

Paoletti, X., Oba, K., Bang, Y.J., Bleiberg, H., Boku, N., Bouch, O., Catalano, P., Fuse, N., Michiels, S., Moehler, M., Morita, S., Ohashi, Y., Ohtsu, A., Roth, A., Rougier, P., Sakamoto, J., Sargent, D., Sasako, M., Shitara, K., Thuss-Patience, E., Van Cutsem, E., Burzykowski, T., and Buyse, M. on behalf of the GASTRIC group. (2013). Progression-free survival as a surrogate for overall survival in patients with advanced/recurrent gastric cancer: A meta-analysis. *Journal of the National Cancer Institute*, **5**, 1608–1612.

Pardo, O.E., Lesay, A., Arcaro, A., Lopes, R., Ng, B.-L., Warne, P.H., McNeish, I.A., Tetley, T.D., Lemoine, N.R., Mehmet, H., Seckl, M.J., and Downward, J. (2003). Fibroblast growth factor 2-mediated translational control of IAPS blocks mitochondrial release of SMAC/DIABLO and apoptosis in small cell lung cancer cells. *Molecular and Cellular Biology*, **23**, 7600–7610.

Pearl, J. (2001). *Causality: Models, Reasoning, and Inference.* Cambridge: Cambridge University Press.

Perl, D.P. (2010). Neuropathology of Alzheimer's disease. *The Mount Sinai Journal of Medicine*, **77**, 32–42.

Petrylak, D.P., Ankerst, D.P., Jiang, C.S., Tangen, C.M., Hussain, M.H.A., Lara, P.N., Jr.,Jones, J.A., Taplin, M.E., Burch, P.A., Kohli, M., Benson, M.C., Small, E.J., Raghavan, D., and Crawford, E.D. (2006). Evaluation of prostate-specific antigen declines for surrogacy in patients treated on SWOG 99–16. *Journal of the National Cancer Institute*, **98**, 516–521.

Peuskens, J. and the Risperidone Study Group (1995). Risperidone in the treatment of chronic schizophrenic patients: A multinational, multicentre, double-blind, parallel-group study versus haloperidol, *British Journal of Psychiatry*, **166**, 712–726.

Pharmacological Therapy for Macular Degeneration Study Group (1997). Interferon α-IIA is ineffective for patients with choroidal neovascularization secondary to age-related macular degeneration. Results of a prospective randomized placebo-controlled clinical trial. *Archives of Ophthalmology*, **115**, 865–872.

Powis, G. and Kirkpatrick, D.L. (2007). Thioredoxin signaling as a target for cancer therapy. *Current Opinion in Pharmacology*, **7**, 392–397.

Prentice, R. L.(1989). Surrogate endpoints in clinical trials: Definitions and operational criteria. *Statistics in Medicine*, **8**, 431–440.

Ray, M.E., Bae, K., Hussain, M.H., Hanks, G.E., Shipley, W.U., and Sandler, H.M. (2009). Potential surrogate endpoints for prostate cancer survival: Analysis of a phase III randomized trial. *Journal of the National Cancer Institute* **101**, 228–236.

Renard, D., Geys, H., Molenberghs, G., Burzykowski, T., and Buyse, M. (2002). Validation of surrogate endpoints in multiple randomized clinical trials with discrete outcomes. *Biometrical Journal*, **44**, 921–935.

Renard, D., Geys, H., Molenberghs, G., Burzykowski, T., Buyse, M., Vangeneugden, T., and Bijnens, L. (2003). Validation of a longitudinally measured surrogate marker for a time-to-event endpoint. *Journal of Applied Statistics*, **30**, 235–247.

Renfro, L.A., Shang, H., and Sargent, D.J. (2015). Impact of copula directional specification on multi-trial evaluation of surrogate endpoints. *Journal of Biopharmaceutical Statistics*, **25**, 857–877.

Renfro, L.A., Shi, Q., Sargent, D.J., and Carlin, B.P. (2012). Bayesian adjusted R^2 for the meta-analytic evaluation of surrogate time-to-event endpoints in clinical trials. *Statistics in Medicine*, **31**, 743–761.

Renfro, L.A., Shi, Q., Xue,Y., Li, J., Shang, H., and Sargent, D.J. (2014). Center-within-trial versus trial-level evaluation of surrogate endpoints. *Computational Statistics and Data Analysis*, **78**, 1–20.

Rizopoulos, D. (2010). JM: An R package for the joint modelling of longitudinal and time-to-event data. *Journal of Statistical Software*, **35**, 1–33.

Rizopoulos, D. (2012). *Joint Models for Longitudinal and Time-to-Event Data with Applications in R.* Boca Raton: Chapman & Hall/CRC.

Rosenfeld, P.J., Brown, D.M., Heier, J.S., Boyer, D.S., Kaiser, P.K., Chung, C.Y., Kim, R.Y., for the MARINA Study Group. (2006). Ranibizumab for neovascular age-related macular degeneration. *New England Journal of Medicine* **355**, 1419–1431.

Saad, E. and Buyse, M. (2015). Endpoints other than survival are vital for regulatory approval of anticancer agents. *Annals of Oncology*, **21**, 7–12.

Sanchez, J.C.H. and Vicente-Villardon, J.L. (2013). Ordinal logistic biplot for ordered polytomous data. R package. http://rpackages.ianhowson.com/cran/OrdinalLogisticBiplot/... .../man/OrdinalLogisticBiplot.html.

Sargent, D.J., Wieand, H.S., Haller, D.G., Gray, R., Benedetti, J., Buyse, M., Labianca, R., Seitz, J.F., O'Callaghan, C.J., Francini, G., Grothey, A., O'Connell, M., Catalano, P.J., Blanke, C.D., Kerr, D., Green, E., Wolmark, N., Andre, T., Goldberg, R.M., and de Gramont, A. (2005). Disease-free survival versus overall survival as a primary end point for adjuvant colon cancer studies: individual patient data from 20,898 patients on 18 randomized trials. *Journal of Clinical Oncology*, **23**, 8664–8670.

Schafer, J.L. (1997). *Analysis of Incomplete Multivariate Data.* New York: Chapman & Hall.

Schatzkin, A. and Gail, M. (2002). The promise and peril of surrogate end points in cancer research. *Nature Reviews Cancer* **2**, 19–27.

Scher, H.I., Heller, G., Molina, A., Attard, G., Danila, D.C., Jia, X., Peng, W., Sandhu, S.K., Olmos, D., Riisnaes, R., McCormack, R., Burzykowski, T., Kheoh, T., Fleisher, M., Buyse, M., and de Bono, J.S. (2015). Circulating tumor cell biomarker panel as an individual level surrogate for survival in metastatic castration-resistant prostate cancer. *Journal of Clinical Oncology*, **33**, 1348–1355.

Serrano-Pozo, A., Frosch, M.P., Masliah, E., and Hyman, B.T. (2011). Neuropathological alterations in Alzheimer disease. *Cold Spring Harbor Perspectives in Medicine*, **1**, a006189.

Shaib, W., Mahajan, R., and El-Rayes, B. (2013). Markers of resistance to anti=EGFR therapy in colorectal cancer. *Journal of Gastrointestinal Oncology*, **4**, 303–318.

Shannon, C. (1948). A mathematical theory of communication. *Bell System Technical Journal*, **27**, 379–423 and 623–656.

Shannon, C.E. and Weaver, W. (1949). *The Mathematical Theory of Communication.* University of Illinois Press.

Shi, Q., de Gramont, A., Grothey, A. Zalcberg, J., Chibaudel, B., Schmoll, H.-J., Seymour, M.T., Adams, R., Saltz, L., Goldberg, R.M., Punt, C.J.A., Douillard, J.-Y., Hecht, J.R., Hurwitz, H., Diaz-Rubio, E., Proschen, R., Tebbutt, N.C., Fuchs, C., Souglakos, J., Falcone, A., Tournigand, C., Kabbinavar, F.F., Heinemann, V., Van Cutsem, E., Bokemeyer, C., Buyse, M. and Sargent, D.J., for the Analysis and Research in CAncers of the Digestive System (ARCAD) Group. (2015). Individual patient data analysis of progression-free versus overall survival as a first-line endpoint for metastatic colorectal cancer in modern randomized trials: Findings from 16,700 patients from the ARCAD database. *Journal of Clinical Oncology*, **33**, 22-28.

Shih, J.H. and Louis, T.A. (1995). Inferences on association parameter in copula models for bivariate survival data. *Biometrics*, **51**, 1384–1399.

Singh, M. and Kay, S. (1975). A comparative study of haloperidol and chlorpromazine in terms of clinical effects and therapeutic reversal with benztropine in schizophrenia. Theoretical implications for potency differences amongst neuroleptics. *Psychopharmacologia*, **43**, 103–113.

Strom, B.L., Buyse, M., Hughes, J., Koppers, B.M. (2014). Data sharing, year 1-Access to data from industry-sponsored clinical trials. *New England Journal of Medicine*, **371**, 2052–2054.

Taichman, D.B., Backus, J., Baethge, C., Bauchner, H., and de Leeuw, P.W. (2016). Sharing clinical trial data – A proposal from the International Committee of Medical Journal Editors. *Annals of Internal Medicine*. doi: 10.7326/M15–2928.

Tassi, E., Henke, R.T., Bowden, E.T., Swift, M.R., Kodack, D.P., Kuo, A.H., Maitra, A., and Wellstein, A. (2006). Expression of a fibroblast growth factor-binding protein during the development of adenocarcinoma of the pancreas and colon. *Cancer Research*, **66**, 1191–1198.

Taylor, J.M.G., Wang, Y., and Thiébaut, R. (2005). Counterfactual links to the proportion of treatment effect explained by a surrogate marker. *Biometrics*, **61**, 1102–1111.

Taylor, R.S., and Elston, J. (2009). The use of surrogate outcomes in model-based cost-effectiveness analyses: A survey of UK Health Technology Assessment reports. *Health Technology Assessment*, **13**, Paper 8.

Tibaldi, F. S, Cortiñas Abrahantes, J., Molenberghs, G., Renard, D., Burzykowski, T., Buyse, M., Parmar, M., Stijnen, T., and Wolfinger, R. (2003). Simplified hierarchical linear models for the evaluation of surrogate endpoints. *Journal of Statistical Computation and Simulation*, **73**, 643–658.

Tilahun, A., Lin, D., Shkedy, Z., Geys, H., Alonso, A., Peeters, P., Talloen, W., Drinkenburg, W., Göhlmann, H., Gorden, E., Bijnens, L., and Molenberghs, G. (2010). Genomic biomarkers for depression: Feature-specific and joint biomarkers. *Statistics in Biopharmaceutical Research*, **2**, 419–434.

Urig, S. and Becker, K., (2006). On the potential of thioredoxin reductase inhibitors for cancer therapy. *Seminars in Cancer Biology*, **16**, 452–465.

Valicenti, R.K., DeSilvio, M., Hanks, G.E., Porter, A., Brereton, H., Rosenthal, S.A., Shipley, W.U., and Sandler, H.M. (2006). Post-treatment prostatic-specific antigen doubling time as a surrogate endpoint for prostate cancer-specific survival: An analysis of Radiation Therapy Oncology Group Protocol 92-02. *International Journal of Radiation Oncology Biology Physics*, **66**, 1064–1071.

Van der Elst, W., Hermans, L., Verbeke, G., Kenward, M. G., Nassiri, V., and Molenberghs, G. (2015). Unbalanced cluster sizes and rates of convergence in mixed-effects models for clustered data. *Journal of Statistical Computation and Stimulation*, **00**, 000–000.

van Houwelingen, J.C., Arends, L.A., and Stijnen, T. (2002). Advanced methods in meta-analysis: Multivariate approach and meta-regression. *Statistics in Medicine*, **21**, 589–624.

van Krieken, J.H., Jung, A., Kirchner, T., Carneiro, F., Seruca, R., Bosman, F.T., Quirke, P., Fléjou, J.F., Plato, H.T., de Hertogh, G., Jares, P., Langner, C., Hoefler, G., Ligtenberg, M., Tiniakos, D., Tejpar, S., Bevilacqua, G., and Ensari, A. (2008). KRAS mutation testing for predicting response to anti-EGFR therapy for colorectal carcinoma: Proposal for a European quality assurance program. *Virchows Archives*, **435**, 417–431.

Van Sanden, S., Shkedy, Z., Burzykowski, T., Göhlmann, H.W., Talloen, W., and Bijnens, L. (2012). Genomic biomarkers for a binary clinical outcome in early drug development microarray experiments. *Journal of Biopharmaceutical Statistics*, **22**, 72–92.

Veraart, J., Poot, D.H.J., Van Hecke, W., Blockx, I., Van der Linden, A., Verhoye, M., and Sijbers, J. (2011). More accurate estimation of diffusion tensor parameters using diffusion kurtosis imaging. *Magnetic Resonance in Medicine*, **65**, 138–145.

Veraart, J., Rajan, J., Peeters, R.R., Leemans, A., Sunaert, S., and Sijbers, J. (2013). Comprehensive framework for accurate diffusion MRI parameter estimation. *Magnetic Resonance in Medicine*, **70**, 972–984.

Verbeke, G. and Molenberghs, G. (2000). *Linear Mixed Models for Longitudinal Data.* New York: Springer.

Verbist, B., Klambauer, G., Vervoort, L., Talloen, W., QSTAR Consortium, Shkedy, Z., Thas, O., Bender, A., Göhlmann, H., and Hochreiter, S. (2015). Using transcriptomics to guide lead optimization in drug discovery projects: Lessons learned from the QSTAR project. *Drug Discovery Today*, **20**, 505–551.

Verma, J., Khedkhar, V.M., and Coutinho, E.C. (2010). 3d-QSAR in drug design – A review. *Current Topics in Medicinal Chemistry*, **10**, 95–115.

West, B.T., Welch, K.B., and Galecki, A.T. (2007). *Linear Mixed Models: A Practical Guide Using Statistical Software*. New York: Chapman & Hall/CRC.

Woodburn, J.R. (1999). The epidermal growth factor receptor and its inhibition in cancer therapy. *Pharmacology & Therapeutics*, **822**, 241–250.

Zimmermann, G., Papke, B., Ismail, S., Vartak, N., Chandra, A., Hoffmann, M., Hahn, S.A., Triola, G., Wittinghofer, A., Bastiaens, P.I.H., and Waldmann, H. (2013). Small molecule inhibition of the KRAS-PDEδ interaction impairs oncogenic KRAS signalling. *Nature*, **497**, 638–642.

Index